VOLUME SEVENTY FIVE

ADVANCES IN PHARMACOLOGY

VOLUME SEVENTY FIVE

ADVANCES IN PHARMACOLOGY

Pharmacological Mechanisms and the Modulation of Pain

Edited by

JAMES E. BARRETT

Department of Pharmacology and Physiology, Drexel University College of Medicine, Philadelphia, Pennsylvania, USA

Serial Editor

S. J. ENNA

Department of Molecular and Integrative Physiology, Department of Pharmacology, Toxicology and Therapeutics, University of Kansas Medical Center, Kansas City, Kansas, USA

Managing Editor

LYNN LECOUNT

University of Kansas Medical Center School of Medicine, Kansas City, Kansas, USA

ELSEVIER

AMSTERDAM • BOSTON • HEIDELBERG • LONDON
NEW YORK • OXFORD • PARIS • SAN DIEGO
SAN FRANCISCO • SINGAPORE • SYDNEY • TOKYO

Academic Press is an imprint of Elsevier

Academic Press is an imprint of Elsevier
50 Hampshire Street, 5th Floor, Cambridge, MA 02139, USA
525 B Street, Suite 1800, San Diego, CA 92101-4495, USA
The Boulevard, Langford Lane, Kidlington, Oxford OX5 1GB, UK
125 London Wall, London, EC2Y 5AS, UK

First edition 2016

Notices
Knowledge and best practice in this field are constantly changing. As new research and experience broaden our understanding, changes in research methods, professional practices, or medical treatment may become necessary.

Practitioners and researchers must always rely on their own experience and knowledge in evaluating and using any information, methods, compounds, or experiments described herein. In using such information or methods they should be mindful of their own safety and the safety of others, including parties for whom they have a professional responsibility.

To the fullest extent of the law, neither the Publisher nor the authors, contributors, or editors, assume any liability for any injury and/or damage to persons or property as a matter of products liability, negligence or otherwise, or from any use or operation of any methods, products, instructions, or ideas contained in the material herein.

ISBN: 978-0-12-803883-3
ISSN: 1054-3589

For information on all Academic Press publications
visit our website at http://store.elsevier.com/

CONTENTS

CONTRIBUTORS

Seena K. Ajit
Department of Pharmacology and Physiology, Drexel University College of Medicine, Philadelphia, Pennsylvania, USA

James E. Barrett
Department of Pharmacology and Physiology, Drexel University College of Medicine, Philadelphia, Pennsylvania, USA

Geoffrey Burnstock
Autonomic Neuroscience Centre, Royal Free and University College Medical School, London, United Kingdom; Department of Pharmacology and Therapeutics, The University of Melbourne, Melbourne, Australia

Santina Chiechio
Department of Drug Sciences, University of Catania, Catania, Italy

Huiping Ding
Department of Physiology and Pharmacology, Wake Forest University School of Medicine, Winston-Salem, North Carolina, USA

Guan-hua Du
State Key Laboratory of Bioactive Substances and Functions of Natural Medicines; Beijing Key Laboratory of Drug Targets Identification and Drug Screening, Institute of Materia Medica, Chinese Academy of Medical Sciences and Peking Union Medical College, Beijing, PR China

Li-da Du
School of Biomedical Sciences, Chinese University of Hong Kong, Hong Kong, PR China

Derick A. Haas
Department of Pharmacology and Physiology, Drexel University College of Medicine, Philadelphia, Pennsylvania, USA

Huijuan Hu
Department of Pharmacology and Physiology, Drexel University College of Medicine, Philadelphia, Pennsylvania, USA

Anthony C. Johnson
Oklahoma Center for Neuroscience, University of Oklahoma Health Sciences Center, Oklahoma City, Oklahoma, USA

Jeffrey D. Kennedy
JK Associates BioPharma Consulting, LLC, Carmel, Indiana, USA

Bradley J. Kerr
Neuroscience and Mental Health Institute; Department of Pharmacology; Department of Anesthesiology and Pain Medicine, University of Alberta, Edmonton, Alberta, Canada

Norikazu Kiguchi
Department of Physiology and Pharmacology, Wake Forest University School of Medicine, Winston-Salem, North Carolina, USA

Mei-Chuan Ko
Department of Physiology and Pharmacology, Wake Forest University School of Medicine, Winston-Salem, North Carolina, USA

Ana Paula Luiz
Molecular Nociception Group, Wolfson Institute for Biomedical Research, University College London, London, United Kingdom

Beverley Greenwood-Van Meerveld
Oklahoma Center for Neuroscience; Veterans Affairs Medical Center; Department of Physiology, University of Oklahoma Health Sciences Center, Oklahoma City, Oklahoma, USA

Manuel Merlos
Drug Discovery and Preclinical Development, ESTEVE, Parc Científic de Barcelona, Baldiri Reixac 4-8, Barcelona, Spain

Frances Munoz
Department of Pharmacology and Physiology, Drexel University College of Medicine, Philadelphia, Pennsylvania, USA

James D. Pomonis
American Preclinical Services, LLC, Minneapolis, Minnesota, USA

Sujay Ramanathan
Department of Pharmacology and Physiology, Drexel University College of Medicine, Philadelphia, Pennsylvania, USA

Luz Romero
Drug Discovery and Preclinical Development, ESTEVE, Parc Científic de Barcelona, Baldiri Reixac 4-8, Barcelona, Spain

José Miguel Vela
Drug Discovery and Preclinical Development, ESTEVE, Parc Científic de Barcelona, Baldiri Reixac 4-8, Barcelona, Spain

Garth T. Whiteside
Discovery Research, Purdue Pharma L.P., Cranbury, New Jersey, USA

John N. Wood
Molecular Nociception Group, Wolfson Institute for Biomedical Research, University College London, London, United Kingdom

Muhammad Saad Yousuf
Neuroscience and Mental Health Institute, University of Alberta, Edmonton, Alberta, Canada

Tian-yi Yuan
State Key Laboratory of Bioactive Substances and Functions of Natural Medicines; Beijing Key Laboratory of Drug Targets Identification and Drug Screening, Institute of Materia Medica, Chinese Academy of Medical Sciences and Peking Union Medical College, Beijing, PR China

Yong-xiang Zhang
Department of Neuroimmunopharmacology, Beijing Institute of Pharmacology and Toxicology; State Key Laboratory of Toxicology and Medical Countermeasures, Beijing, PR China

PREFACE

Despite our long-standing intimacy with the experience of pain, it continues to be a significant health burden, often disabling, frequently intrusive, and with restrictive treatment options. Associated with many psychiatric and neurological conditions, the many different facets of pain are poorly understood, very heterogeneous, etiologically diverse, and often progressive with the link between acute and chronic pain remaining enigmatic. Current treatments are all too frequently ineffective or are associated with considerable side effects and, in the case of opioids, significant abuse liability. The challenges of addressing these complex issues are widely acknowledged, and a number of new approaches are being taken to address perceived shortcomings that have thwarted the development of new therapeutics. One of the major shortcomings is the lack of understanding of the molecular and cellular bases of pain pathophysiology which are needed to reveal new validated targets for pharmacological intervention. Our understanding of pain requires approaches from many different perspectives, a much better knowledge of the genetic, epigenetic, and systems-level approaches, and includes the need for new tools for more insightful clinical diagnosis and, eventually, adoption of stratified treatment interventions. The chapters in this volume cover many of these areas and provide a rich overview of interesting pharmacological targets that include voltage-gated sodium channels, purinergic receptors, store-operated calcium channels, metabotropic glutamate receptors, Sigma-1 inhibitors, transporter systems, and the nociceptin/orphanin FQ–NOP receptor system. These targets are involved in a wide variety of pain conditions that include cancer, neuropathic, and inflammatory pain. The focus on the pharmacological modulation of pain is complemented by chapters on visceral pain and stress, an overview of animal models of pain, and their translational alignment with the clinic, and a chapter on the development of miRNA-based biomarkers for pain. Finally, we have attempted to provide an initial perspective of some trends in pain research to set a foundation for subsequent opportunities in the area of comorbid disorders associated with pain, substance abuse, and model systems.

James E. Barrett
Department of Pharmacology and Physiology,
Drexel University College of Medicine, Philadelphia,
Pennsylvania, USA

S. J. Enna
Department of Molecular and Integrative Physiology,
Department of Pharmacology, Toxicology and Therapeutics,
University of Kansas Medical Center, Kansas City,
Kansas, USA

CHAPTER ONE

Perspectives and Trends in Pharmacological Approaches to the Modulation of Pain

James E. Barrett[1], Derick A. Haas
Department of Pharmacology and Physiology, Drexel University College of Medicine, Philadelphia, Pennsylvania, USA
[1]Corresponding author: e-mail address: jbarrett@drexelmed.edu

Contents

Abstract

Pharmacological approaches to our understanding and treatment of pain have had a long history and have traditionally relied on very few drugs that either have significant side effects and abuse liability, such as the nonsteroidal anti-inflammatory drugs or the opioids, respectively, or those that have been developed for other conditions such as the tricyclic antidepressants. The pathophysiology of pain is undoubtedly complex, complicated in part by the fact that it is not a singular condition, and has a variety of etiologies and a number of associated comorbidities that make treatment interventions challenging. Moreover, there are changes in the central nervous system during the course of the development of chronic pain that, in a manner parallel to

Advances in Pharmacology, Volume 75
ISSN 1054-3589
http://dx.doi.org/10.1016/bs.apha.2015.12.004

neurodegenerative disorders, likely require different pharmacological approaches in the early stages of acute pain compared to those that would be effective when pain has become chronic. This chapter reviews the current status of the field of pain research focusing on some relatively underdeveloped areas, such as pain and its associated comorbidities, and the use of transgenic animals and drug self-administration procedures in the context of analgesic assessment. This chapter also incorporates more recent developments and emerging trends in the area of epigenetics, biomarkers, and the use of induced pluripotent stem cells for pharmacological evaluation, target identification, and validation. Recent progress in the study of "organs-on-a-chip" will also be included in this overview, setting expectations for future progress that integrates these advances for deeper insights into mechanisms, novel treatments, and facilitated efforts in drug discovery.

1. INTRODUCTION

1.1 Epidemiology and Incidence of Pain

Efforts to understand the complex and multifaceted nature of pain have challenged researchers for decades. Estimates of the prevalence and severity of pain vary considerably depending on several factors such as the manner in which pain has been defined, whether the focus is on acute or chronic pain, whether it is associated with other pathologies, and how it is measured or defined in terms of onset, duration and/or relief (Nahin, 2015). There are also noteworthy differences in the influence of gender, age, and ethnicities that have not been clearly addressed. It is increasingly acknowledged that pain has several other effects that impact the well-being and quality of life issues for individuals that, when not effectively managed, lead to the development of other, often incapacitating, conditions such as depression and anxiety. The transition from acute to chronic pain results in complex progressive changes in and reorganization of the central nervous system, thereby posing significant challenges for pharmacological intervention as the potential targets for treatment may well depend on the stage in which these transitions take place (Henry, Chiodo, & Yang, 2011; Mifflin & Kerr, 2014). In this sense, pain shares some features with a number of neurodegenerative disorders such as Alzheimer's disease, amyotrophic lateral sclerosis, and Parkinson's disease where the progression of the disorder results in significant changes in the central nervous system and where the quest for new drugs is currently directed at delaying or stopping the progression of the disease. With these conditions, it may well be too late in the process to restore the progressive destruction and neuronal loss, whereas in pain, it is not currently know whether it is possible to restore normal homeostatic processes once chronic pain has been established. With the many variations in the assessment and characterization of pain and its associated comorbidities, and with the findings that the development and chronicity of pain is not static, it is perhaps not surprising that pain remains poorly managed and that the identification of pathophysiological mechanisms that precede the introduction of new drugs to treat pain has been so problematic (Woolf, 2010).

What is clear, however, is that pain represents a significant health burden that, by any estimate, affects a significant number of individuals worldwide and at an economic cost in the hundreds of billions of dollars. These costs exceed the combined costs of cancer, heart disease, and diabetes (Gaskin & Richard, 2012; Institute of Medicine Report, 2011). Gereau et al. (2014), in characterizing the status of pain research together with the development of an agenda for the twenty-first century in America, referred to "the desperate status of pain research in America" which is a poignant and forthright acknowledgment of the challenges as well as the opportunities for basic research and for the development and introduction of new therapeutics. Despite these alarming facts on the impact of chronic pain on both individuals and society, NIH expenditures per affected person in the United States are the lowest of those listed as major chronic conditions, with a 10- to 250-fold separation in expenditures for those conditions relative to pain (Gereau et al., 2014; see also Max & Stewart, 2008).

1.2 Unmet Need and Challenges

For decades, the development of novel and effective analgesics has remained largely stagnant. Most analgesic development efforts have concentrated on various reformulations of existing opioids, with these formulations incorporated into existing treatments that, for decades, have involved anticonvulsants, amine reuptake inhibitors, nonsteroidal anti-inflammatory drugs (NSAIDs), and cyclooxygenase inhibitors. It has been all too common over the past few years to lament the lack of progress in developing drugs for the treatment of a wide variety of central nervous system disorders as well as for pain. Kissin (2010), for example, has commented that morphine and aspirin, both introduced more than a century ago (morphine in 1827 by Merck and aspirin in 1897 by Bayer), continue to dominate biomedical publications on pain despite their serious side effects and limited efficacy for a number of painful conditions. Kissin also points out that between 1960 and 2009,

59 drugs were identified as analgesics that remain in use today. However, only seven of these were considered to be drugs directed against novel molecular targets, and only one class, the triptans, was viewed as having sufficient efficacy to spawn the development of similar drugs acting at the same target. Clearly, despite considerable efforts and significant advances in a wide variety of areas, a great deal remains to be accomplished to better understand the pathophysiology and heterogeneity underlying chronic pain, along with the nature of the variability in response by different individuals to pain treatments.

A number of relatively novel pharmacological mechanisms have been evaluated in recent years but, for the most part, with little success in yielding new medications (Hayes, Arendt-Nielsen, & Tate, 2014). The challenges are unquestionably considerable. Suggestions for increasing the probability of success have ranged from the need to better understand the underlying pathophysiology of acute and chronic pain, to the need to develop better diagnostic tools. Other proposals have included the need to pursue human genome-wide association studies for identifying novel analgesic targets along with the very frequent call for developing more predictive and translational animal as well as human experimental pain models. Additional suggestions have included the need to expand epidemiological studies, improve clinical trial design, and expand epigenetic studies addressing the mechanisms of chronic pain, proof of target engagement, and the development of genetic- and imaging-based biomarkers (Crow, Denk, & McMahon, 2013; Descalzi et al., 2015; Hayes et al., 2014; Max & Stewart, 2008; Seo et al., 2013; Woolf, 2010). Individually, these are significant challenges and, collectively, these proposals amount to a considerable undertaking. The objective of this chapter is to cover some emerging areas that may help to shed new light on the ability to better differentiate pain conditions, identify a means for developing more appropriate animal models or *in vivo* assay systems, and focus on the issues of comorbidity where pain is associated with a range of other conditions and disorders. In addition, some attention will be given to the issue of substance abuse assessment in the context of pain and analgesic drug development. We will then summarize current efforts to identify appropriate biomarkers, highlighting the need to better understand epigenetic mechanisms in pain, and will conclude with an overview of recent developments in the use of *in vitro* approaches that include the use of stem cells and organs-on-chips to aid in the identification of new targets and to provide other means of understand signaling pathways and potentially toxicities.

2. ANIMAL MODELS AND TRANSLATIONAL PAIN RESEARCH

There are several accounts and descriptions of the various animal models that have been used in pain research along with extensive analyses of their use and limitations (e.g., Barrett, 2015; Berge, 2014; Gregory et al., 2013; King & Porreca, 2014; Yaksh, Woller, Ramachandran, & Sorkin, 2015). The chapter "Preclinical Pharmacological Approaches in Drug Discovery for Chronic Pain" by Whiteside, Pomonis, and Kennedy supplements these articles by focusing on the use of animal models of pain in the pharmaceutical industry. Although a few new approaches have been developed to examine pain in preclinical procedures, it is striking that one of the more frequently used procedures continues to be the method first introduced by von Frey (1896). This procedure, used extensively in rodent pain assays, measures reflexive withdrawal responses of the hind paw following various procedures that induce pain (e.g., spinal nerve ligation). A measure of mechanical allodynia, the von Frey method, uses fibers or filaments of different strengths to determine sensory withdrawal thresholds to the application of different forces applied to the sensitive regions of the hind paw. The Hargreaves method is another procedure based on reflexive responses to heat. Despite their relative ease and widespread use, these procedures have not reliably predicted clinical utility nor have they translated well to clinical assessments where the assessments of analgesia are typically not measured as reflexive responses but rely more on spontaneous behavior and subjective assessments. We will not review these various models here (refer to references above for more detail on animal models and alternative approaches) but will instead concentrate on selected procedures using animals that warrant particular emphasis in this context and where there appear to be further opportunities for advancing pain research.

2.1 Transgenic Animals in Pain Research

Insights into genetic factors associated with pain and pain syndromes have emerged from both human genetic studies as well as from animal models. These developments have provided new tools and targets as well as approaches to validate those targets and yield potentially novel pain therapeutics. Over 15 years ago, Mogil and Grisel (1998) provided one of the first reviews of the use of transgenic animals for the study of pain. Advances in molecular biology for the study of pain at the genetic level were heralded as a significant improvement, providing another tool to complement the techniques of pharmacology, electrophysiology, biochemistry, and behavior. Mogil and Grisel (1998) provided a very thorough and balanced assessment of the various approaches, advantages, cautionary points, and limitations of this relatively new technology for use in pain research that helped to set the stage for more extensive studies that have occurred in the interim. Subsequently, LaCroix-Fralish, Ledoux, and Mogil (2007) provided a *Pain Genes Database* for transgenic knockout studies. Several recent reviews have highlighted and described the contributions of gene-based approaches to explore and validate novel targets, guide translational research (e.g., Foulkes & Wood, 2008; Molet & Pohl, 2013; Sikandar et al., 2013), and combine functional magnetic resonance imaging with mouse genomics in pain research (Heindl-Erdmann et al., 2010).

Recent insights have been gained from human and nonhuman genetic studies for understanding pain pathways and novel mechanisms. The introduction and utilization of transgenic mouse models to validate potential pain targets derived from human genetic studies have added new dimensions and opportunities for focusing on novel pharmacological approaches (see reviews by Hatcher & Chessell, 2006; Nissenbaum, 2012). Rare instances of individuals with congenital insensitivity to pain have been reported in the literature for more than 30 years but, until recently, the precise underlying etiology of these conditions has remained a mystery (Manfredi et al., 1981). The breakthrough came with the creation of inducible knockout mice for the Nav1.7, 1.8, and 1.9 voltage-gated sodium channels. These models demonstrated that removal of exons 14 and 15 in the Nav1.7 gene, for example, significantly reduced or abolished acute and inflammatory pain (Nassar et al., 2004). Shortly thereafter, researchers published a genetic study on three families in northern Pakistan with a congenital defect in their ability to sense pain. Chromosomal mapping of their genome revealed a loss of function in the SCN9A gene on chromosome 2q24.3, which encodes for the α-subunit of Nav1.7 (Cox et al., 2006). Taken together, these findings created a translational link between the animal model and the patients, which drove Goldberg et al. (2012) to create XEN402 (now TV-45070), and a specific pharmacological inhibitor of Nav1.7. XEN402 has completed phase I and phase II clinical trials for the treatment of erythromelalgia, a spontaneous pain condition resulting from a gain-of-function mutation in the Nav1.7 that results in the hyperexcitability of dorsal root ganglion neurons. Recently, however, it has been demonstrated that deletion of Nav1.7 resulted in increased transcription of *Penk* messenger RNA, the precursor of Leu- and Met-enkephalin (Minett et al., 2015). This finding has suggested that the congenital insensitivity to pain in both null mutant mice and humans could be mediated by enkephalins. This relationship was confirmed when, following the administration of the μ-opioid receptor antagonist naloxone to the Nav1.7 mutant mice, there was a reversal of the analgesia and a restoration of both thermal and mechanical pain thresholds. Naloxone was also administered to a human Nav1.7-null individual insensitive to pain. In this individual, there was also a reversal of the analgesia following intravenous administration of naloxone. Minett et al. (2015) conclude that the loss of Nav1.7 leads to an upregulation of an endogenous opioid system that contributes significantly to the absence of pain associated with the loss of Nav1.7-null mice and humans. Importantly, this study further characterizes the complex interrelationship between systems involved in pain.

The knockout studies involving the transient receptor potential (TRP) channels have provided a wealth of information into the receptor's role in inflammatory and noxious heat pain. TRPV1 channels are nonselective cation channels that normally open in response to capsaicin or temperatures >43 °C and their action can be modulated by the presence of protons (Caterina et al., 1997), such as the acidic environment surrounding bone metastases (Lozano-Ondoua, Symons-Liguori, & Vanderah, 2013). TRPV1 knockout mice show a significant reduction in the detection of painful heat and thermal hypersensitivity in response to inflammation, while there is no impact on their sensitivity to mechanical allodynia (Caterina et al., 2000). Alternatively, TRPV1 knockout mice that undergo a partial lesion of the sciatic nerve to induce neuropathic pain show no alterations in thermal hyperalgesia or mechanical allodynia, indicating that TRPV1 does not have a role in neuropathic pain (Bolcskei et al., 2005). However, TRPV1-selective antagonists have been shown to inhibit mechanical allodynia in models of both inflammatory and neuropathic pain (Honore et al., 2005), which indicates that acute pharmacological blockade of TRPV1 can produce results that differ from lifelong absence of a particular gene product.

Voltage-dependent calcium channel knockout mice have implicated both N- and T-type channels in the development of chronic pain. Saegusa et al. (2001) showed that N-type Cav2.2 knockout mice had a significantly reduced mechanical allodynia and thermal hyperalgesia in a neuropathic pain model, but the absence of Cav2.2 had no effect in several inflammatory models of pain (Saegusa et al., 2001). In T-type knockout studies, Cav3.2 mice showed a significant decrease in calcium currents in the dorsal root ganglion (Chen et al., 2003) and attenuation of chemically induced inflammatory pain (Choi et al., 2007). Furthermore, T-type

Cav3.1 knockout mice have been shown to have significantly reduced mechanical allodynia and thermal hyperalgesia in neuropathic pain (Na, Choi, Kim, Park, & Shin, 2008).

P2X7 receptors are found on macrophages and monocytes, where they play an important role in triggering the release of the proinflammatory cytokine IL-1β (Solle et al., 2001). P2X7 receptor knockout mice exhibited abolished mechanical allodynia and thermal hyperalgesia associated with neuropathic pain, and differences in weight bearing were also eliminated in the chronic inflammatory model using Freund's complete adjuvant injection (Chessell et al., 2005). Furthermore, intrathecal injection of lipopolysaccharide into the lumbar spinal cord was able to induce mechanical hypersensitivity in the hind paw of wild-type mice but not in the P2X7 knockout mice (Clark et al., 2010). Clark et al. (2010) were able to mirror the findings in the knockout mice using A-438079, a selective P2X7 small-molecule antagonist.

In addition to removing the gene of interest, knock-in mice have also been utilized. By selectively mutating a single histidine residue in the four subtypes of the $GABA_A$ receptor (α1, α2, α3, or α5), Knabl et al. (2008) were able to show that the α2 and α3 subunits were responsible for diazepam-induced analgesia seen in both neuropathic and inflammatory pain (Knabl et al., 2008). Additionally, the authors determined that the sedative effects of diazepam were a result of activation of $GABA_A$ receptors containing the α1 subunit. Furthermore, they demonstrated that the use of L-838,417, an α1-sparing ligand, diminished the nociceptive input to the brain while simultaneously decreasing brain activity in regions linked to the associative-emotional components of pain.

Transgenic "ZW" mice can also be utilized to trace the neuronal pathways associated with pain processing from a particular region of the body (Basbaum & Braz, 2010). This transgenic mouse is a combination of a floxed *lacZ* gene followed by the neuronal tracer wheat germ agglutinin (WGA), hence "ZW". In normal neurons, only lacZ is expressed, but in Cre recombinase-expressing neurons, the lacZ coding sequence is excised, allowing for both a temporally and spatially inducible expression of the WGA tracer. Insertion of tracer genes into Cre-positive subtypes of neurons in these mice allows for significant accumulation of fluorescent proteins that are then synaptically transferred up to fourth-order synaptically connected neurons. Basbaum and Braz (2010) used this technique in Nav1.8-Cre ZW mice and made an interesting discovery when they found no transneuronal labeling in the parabrachial nuclei or in the thalamus, even though the spinoparabrachial and spinothalamic pathways are the main ascending pathways for the transmission of nociceptive information from the spinal cord. The data from these studies provide new insights into how the central nervous system may route different types of pain signals through different channels. Additionally, Basbaum and Braz created a version of the ZW mouse where WGA expression was driven by the neuropeptide Y promoter, which allowed them to trace the activated pathway following peripheral nerve injury. As the stability of the tracers improves and new critical subpopulations of Cre-positive neurons are created, this technique will allow for even greater downstream mapping of the neuronal circuitry associated with pain.

Transgenic mice can provide a great deal of insight into the functions of specific genes in differing types of pain, but they also present some disadvantages that require consideration. The majority of these models are produced by injecting mutated embryonic stem cells (ESCs) of 129 mice into the blastocyst of C57BL/6 mice which, when compared to nine other mice strains, actually have some of the greatest deviations from the mean phenotypic response across 12 different measures of nociception (Lariviere, Chesler, & Mogil, 2001; Mogil et al., 1999). To further complicate the issue, there is carryover of the genetic code surrounding the gene of interest from the 129 donor mouse, which may potentially have confounding effects when comparing the transgenic C57BL/6 mice to their wild-type littermates (Lariviere et al., 2001).

Additionally, only a few human pain conditions have been shown to be the result of a monogenetic defect (Mogil, 2012). Pain is extremely complex from its etiology to its emotional processing components, and the current understanding of the genetic and epigenetic alterations in common clinical pain conditions such as fibromyalgia is too cursory to make a representative transgenic model of the disorder (Mogil, 2009). This complexity may limit the scope to which the pain data from a particular experiment can be applied, i.e., inflammatory or neuropathic pain. Finally, knocking out a gene in a mouse at the time of conception will likely result in compensatory mechanisms to buffer the effect of the missing component. Nassar, Levato, Stirling, and Wood (2005) showed that Nav1.8 knockout mice upregulated Nav1.7 channels to functionally compensate for the deletion. As mentioned previously, deletion of the Nav1.7 channel produced an upregulation of endogenous enkelphalins (Minett et al., 2015). These compensatory mechanisms make it difficult for researchers to be certain that the effect seen in the mouse is a result of the gene knockout and not caused by the compensatory responses to enable the animal to survive.

While the aforementioned disadvantages should be acknowledged when considering the use of transgenic animals to study pain, these models can provide undeniable advantages. First, genetic knockout animals allow for testing of the effects of a specific gene target when there are no selective pharmacological agents available, thereby pinpointing the specific protein source of an effect. Second, inducible knockout genes allow the animals to develop normally without the presence of compensatory mechanisms. The administration of a drug can induce the CRE-lox gene, which can inactivate the gene of interest in a temporal, spatial, and even cell subtype-specific manner (Molet & Pohl, 2013). The application of the bacterial CRISPR/Cas9 system for knockout of genes in fully developed animals has more recently helped to eliminate the worry that the effect of the deletion is purely a compensatory mechanism (Cong et al., 2013). In this system, the CRISPR protein uses RNA segments to target a specific gene anywhere in the genome. Once the guide RNA binds the target, the associated Cas9 endonuclease makes a double-stranded break to cleave out that particular section of DNA. The cell repairs the break by nonhomologus end joining, rendering the gene inactive. This technology also has the ability to replace the cleaved gene with an alternative variant, allowing researchers to introduce the gene of their choice (for further reviews, see Hsu, Lander, & Zhang, 2014; Sander & Joung, 2014).

Finally, knockout mice have provided valuable insight for evaluating the behavioral assays used to evaluate pain response. Minett, Eijkelkamp, and Wood (2014) have shown that pain sensitivity can vary based on the type of skin on which the test is performed. The researchers also indicated that circadian rhythm could alter behavioral responses by 80% throughout the course of the day. Their work demonstrates that different tissues have different types of nociceptors and to replicate the results researchers must test the target behaviors at the same point during the day. These details may account for some of the conflicting results obtained from different laboratories working with the same knockout model.

Advances in transgenic models of pain continue to provide valuable information to identify new potential gene targets and to confirm that a hypothesized gene target for a new pharmaceutical is responsible for its mechanism of action. Inducible knockouts and CRISPR models have greatly reduced the concern of compensatory mechanisms that result from a lifelong absence of a particular gene. Additionally, the use of CRISPR to insert new genes might allow researchers to analyze specific configurations of heteromeric receptors, such as the GABA, Cav, or NMDA receptors, leading to a better understanding of each subunit's role in pain. Another potential tool could be the combination of CRISPR gene knockout and ZW mice driven by a pain-specific promoter to illustrate which specific genes are responsible for activation and alteration of the pain pathway in response to different types of pain. Furthermore, a version of this tool could be used to evaluate the efficacy of new analgesics for each type of pain by looking for the absence of pain pathway activation. Whatever the application, transgenic models will continue to be an invaluable aid in the development of new pharmacological therapies for the treatment of pain.

2.2 Drug Self-administration in the Context of Pain and Analgesia

Despite their beneficial analgesic effects, the use of opioids for pain relief has a number of liabilities that range from the physiological impact of constipation and respiratory depression to the considerable risk of abuse liability. Drug self-administration procedures in animals that are provided with intravenous catheters and allowed to perform an operant response such as the depression of a lever to administer a drug have been used extensively as a means to evaluate a drug's propensity for abuse (Ator & Griffiths, 2003; Horton, Potter, & Mead, 2013; Teuns, Geys, Geuens, Stinissen, & Meert, 2014) and have been quite reliable predictors of abuse potential. The quest for an effective analgesic devoid of abuse potential and without the wide range of side effects characteristic of the opiates has been long standing. There has been some anticipation that opioid receptors other than mu receptor agonists such as kappa or delta compounds may fulfill this expectation, but at least at the present, these approaches have not yielded appropriate therapeutics (but see chapter "Central N/OFQ-NOP Receptor System in Pain Modulation" by Ho for research summarizing nociception-ORL and points later in this chapter regarding nociception/orphanin FQ and pain associated with posttraumatic stress disorder (PTSD) and anxiety). Due to the close association of pain relief with abuse liability, there have been a number of efforts to assess whether pain-inducing procedures in animals would result in the self-administration of an analgesic to alleviate the pain (Wade & Fairbanks, 2014). Of particular interest are those drugs that may have analgesic properties but which may not have the potential for abuse. There are a few studies that have used drug self-administration procedures in animals that have been exposed to a painful procedure. The primary objective of these studies has been to address the question of whether an experimental compound with putative analgesic effects would be self-administered in a control animal in the absence of pain, suggesting potential abuse liability or, alternatively, whether that compound would be self-administered when pain is present. Other methods to evaluate the relief from pain have used conditioned place preference procedures that have been reviewed extensively (King & Porreca, 2014; Navratilova, Xie, King, & Porreca, 2013) and will not be covered in this chapter.

Early studies by Colpaert using a two-bottle choice procedure reported that rats with adjuvant arthritis, induced by *Mycobacterium butyricum* which produces a syndrome of paw edema, inflammation, and heightened sensitivity to touch, demonstrated a preference for the bottle containing a solution of the NSAID suprofen (no longer available) over one containing a saccharin–glucose sweet solution (Colpaert et al., 1980). Control animals, however, showed a strong preference for the alternative sweet solution over that containing the NSAID. This relatively straightforward experiment suggested that it is possible to induce consumption of an analgesic when pain is present even though the analgesics appear to have no abuse liability as it was not ingested in control animals that were pain free. It is noteworthy that the consumption of suprofen decreased as the pathology (changes in joints and paws) decreased, a finding that might not be expected if the drug had both analgesic effects and abuse liability.

Lyness, Smith, Heavner, Iacono, and Garvin (1989) were among the first to examine the effects of intravenous morphine self-administration in rats following CFA injections in a model that also assessed responses to tail pressure as a measure of pain. Control animals that did not receive CFA rapidly escalated the self-administration of morphine over a 30-day period, whereas those rats that received CFA maintained much lower levels of morphine self-administration. Separate tests with these animals demonstrated that those self-administering morphine were similar to control pain-free animals in their sensitivity to tail pressure, indicating that the self-administered morphine was having an analgesic effect. As the effects of the pain began to dissipate in the CFA animals, however, morphine self-administration began to drift upward, suggesting that the maintenance of responding in pain differs from that in pain-free conditions.

The self-administration of a compound in animal models of pain has been used as a means to supplement the more reflex withdrawal methods that have been so widely used. For example, Martin, Kim, Buechler, Porreca, and Eisenach (2007) studied intravenous self-administration of a number of opioids (e.g., heroin, morphine, and fentanyl) in spinal nerve-ligated rats and compared the effects of these drugs to those obtained in sham-operated control animals. Across a broad range of doses for each drug, the nerve-injured animals self-administered less of each of these drugs at the lower doses than the sham-operated animals. Self-administration at intermediate to higher doses of these drugs was comparable in these two groups, but these effects were characteristically observed at the medium to higher doses on the descending limb of the dose–response curves. Most of the dose–response curves for the sham-operated animals were shifted to the left, possibly suggesting either that lower doses were more reinforcing in these animals than in those with pain or that the animals with the nerve ligation were titrating opioid doses for pain relief and not for the reinforcing aspects of the drug. Although these drugs were able to reverse the tactile allodynia following nerve ligation, the fact that responding was not as well maintained at the lower doses in the nerve-injured animals suggests that this differential sensitivity warrants further study. The effect was also obtained in an extensive study that examined fentanyl self-administration in three animal models of chronic pain, including inflammatory pain, peripheral nerve injury, and chemotherapy-induced pain (Wade et al., 2013). Under all conditions, self-administration of fentanyl was lower in those animals with pain than in control animals. Although there has been some concern about the effects of these drugs producing a diminished ability to respond due to pain, this issue was addressed by evaluating food-maintained responding which was not affected and did not differ between the control and experimental pain conditions. Thus, it seems to be a generally reproducible finding that the level of opioid self-administration is lower in those animals with induced pain, that this result cuts across different painful conditions, and that factors governing the self-administration of opiates differ between these groups.

A few studies in nerve-injured animals have examined drug self-administration of compounds that have analgesic effects but which have not been shown to have an associated abuse liability. For example, intrathecal self-administration of clonidine was examined in rats after spinal nerve ligation and in control animals (Martin, Kim, & Eisenach, 2006). Control animals in this study did not self-administer clonidine, whereas those with nerve injury engaged in high levels of clonidine self-administration. However, the nerve-injured animals did not continue to make lever responses when saline replaced the clonidine solution. In addition, the nerve-injured animals responded to changes in doses of clonidine such that when lower clonidine doses were made available, those doses were administered more frequently than the higher doses, suggesting that the animals were titrating the analgesic effects. Finally, this study also demonstrated that self-administration of clonidine, as well as the analgesic effects of clonidine, could be blocked by the α2-adrenoreceptor antagonist idazoxan, providing a clear indication of receptor specificity in mediating these effects.

Drug self-administration procedures also have been used to examine drugs from other pharmacological classes. For example, the sigma-1 antagonist S1RA was studied in a neuropathic pain model in mice and was found to maintain self-administration in nerve-injured animals at higher levels than those of the control mice (Bura, Guegan, Zamanillo, Vela, & Maldonado, 2013). In addition, S1RA also attenuated the reduction in sucrose consumption in the nerve-injured animals where the decrease in consumption of this palatable substance was believed to reflect an anhedonic state associated with the neuropathic pain. Gutierrez, Crystal, Zvonok, Makriyannis, and Hohmann (2011) studied the effects of the cannabinoid CB_2 receptor agonist (*R*,*S*)-AM1241 in a drug self-administration procedure with rats using a spared nerve injury model of neuropathic pain. In this study, drug self-administration and assessment of mechanical hypersensitivity were evaluated in the same animals. The self-administration procedure used a two-lever methodology in which a response on only one of the levers produced drug infusions. There were no differences in the percentage of responses on the two levers when each depression of the lever produced a drug infusion (fixed-ratio 1 or FR 1 schedule). However, when the response requirement for drug administration was increased from 1 to 3, 6, and then 9, the percentage of responses on the active lever that produced the drug increased for the injured animals up to the FR 6 response requirement but did not do so for the sham-operated subjects. In this study, the self-administration of (*R*,*S*)-AM1241 was sufficient in the spared nerve injury animals to reduce mechanical allodynia but had no effect on the sham or naïve animals.

Taken as a whole, the combined study of drug self-administration and the simultaneous assessment of analgesic effects is an exceptionally useful procedure for examining the potential abuse liability of a drug in the context of pain assessment. Using a within-subjects approach together with the appropriate control procedures and experimental paradigms offers unique opportunities not otherwise available with simple reflex models. In some respects, this procedure is similar to the many studies that have examined an escape response from a noxious stimulus such as an electric shock where the response terminates that stimulus. A major difference between these two procedures is that it is possible in the latter situation to repeatedly expose subjects to the noxious stimulus, whereas this is not possible under the self-administration procedure. However, it is possible to evaluate different doses, to assess titration levels, to explore a variety of schedules, and to simultaneously expose the animals to other conditions known to play a role in pain sensitivity, which are otherwise difficult using other methods. It is clear that this approach has much to offer and warrants greater attention and use in the future.

3. COMORBIDITIES WITH PAIN OR MULTISYMPTOM DISORDERS

The pathophysiology of pain is unquestionably complex and occurs at different levels that include peripheral nociceptors, the spinal cord, and in the brain where there is a further complex integration of pain transmission that involves different brain regions as well as responses that often lead to cognitive, emotional, and affective responses mediated by a variety of neurotransmitters. It is clear that pain is not a unidimensional condition and that there are frequently other coexisting features, particularly in the case of chronic pain. These can include cognitive impairment, insomnia, depression, PTSD, and anxiety (Burke, Finn, & Roche, 2015; Defrin et al., 2008; Li, 2015; Moriarty, McGuire, & Finn, 2011). Whether these conditions existed prior to the onset of pain or whether they ensue from, or are exacerbated by, chronic pain states adds to the difficulty in treatment approaches and to the design and conduct of clinical trials (Fishbain, Cutler, Rosomoff, & Rosomoff, 1997). The spectrum of pain comorbidities is quite heterogeneous and, at the present time, very little is known about the neurobiological relationships or the underlying pathophysiology of these conditions and how they may interact.

There are a number of very comprehensive reviews of preclinical research on the comorbidity of pain with affective disorders that clearly indicate that it is possible to induce some of those behaviors in rodent models that are seen in clinical populations where there is, for example, heightened anxiety and depression associated with chronic pain (e.g., Liu & Chen, 2014; Yalcin, Barthas, & Barrot, 2014). These reviews also include a survey of the various procedures that have been used to examine preclinical models of depression and anxiety, along with a focus on the neuroanatomical and neurobiology of CNS plasticity associated with the consequences of pain. These preclinical assays of depression and anxiety are usually quite similar to those assays that have been used to screen or evaluate new medical entities for their potential effects in these models to gauge potential therapeutic activity. They include the forced swimming test, tail suspension, and the Wistar–Kyoto strain of rats that manifest depression-like physiological and behavioral patterns, along with other models that produce immobility as an index of depressive-like behaviors. Although there has been less focus on animal models of anxiety, these have included the social defeat procedure (Andre et al., 2005), the elevated plus maze, as well as the light–dark apparatus.

There are many potential confounding factors in studies of comorbid pain and affective disorders that must be considered when evaluating the results. Several authors have pointed out the potential issues surrounding the possible motor impairment that results from spinal nerve ligation procedures if the behavioral assessment involves changes in locomotor behavior. Some have conducted studies to include roto-rod performances in control and experimental animals and have not reported impairments that could have confounded the results. In addition to these considerations, it must be determined whether the comorbid disorder of interest is specifically related to pain or is a possible pathophysiological characteristic or byproduct of the disease itself. For example, streptozotocin injections, used to examine diabetes and peripheral diabetic neuropathies, are known to produce a number of biochemical changes and modification of synaptic function that not only produce hyperalgesia but which might also directly affect behavior that is indirectly related to pain (Liu & Chen, 2014).

3.1 Clinical Studies

Clinical studies have recognized for some time that pain quite frequently coexists with other conditions, particularly depression and anxiety. The coexistence of pain with other conditions frequently leads to significant emotional lability and attentional biases with these conditions often leading to further impairment, incapacitation, and other disabilities. It has been estimated that, on average, roughly 65% of patients with depression have clinically significant pain and that this varies little across different settings (Bair, Robinson, Katon, & Kroenke, 2003). One clinical study, for example, reported that in a large randomized controlled trial of depressed patients being treated with one of the three selective serotonin reuptake antidepressants (sertraline, fluoxetine, and paroxetine), more than two-thirds of the patients reported varying degrees of pain from mild to severe at the baseline assessment period (Bair et al., 2004). Treatment response to depression was less likely to improve in patients suffering from pain than in those patients that reported no ongoing pain, with the severity of pain also affecting the outcome on measures of quality of life (Bair et al., 2004). Pain is also associated with a number of other clinical conditions. For example, chronic pain is also relatively common in HIV-infected patients, with coexistent elevated symptoms of depression (Uebelacker et al., 2015). Patients with greater anxiety and depression at the initial assessment are more likely to develop chronic pain from herpes zoster such that depressive symptoms significantly predict the development of chronic pain (Dworkin et al., 1992). Conversely, patients suffering from chronic pain are at an increased risk for depression. The interplay between psychological symptoms and chronic pain is evident in complex regional pain syndromes (CRPSs), for example, where symptoms, such as anxiety and depression as well as personality disorders, are not uncommon (Gierthmühlen, Binder, & Baron, 2014). CRPS is a condition with a complex pathophysiology and often unclear etiology that is associated with a number of symptoms that include sensory, autonomic, and motor abnormalities that are poorly managed and without definitive treatment options. Psychological comorbidities, including stress, can exacerbate CRPS and could be related to increased catecholamine release and higher levels of circulating epinephrine and norepinephrine (e.g., Bruehl, 2010; Harden et al., 2004). A more detailed analysis of the relationship of stress to pain is provided in a recent review by Johnson and Greenwood-Van Meerveld (2014).

3.2 Preclinical Studies of Coexisting Morbidities

It has also been demonstrated that, while depression can lead to emotional dysfunction in patients suffering from chronic pain, induced depression in animal models enhances the perception of selected sensory modalities such as cold allodynia while having little influence on mechanical threshold sensitivities (Bravo et al., 2012). Both pain and depression produce structural changes in several brain regions and systematic studies of the relationship between these conditions and how they may interact with pain currently is not known. Carefully conducted animal studies can yield insight into the relationship between pain and other comorbidities, particularly when it comes to "staging" the sequence of each condition, thereby providing potential insight into the genesis of how those comorbidities are established. An effort in this direction has been taken by Suzuki et al. (2007) who used a spared nerve injury model of neuropathic pain. These investigators found that both mechanical and thermal sensitivity were evident within 2 days following the surgery, and these sensitivities remained for at least a 3-month period. Depression- and anxiety-like behaviors, however, did not appear until 15 days following the nerve ligation, and both of these behaviors were also evident 30 days following the surgery. Since there was no indication of impaired motor abilities or alterations in circadian rhythms in the ligated mice, it was suggested that the changes in affective behaviors were not related to any motor dysfunctions or biological rhythms stemming from the surgical procedure. Although there are some exceptions, several other studies using a variety of pain models have generally replicated these results under conditions where pain has been demonstrated to induce or exacerbate depression or where depression induces or exacerbates the sensitivity to pain with findings somewhat more variable in the latter procedure (see review by Li, 2015). Several studies have demonstrated a relationship between impaired neurogenesis and depression, with these findings also demonstrated in animal models of pain and depression. The changes associated with nerve injury, depression-like behavior, and neurogenesis have been shown to occur in an interesting manner as was obtained in a study that examined tactile hypersensitivity, behavioral changes related to anxiety- and depression-like behaviors, and neurogenesis (Dimitrov, Tsuda, Cameron, & Usdin, 2014). In this study, tactile allodynia was produced in rats by placing a plastic cuff around the sciatic nerve. When subsequently removed, pain sensitivity resolved within several days. However, changes in behaviors indicative of anxiety, depression, and cognition, as measured by the elevated O-maze, forced swim, and novel object recognition procedure, respectively, persisted for at least 3 weeks following removal of the cuff. Furthermore, hippocampal neurogenesis, which was suppressed following the placement of the cuff, did not return within that same time period. It seems clear that the pathophysiological consequences of neuropathic pain as well as its resolution follow a different time course and are reflective of different processes.

An example of a depression model that has not been examined for its sensitivity to pain is shown in Fig. 1. In this study (B. Platt et al., unpublished data), animals were injected with BCG which induces sickness in rats that is then followed by a period of depressive-like behaviors such as decreases in locomotor behavior and reduced struggling in the tail-suspension test. When these behaviors were reduced, von Frey and Hargreaves assessments were conducted to examine sensitivity to mechanical and thermal stimuli, respectively. Compared to control (sham) animals that had not received BCG, there was a heightened sensitivity to these stimuli in the BCG-treated animals, showing that during the depressive-like condition, thresholds for mechanical and thermal pain were reduced.

A number of studies have examined the effects of different drugs on comorbid pain and depression in animal systems. Since the antidepressant

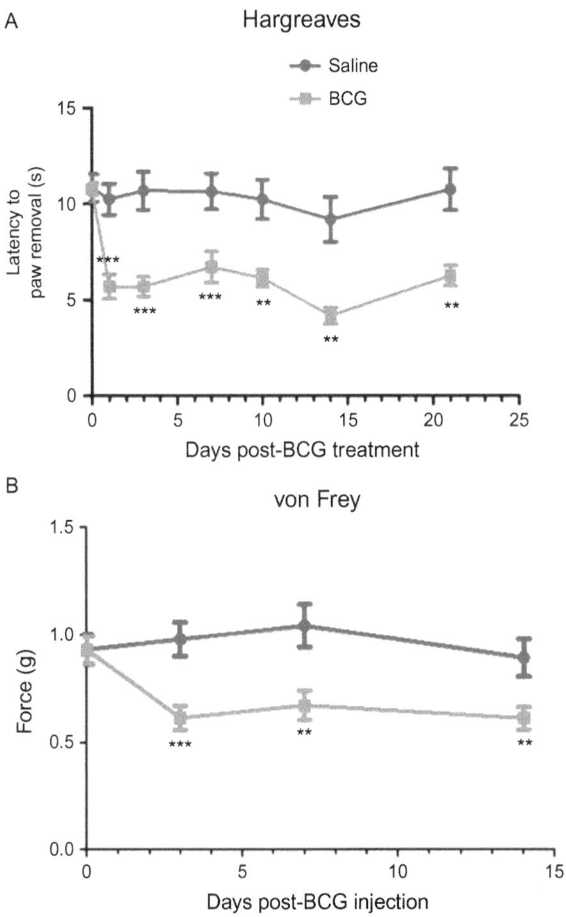

Figure 1 Thermal and tactile sensitivity of BCG-treated mice. Mice were tested for thermal sensitivity to pain using the Hargreaves test (A). A significant increase in thermal sensitivity was observed in BCG-treated mice with a 44% reduction in latency to paw removal observed 1 day post-BCG treatment that was maintained out to 21 days where a 42% reduction was observed. Saline $n=10$, BCG $n=9$. Mice were tested for tactile sensitivity to pain using the von Frey test (B). There was a significant 37% increase in tactile sensitivity in BCG-treated mice observed 3 days post-BCG that was maintained out to 14 days where a 31% increase was measured. (A) $n=9$–10. (B) $n=19$. UNIANOVA and post hoc *t*-tests used. $^{***}p \leq 0.001$, $^{**}p \leq 0.01$.

amitriptyline was developed to treat depression and has shown efficacy in a variety of clinical studies of depression as well as pain, it is not surprising that this drug has been shown to be effective in conditions where pain and depression coexist (Burke et al., 2015). In a chronic constriction injury model with mice subjected to the forced swim test, amitriptyline, fluoxetine, and bupropion produced antiallodynic effects but only amitriptyline produced significant antidepressant-like effects in the forced swim test (Jesse, Wilhelm, & Nogueria, 2010). These few studies suggest that it is possible to examine both the pharmacological and neurobiological aspects of pain and associated comorbidities. However, despite the prevalence of comorbid pain and mood disorders, it is clear that additional research is needed to yield better insight into the coexistence of these conditions in an effort to pursue more effective mediations.

3.3 Pain and Posttraumatic Stress Disorder

PTSD is typically the result of exposure to a traumatic event that posed actual or threatened death or injury. A consequence of these traumatic events is the development of fear, helplessness, and anxiety, as well as substance abuse. PTSD is estimated to have a prevalence rate of approximately 7–8% in the general population (Keane, Marshall, & Taft, 2006). A number of studies have reported a high degree of the co-occurrence of chronic pain and PTSD with the prevalence of chronic pain higher in patients with PTSD than in individuals without PTSD and the prevalence of PTSD in chronic pain patients greater than that in the rest of the population (Asmundson, Coons, Taylor, & Katz, 2002; Stam, 2007). PTSD has been associated frequently with combat veterans, where it has been estimated that between 66% and 80% of veterans that experienced combat-related PTSD also suffer from chronic pain (Beckham et al., 1997). Chronic pain has been reported by 25–93% of noncombat patients with PTSD; the severity of pain as well as pain-related disability is reported to be significantly greater in those individuals with current PTSD (Morasco et al., 2013; Outcalt et al., 2014). PTSD and chronic pain share many features that include hypervigilance and anxiety, as well as cognitive impairment and other physiological and psychological responses (Sharp & Harvey, 2001). It has been reported that individuals with pain and a current diagnosis of PTSD were significantly more likely to report having a prescription for opioid medication compared to those without a diagnosis of PTSD (Phifer et al., 2011). Individuals using opioid pain medications also had higher overall total PTSD symptoms, leading these authors to suggest that the comorbidity of pain and PTSD may share a vulnerability pathway related to the dysfunction of endogenous opioid neurotransmitter systems. The relationship between comorbid pain and PTSD, as well as the relationship of these conditions to those of depression and substance abuse clearly warrant further investigation as there remain multiple unanswered questions as to whether PTSD sensitizes individuals to pain, whether it induces or exacerbates an existing pain-related condition, and whether these coexisting conditions heighten susceptibility to substance abuse disorders.

Because of the complexity of comorbid pain and PTSD and the likely involvement of several neurobiological and neuropharmacological systems, efforts to treat individuals with these disorders have typically focused on antidepressant drugs. There have been few preclinical studies to examine the pharmacology of comorbid PTSD and pain. Recently, with growing evidence for a role of the nociception/orphanin FQ receptor in pain (Mannelli, Micheli, & Ghelardini, 2015), it has been shown that the nociception/orphanin FQ peptide receptor antagonist, JTC-801, reversed mechanical allodynia and thermal analgesia in a rat model of PTSD (Zhang, Simpson-Durand, & Standifer, 2015). In addition to reducing responses to painful stimuli and demonstrating a clear analgesic effect, JTC-801 also attenuated anxiety-like behavior and produced a significant reversal of corticosterone levels, which were reduced following exposure to the stressors. The finding in the Zhang et al. (2015) study that endogenous levels of nociception/orphanin FQ were increased following the induction of stress and also were reversed by JTC-801 provides further evidence, as mentioned above, that the opioid receptor system is involved in the comorbidities of pain and anxiety associated with PTSD. Clearly, there is much additional work to be pursued to clarify the pathobiology underlying PTSD, the molecular and epigenetic contributions to this condition, along with a better understanding of the development of comorbidities that would allow for the pursuit of effective pharmacological treatment approaches (see also Pitman et al., 2012 for an excellent review of these and other issues related to PTSD).

3.4 Pain and Cognition

The evidence for pain affecting a variety of cognitive functions in humans, including learning and executive function, is quite clear (review by Moriarty et al., 2011). Chronic pain often activates brain regions involved in cognitive processing (Henry et al., 2011; May, 2007). Several preclinical studies have demonstrated impaired learning in a variety of pain models and in a number of different cognitive domains such as spatial learning and attention. These effects have been evaluated in a number of different procedures such as operant nose poke, novel object recognition, and the Morris water maze (Moriarty et al., 2011). Of note is that the alleviation of pain in these procedures has been shown to also reverse the deficits in cognition. For example, Boyette-Davis, Thompson, and Fuchs (2008) examined the effects of inflammatory pain induced by formalin injections on attentional behavior in the five-choice serial reaction time task. These investigators reported that performances were impaired following the injection of formalin and that a dose of morphine attenuated the pain and improved performance. In an experimental model of colitis, Millecamps, Etienne, Jourdan, Eschalier, and Ardid (2004) found impaired attentional behavior in rodents experiencing chronic inflammatory pain, when this behavior was evaluated in a modified novel object recognition test. Both the effects on pain and cognition were attenuated by morphine and acetaminophen but not by aspirin and ibuprofen. The interactions of pain, depression anxiety, and cognition may be difficult to untangle, but the pursuit of answers to these comorbidities may yield considerable insight into the pathogenesis of these disorders.

4. RECENT TRENDS IN PAIN RESEARCH AND NEW APPROACHES TO DRUG DISCOVERY

4.1 Epigenetics and miRNAs

There are a number of relatively recent and exciting trends in pain research that hold considerable promise for helping to move the field forward. These include the emergence of pain epigenetics (e.g., Descalzi et al., 2015; Doehring, Geisslinger, & Lötsch, 2011; Seo et al., 2013) along with the effort to develop microRNA-based biomarkers for pain (see Kynast, Russe, Geisslinger, & Niederberger, 2013; Orlova et al., 2011; Von Schack et al., 2011; chapter "MicroRNA-Based Biomarkers in Pain" by Ramanathan and Ajit). It is widely acknowledged that sensitivity to pain as well as to analgesics can differ considerably between individuals. There are a number of factors that undoubtedly contribute to the differential sensitivity to pain and the effects of analgesics. These include genetic and epigenetic mechanisms, gender, as well as other environmental conditions. The study of epigenetics in the context of pain refers to enduring changes in gene expression that produce functional changes in cellular activity that can contribute to the development and chronicity of pain and to the variability in response to treatment interventions. The pursuit of epigenetic mechanisms that include detailed analyses of miRNAs and their target genes, along with an elucidation of their functional role, should help to stratify patients for clinical trials and treatment approaches, allow the field to move away from more subjective assessments of pain, differentiate the various heterogeneous disorders collectively referred to as "pain," and facilitate the identification of new therapeutic targets. The investigation and exploration of potential biomarkers for pain can also contribute to our knowledge of the epigenetics of pain, with these developments having potential utility in patient stratification and in novel treatment approaches (Douglas et al., 2015). In addition, in the quest for more translational and predictive animal models, the comparison of microRNA analyses from pain patients with various animal models may provide added insight into some of the potential differences between animal models and patients and may offer advantages for greater predictive value when these efforts are directed at back translation (Qureshi et al., 2015).

Both twin studies in humans and genetic–environmental interaction studies in mice have indicated that the environment can have a significant and lasting impact on pain prevalence and perception (Crow et al., 2013; Mogil et al., 2011; Nahorski, Chen, & Woods, 2015). For example, Nielsen et al. (2008), studying monozygotic and dizygotic twin pairs, reported large individual differences in pain sensitivity to cold and to heat pain with genetic factors contributing to an estimated 60% of the variance in cold pain and 26% for pain associated with heat. In this study, women reported more pain sensitivity to cold than to heat, whereas there were no differences between men and women in their sensitivity to heat stimuli. The demonstration that genetic effects are stimulus- or modality-dependent places a strong emphasis on the need for further studies that explore pain genes to play close attention to the phenotypic variations in response to different types of pain. Since it has been suggested that environmentally induced changes that occur throughout an organism's lifetime may account for at least half of the variance in pain perception and prevalence (Crow et al., 2013), it will be particularly important to carefully examine environment conditions as well. As one example of the long-term persistence of pain, it has been shown that physical and social adversity prior to 7 years of age can result in an increase in the risk of chronic widespread pain some 40 years later (Jones, Power, & Macfarlane, 2009). The impact of the environment on the response to pain, and likely to the response to drugs, emphasizes the need for a better understanding of the complex interaction between genetic and epigenetic factors as well as the need to include the role of the environment.

4.2 Stem Cell Approaches

Most pain research has relied on rodent cellular and *in vivo* animal models, leading many to suggest that the almost exclusive reliance on these approaches has been a significant factor in why the development of novel, effective, and safe pain therapeutics has been so difficult. There has been a recent effort to incorporate phenotypic assays that use mature human cells derived from ESCs along with induced pluripotent stem cells (iPSCs) to study disease relevant phenotypes such as autism, amyotrophic lateral sclerosis, and Parkinson's disease (McNeish, Gardner, Wainger, Woolf, & Eggan, 2015). The incorporation of differentiated cells from pluripotent stem cells has been used to screen drugs, to aid in target validation, and to provide an adjunct to the use of whole animal models. The process of generating iPSCs for therapeutic use in neurodegenerative diseases also has prompted new approaches for biomanufacturing iPSCs on a scalable level for commercialization (Silva et al., 2015). The investigational use of iPSCs has the potential also to identify new drug targets as well as to aid in the selection of patients where it may be possible to align a patient's genotype and cellular physiology with the appropriate drug. Advances in stem cell biology using pluripotent methodology have enabled the development of neurons from human embryonic stem cells (hESCs) as well as from fibroblasts that have resulted in the differentiation of nociceptor-like phenotypes. Chambers et al. (2012), for example, used a small-molecule screen and identified a combination of five small-molecule pathway inhibitors that overcame the relatively slow, stepwise process and produced human pluripotent stem cell (hPSC)-derived neurons with greater than 75% efficiency within 10 days of differentiation. Of interest in the present context, the resulting neurons expressed functional properties along with canonical markers of human nociceptor sensory neurons. In other studies, the differentiation of hPSCs and human induced pluripotent stem cells has been shown to produce functional neurons that express canonical markers of nociceptors such as Nav1.7 and Nav 1.8. These nociceptor-like neurons exhibit currents mediated by acid-sensing ion channels, TRPV1, and other targets known to be involved in pain (Chambers et al., 2012; Young et al., 2014). The functionality of some of these channels was confirmed using electrophysiology. In a separate study, Eberhardt et al. (2015) generated nociceptive sensory neurons from hESCs and also examined retrovirally reprogrammed iPSCs derived from fibroblasts. These neurons expressed markers of tetrodotoxin voltage-gated sodium currents (Nav1.8 and Nav1.9) that, using patch clamp experiments, were significantly more hyperpolarized than those obtained from rodent dorsal root ganglia. The difference in results was attributed to the expression of the developmentally important sodium channel Nav1.5.

Although promising and offering many advantages, several questions remain about this emerging area of research within the context of pain. For example, it is not clear how iPSCs will reflect epigenetic and environmental factors that appear to be so important in the development of chronic pain and in pain comorbidities. Nor is it clear how important the idiosyncratic history of the donor may be in the development of these model cell systems. However, the promise of these stem cell systems for probing signaling pathways, identifying drug target interactions, and exploring the role of the microenvironment, along with the exploration of iPSCs from patients suffering from different types of pain, may add new dimensions, insights, and opportunities for exploring new targets and enhancing the predictive validity of preclinical models.

4.3 Organs-on-a-Chip

Another development that will likely have an impact on pain research comes from the relatively recent advent of technologies that have combined cell biology, microfabrication, and microfluidics to produce microengineered models of human organs. These developments have provided new opportunities that are likely to have a significant future impact in several areas of drug discovery and development, including pain. Though somewhat early in the application of these technologies to pain, organs-on-chips hold the promise of introducing marked improvements in the study of drug effects on organ toxicity, pharmacokinetics and drug metabolism, biomarker development, as well as aiding in the more complicated areas such as target identification and validation (reviews by Bhatia & Ingber, 2014; Esch, Bahinski, & Huh, 2015). Organs-on-chips are devices using microchip manufacturing methods that permit the culturing of living cells to create model physiological functions of tissues and cells in a microfluidic environment. These microengineered cell culture organ system models are continuously perfused and permit the application of added physiological features such as mechanical or physical forces (e.g., stretch or compression) and fluidic flow parameters, thereby mimicking the cellular microenvironment and closely approximating organ functionality. The studies conducted thus far do not recreate the entire organ of interest but incorporate those cells that essentially recapitulate tissue- and organ-level physiological functions. Most studies to date have used established cell lines or primary cells, but it has also been demonstrated that the technology can be applied to ESCs and iPSCs isolated from different genetic populations and disease subgroups. The ability to study human molecular and cellular targets under conditions where they exist in their more physiological microenvironment offers great advantages for studying pain. Although not well suited at the present time for the study of more complex systems, there are possibilities of creating more integrated approaches through linkages and interconnected cell culture microchambers. Continued development of these approaches, particularly as they integrate stem cells with other techniques traditional to pain research, will help to address some of the challenges that have provided a barrier to the translation of pain research and the development of new therapeutics.

5. CONCLUSION

We have emphasized some of the perspectives and directions in the field of pain research that appear to warrant further attention. Several perspectives surrounding pain have evolved significantly in recent years. It has become clear that pain is not a unitary condition and that a single drug will not be effective in treating all forms of pain. There is considerable urgency to develop new nonopioid medications in light of the current epidemic with regard to opioid abuse and the high levels of overdose mortalities associated with these drugs. The coalescence and integration of different approaches are essential for better understanding the different types of pain and the underlying molecular mechanisms that will hold promise for identifying new targets for drug development. There is a need to move away from the excessive reliance on preclinical reflex models of hypersensitivity toward more translational models that include models of comorbid conditions associated with pain. Although we have not devoted much attention in this chapter to the issue of gender differences in pain, included in this shifting emphasis is the pressing need to better understand the underlying bases of sex differences in pain which will also likely involve different treatment approaches. Similarly, there is a need for the development of better biomarkers to allow for patient assessment and stratification and to evaluate treatment outcome. The more recent advances in the use of hESCs and iPSCs to complement these approaches for more effective translation of basic research findings into novel therapeutics hold considerable potential in many areas of pain research and clinical development. Although early in their development, these approaches will be complemented by further progress in the genetics and genomics of pain that will permit deeper insight into new diagnostic criteria, patient stratification, and more focused clinical trials (Dib-Hajj & Waxman, 2014). While these developments are promising, there are many questions that remain and it is hopefully clear that at the present time much additional work is required to further advance the field of pain research and therapeutics. One area of growing emphasis, and not addressed in this chapter, is the likely need for multitarget drugs to address the heterogeneity of pain disorders. There is also a clear need to better understand the pathophysiology and neuromolecular biology underlying the transition from acute to chronic pain. While we have concentrated mainly on certain aspects of emerging trends, we have not addressed the potential role of imaging, potential ways to improve human experimental pain models, or ways to improve the conduct and success of clinical trials and translation in pain research; these have been addressed by others (e.g., Arendt-Nielsen, Nielsen, & Gazerani, 2014; Borsook, Hargreaves, Bountra, & Porreca, 2014; Hayes et al., 2014; Lötsch, Oertel, & Ultsch, 2014; Oertel & Lötsch, 2012; Percie du Sert & Rice, 2014). Taken together, these new developments and technologies offer considerable potential to move our understanding of pain to new levels and to provide the foundation for novel approaches to therapeutic treatments.

CONFLICT OF INTEREST

The authors have no conflicts of interest to declare.

REFERENCES

Andre, J., Zeau, J., Pohl, M., Cesselin, F., Benoliel, J. J., & Becker, C. (2005). Involvement of cholecystokininergic systems in anxiety-induced hyperalgesia in male rats: Behavioral and biochemical studies. *Journal of Neuroscience*, *25*, 7896–7904.

Arendt-Nielsen, L., Nielsen, T., & Gazerani, P. (2014). Translational pain biomarkers in the early development of new neurotherapeutics for pain management. *Expert Reviews in Neurotherapeutics*, *14*, 241–254.

Asmundson, G. J. G., Coons, M. J., Taylor, S., & Katz, J. (2002). PTSD and the experience of pain: Research and clinical implications of shared vulnerability and mutual maintenance models. *Canadian Journal of Psychiatry*, *47*, 930–937.

Ator, N. A., & Griffiths, R. R. (2003). Principles of drug abuse liability assessment in laboratory animals. *Drug and Alcohol Dependence*, *70*(Suppl.), S55–S72.

Bair, M. J., Robinson, R. L., Eckert, G. J., Stang, P. E., Croghan, T. W., & Kroenke, K. (2004). Impact of pain on depression treatment response in primary care. *Psychosomatic Medicine*, *66*, 17–22.

Bair, M. J., Robinson, R. L., Katon, W., & Kroenke, K. (2003). Depression and pain comorbidity. *Archives of Internal Medicine*, *163*, 2433–2445.

Barrett, J. E. (2015). The pain of pain. *European Journal of Pharmacology*, *753*, 183–190.

Basbaum, A. I., & Braz, J. M. (2010). Transgenic mouse models for the tracing of "pain" pathways. In L. Kruger & A. R. Light (Eds.), *Translational pain research: From mouse to man*. Boca Raton, FL: CRC Press/Taylor & Francis.

Beckham, J. C., Crawford, A. L., Feldman, M. E., Kirby, A. C., Hertzberg, M. A., et al. (1997). Chronic posttraumatic stress disorder and chronic pain in Vietnam combat veterans. *Journal of Psychosomatic Research*, *43*, 379–389.

Berge, O.-G. (2014). Behavioral pharmacology of pain. *Current Topics in Behavioral Neurosciences*, *20*, 33–56.

Bhatia, S. N., & Ingber, D. E. (2014). Microfluidic organs-on-chips. *Nature Biotechnology*, *32*, 760–772.

Bolcskei, K., Helyes, Z., Szabo, A., Sandor, K., Elekes, K., Nemeth, J., et al. (2005). Investigation of the role of TRPV1 receptors in acute and chronic nociceptive processes using gene-deficient mice. *Pain*, *117*(3), 368–376.

Borsook, D., Hargreaves, R., Bountra, C., & Porreca, F. (2014). Lost but making progress—Where will new analgesic drugs come from? *Science Translational Medicine*, *6*, 249sr3.

Boyette-Davis, J. A., Thompson, C. D., & Fuchs, P. N. (2008). Alterations in attentional mechanisms in response to acute inflammatory pain and morphine administration. *Neuroscience*, *151*, 558–563.

Bravo, L., Mico, J. A., Rey-Brea, A. S., Pérez-Nievas, B., Leza, J. C., & Berrocoso, E. (2012). Depressive-like states heighten the aversion to painful stimuli in a rat model of comorbid chronic pain and depression. *Anesthesiology*, *117*, 613–625.

Bruehl, S. (2010). An update on the pathophysiology of complex regional pain syndrome. *Anesthesiology*, *113*, 713–725.

Bura, A. S., Guegan, T., Zamanillo, D., Vela, J. M., & Maldonado, R. (2013). Operant self-administration of a sigma ligand improves nociceptive and emotional manifestations of neuropathic pain. *European Journal of Pain*, *17*, 832–843.

Burke, N. N., Finn, D. P., & Roche, M. (2015). Chronic administration of amitriptyline differentially alters neuropathic pain-related behavior in the presence and absence of a depressive phenotype. *Behavioural Brain Research*, *278*, 193–201.

Caterina, M. J., Leffler, A., Malmberg, A. B., Martin, W. J., Trafton, J., Petersen-Zeitz, K. R., et al. (2000). Impaired nociception and pain sensation in mice lacking the capsaicin receptor. *Science*, *288*, 306–313.

Caterina, M. J., Schumacher, M. A., Tominaga, M., Rosen, T. A., Levine, J. D., & Julius, D. (1997). The capsaicin receptor: A heat-activated ion channel in the pain pathway. *Nature*, *389*, 816–824.

Chambers, S. M., Qi, Y., Mica, Y., Lee, G., Niu, L., Bilsland, J., et al. (2012). Combined small-molecule inhibition accelerates developmental timing and converts human pluripotent stem cells into nociceptors. *Nature Biotechnology*, *30*, 715–720.

Chen, C. C., Lamping, K. G., Nuno, D. W., Barresi, R., Prouty, S. J., Lavoie, J. L., et al. (2003). Abnormal coronary function in mice deficient in alpha1H T-type Ca^{2+} channels. *Science*, *302*, 1416–1418.

Chessell, I. P., Hatcher, J. P., Bountra, C., Michel, A. D., Hughes, J. P., Green, P., et al. (2005). Disruption of the P2X7 purinoceptor gene abolishes chronic inflammatory and neuropathic pain. *Pain*, *114*, 386–396.

Choi, S., Na, H. S., Kim, J., Lee, J., Lee, S., Kim, D., et al. (2007). Attenuated pain responses in mice lacking Ca(V)3.2 T-type channels. *Genes, Brain, and Behavior*, *6*, 425–431.

Clark, A. K., Staniland, A. A., Marchand, F., Kaan, T. K., McMahon, S. B., & Malcangio, M. (2010). P2X7-dependent release of interleukin-1beta and nociception in the spinal cord following lipopolysaccharide. *Journal of Neuroscience*, *30*, 573–582.

Colpaert, F. C., De Witte, P., Maroli, A. N., Awouters, F., Niemegeers, C. J. E., & Janssen, P. A. J. (1980). Self-administration of the analgesic suprofen in arthritic rats:

Evidence of Mycobacterium butyricum-induced arthritis as an experimental model of chronic pain. *Life Sciences*, *27*, 921–928.

Cong, L., Ran, F. A., Cox, D., Lin, S., Barretto, R., Habib, N., et al. (2013). Multiplex genome engineering using CRISPR/Cas systems. *Science*, *339*, 819–823.

Cox, J. J., Reimann, F., Nicholas, A. K., Thornton, G., Roberts, E., Springell, K., et al. (2006). An SCN9A channelopathy causes congenital inability to experience pain. *Nature*, *444*, 894–898.

Crow, M., Denk, F., & McMahon, S. B. (2013). Genes and epigenetic processes as prospective pain targets. *Genome Medicine*, *5*, 12.

Defrin, R., Ginzburg, K., Solomon, Z., Polad, E., Bloch, M., Govezensky, M., et al. (2008). Quantitative testing of pain perception in subjects with PTSD—Implications for the mechanism of the coexistence between PTSD and chronic pain. *Pain*, *138*, 450–459.

Descalzi, G., Ikegami, D., Ushijima, T., Nestler, E. J., Zachariou, V., & Narita, M. (2015). Epigenetic mechanisms of chronic pain. *Trends in Neurosciences*, *38*, 237–246.

Dib-Hajj, S. D., & Waxman, S. G. (2014). Translational pain research: Lessons from genetics and genomics. *Science Translational Medicine*, *6*, 249sr4.

Dimitrov, E. L., Tsuda, M. C., Cameron, H. A., & Usdin, T. B. (2014). Anxiety- and depression-like behavior and impaired neurogenesis evoked by peripheral neuropathy persist following resolution of prolonged tactile hypersensitivity. *Neurobiology of Disease*, *34*, 12304–12312.

Doehring, A., Geisslinger, G., & Lötsch, J. (2011). Epigenetics in pain and analgesia: An imminent research field. *European Journal of Pain*, *15*, 11–16.

Douglas, S. R., Shenoda, B. B., Qureshi, R. A., Sacan, A., Alexander, G. M., Perreault, M., et al. (2015). Analgesic response to intravenous ketamine is linked to a circulating microRNA signature in female complex regional pain syndrome patients. *Journal of Pain*, *16*, 814–824.

Dworkin, R. H., Hartstein, G., Rosner, H. L., Walther, R. R., Sweeney, E. W., & Brand, L. (1992). A high-risk method for studying psychosocial antecedents of chronic pain: The prospective investigation of herpes zoster. *Journal of Abnormal Psychology*, *101*, 200–205.

Eberhardt, E., Havlicek, S., Schmidt, D., Link, A. S., Neacsu, C., Kohl, Z., et al. (2015). Pattern of functional TTX-resistant sodium channels reveals a developmental stage of human iPSC- and ESC-derived nociceptors. *Stem Cell Reports*, *5*, 305–315.

Esch, E. W., Bahinski, A., & Huh, D. (2015). Organs-on-chips at the frontiers of drug discovery. *Nature Reviews. Drug Discovery*, *14*, 248–260.

Fishbain, D. A., Cutler, R., Rosomoff, H. L., & Rosomoff, R. S. (1997). Chronic pain-associated depression: Antecedent or consequence of chronic pain? A review. *Clinical Journal of Pain*, *13*, 116–137.

Foulkes, T., & Wood, J. N. (2008). Pain genes. *PLoS Genetics*, *4*(7), e1000086.

Gaskin, D. J., & Richard, P. (2012). The economic costs of pain in the United States. *Journal of Pain*, *13*, 715–724.

Gereau, R. W., Sluka, K. A., Maixner, W., Savage, S. R., Price, T. J., Murinson, B. B., et al. (2014). A pain research agenda for the 21st century. *Journal of Pain*, *15*, 1203–1214.

Gierthmühlen, J., Binder, A., & Baron, R. (2014). Mechanism-based treatment in complex regional pain syndromes. *Nature Reviews. Neurology*, *10*, 518–528.

Goldberg, Y. P., Price, N., Namdari, R., Cohen, C. J., Lamers, M. H., Winters, C., et al. (2012). Treatment of Na(v)1.7-mediated pain in inherited erythromelalgia using a novel sodium channel blocker. *Pain*, *153*, 80–85.

Gregory, N. S., Harris, A. L., Robinson, C. R., Dougherty, P. M., Fuchs, P. N., & Sluka, K. A. (2013). An overview of animal models of pain: Disease models and outcome measures. *Journal of Pain*, *14*, 1255–1269.

Gutierrez, T., Crystal, J. D., Zvonok, A. M., Makriyannis, A., & Hohmann, A. G. (2011). Self-medication of a cannabinoid CB_2 agonist in an animal model of neuropathic pain. *Pain, 152*, 1976–1987.

Harden, R. N., Rudin, N. J., Bruehl, S., Kee, W., Parikh, D. K., Kooch, J., et al. (2004). Increased systemic catecholamines in complex regional pain syndrome and relationship to psychological factors: A pilot study. *Anesthesia and Analgesia, 99*, 1478–1485.

Hatcher, J. P., & Chessell, I. P. (2006). Transgenic models of pain: A brief review. *Current Opinion in Investigational Drugs*, 7, 647–652.

Hayes, A. G., Arendt-Nielsen, L., & Tate, S. (2014). Multiple mechanisms have been tested in pain: How can we improve the chances of success? *Current Opinion in Pharmacology, 14*, 11–17.

Heindl-Erdmann, C., Axmann, R., Kreitz, S., Zwerina, J., Penninger, J., Schett, G., et al. (2010). Combining functional magnetic resonance imaging with mouse genomics: New options in pain research. *NeuroReport, 21*, 29–33.

Henry, D. E., Chiodo, A. E., & Yang, W. (2011). Central nervous system reorganization in a variety of chronic pain states: A review. *Physical Medicine and Rehabilitation, 3*, 1116–1125.

Honore, P., Wismer, C. T., Mikusa, J., Zhu, C. Z., Zhong, C., Gauvin, D. M., et al. (2005). A-425619 [1-isoquinolin-5-yl-3-(4-trifluoromethyl-benzyl)-urea], a novel transient receptor potential type V1 receptor antagonist, relieves pathophysiological pain associated with inflammation and tissue injury in rats. *Journal of Pharmacology and Experimental Therapeutics, 314*, 410–421.

Horton, D. B., Potter, D. M., & Mead, A. N. (2013). A translational pharmacology approach to understanding the predictive value of abuse potential assessments. *Behavioural Pharmacology, 24*, 410–436.

Hsu, P. D., Lander, E. S., & Zhang, F. (2014). Development and applications of CRISPR-Cas9 for genome engineering. *Cell, 157*(6), 1262–1278.

Institute of Medicine. (2011). *Relieving pain in America: A blueprint for transforming prevention, care, education and research*. Washington, DC: The National Academies Press.

Jesse, C. R., Wilhelm, E. A., & Nogueria, C. W. (2010). Depression-like behavior and mechanical allodynia are reduced by bis selenide treatment in mice with chronic constriction injury: A comparison with fluoxetine, amitriptyline, and bupropion. *Psychopharmacology, 212*, 513–522.

Johnson, A. C., & Greenwood-Van Meerveld, B. (2014). Stress-induced pain: A target for the development of novel therapeutics. *Journal of Pharmacology and Experimental Therapeutics, 351*, 327–335.

Jones, G. T., Power, C., & Macfarlane, G. J. (2009). Adverse events in childhood and chronic widespread pain in adult life: Results from the 1958 British Birth Cohort Study. *Pain, 143*, 92–96.

Keane, T. M., Marshall, A. D., & Taft, C. T. (2006). Posttraumatic stress disorder: Etiology, epidemiology, and treatment outcome. *Annual Review of Clinical Psychology, 2*, 161–197.

King, T., & Porreca, F. (2014). Preclinical assessment of pain: Improving models in discovery research. *Current Topics in Behavioral Neurosciences, 20*, 101–120.

Kissin, I. (2010). The development of new analgesics over the past 50 years: A lack of real breakthrough drugs. *Anesthesia and Analgesia, 110*, 780–789.

Knabl, J., Witschi, R., Hosl, K., Reinold, H., Zeilhofer, U. B., Ahmadi, S., et al. (2008). Reversal of pathological pain through specific spinal GABAA receptor subtypes. *Nature, 451*, 330–334.

Kynast, K. L., Russe, O. Q., Geisslinger, G., & Niederberger, E. (2013). Novel findings in pain processing pathways: Implications for miRNAs as future therapeutic targets. *Expert Reviews in Neurotherapeutics, 13*, 515–525.

LaCroix-Fralish, M. L., Ledoux, J. B., & Mogil, J. S. (2007). The *Pain Genes Database*: An interactive web browser of pain-related transgenic knockout studies. *Pain, 131*, 1–4.

Lariviere, W. R., Chesler, E. J., & Mogil, J. S. (2001). Transgenic studies of pain and analgesia: Mutation or background genotype? *Journal of Pharmacology and Experimental Therapeutics*, *297*, 467–473.
Li, J.-X. (2015). Pain and depression comorbidity: A preclinical perspective. *Behavioural Brain Research*, *276*, 92–98.
Liu, M.-G., & Chen, J. (2014). Preclinical research on pain comorbidity with affective disorders and cognitive deficits: Challenges and perspectives. *Progress in Neurobiology*, *116*, 13–32.
Lötsch, J., Oertel, B. G., & Ultsch, A. (2014). Human models of pain for the prediction of clinical analgesia. *Pain*, *155*, 2014–2021.
Lozano-Ondoua, A. N., Symons-Liguori, A. M., & Vanderah, T. W. (2013). Cancer-induced bone pain: Mechanisms and models. *Neuroscience Letters*, *557*(Pt. A), 52–59.
Lyness, W. H., Smith, F. L., Heavner, J. E., Iacono, C. U., & Garvin, R. D. (1989). Morphine self-administration in the rat during adjuvant-induced arthritis. *Life Sciences*, *45*, 2217–2224.
Manfredi, M., Bini, G., Cruccu, G., Accornero, N., Berardelli, A., & Medolago, L. (1981). Congenital absence of pain. *Archives of Neurology*, *38*, 507–511.
Mannelli, L. D., Micheli, L., & Ghelardini, C. (2015). Nociceptin/orphanin FQ receptor and pain: Feasibility of the fourth opioid family member. *European Journal of Pharmacology*, *766*, 151–154.
Martin, T. J., Kim, S. A., Buechler, N. L., Porreca, F., & Eisenach, J. C. (2007). Opioid self-administration in the nerve-injured rat: Relevance of antiallodynic effects to drug consumption and effects of intrathecal analgesics. *Anesthesiology*, *106*, 312–322.
Martin, T. J., Kim, S. A., & Eisenach, J. C. (2006). Clonidine maintains intrathecal self-administration in rats following spinal nerve ligation. *Pain*, *125*, 257–263.
Max, M. B., & Stewart, W. F. (2008). The molecular epidemiology of pain: A new discipline for drug discovery. *Nature Reviews. Drug Discovery*, *7*, 647–658.
May, A. (2007). Neuroimaging: Visualizing the brain in pain. *Neurological Sciences*, *28*(Suppl. 2), S101–S107.
McNeish, J., Gardner, J. P., Wainger, B. J., Woolf, C. J., & Eggan, K. (2015). From dish to bedside: Lessons learned while translating findings from a stem cell model of disease to clinical trial. *Cell Stem Cell*, *17*, 8–10.
Mifflin, K. A., & Kerr, B. J. (2014). The transition from acute to chronic pain: Understanding how different biological systems interact. *Canadian Journal of Anaesthesia*, *2014*(61), 112–122.
Millecamps, M., Etienne, M., Jourdan, D., Eschalier, A., & Ardid, D. (2004). Decrease in non-selective, non-sustained attention induced by a chronic visceral inflammatory state as a new pain evaluation in rats. *Pain*, *109*, 214–224.
Minett, M. S., Eijkelkamp, N., & Wood, J. N. (2014). Significant determinants of mouse pain behaviour. *PLoS One*, *9*(8), e104458.
Minett, M. S., Pereira, V., Sikandar, S., Matsuyama, A., Lolignier, S., Kanellopoulos, A. H., et al. (2015). Endogenous opioids contribute to insensitivity to pain in humans and mice lacking sodium channel $Na_v1.7$. *Nature Communications*, *6*, 8967. http://dx.doi.org/10.1038/ncomms9967.
Mogil, J. S. (2009). Animal models of pain: Progress and challenges. *Nature Reviews. Neuroscience*, *10*, 283–294.
Mogil, J. S. (2012). Pain genetics: Past, present and future. *Trends in Genetics*, *28*, 258–266.
Mogil, J. S., & Grisel, J. E. (1998). Transgenic studies of pain. *Pain*, *77*, 107–128.
Mogil, J. S., Sorge, R. E., LaCroix-Fralish, M. L., Smith, S. B., Fortin, A., Sotocinal, S. G., et al. (2011). Pain sensitivity and vasopressin analgesia are mediated by a gene-sex environment interaction. *Nature Neuroscience*, *14*, 1569–1573.
Mogil, J. S., Wilson, S. G., Bon, K., Lee, S. E., Chung, K., Raber, P., et al. (1999). Heritability of nociception I: Responses of 11 inbred mouse strains on 12 measures of nociception. *Pain*, *80*, 67–82.

Molet, J., & Pohl, M. (2013). Gene-based approaches in pain research and exploration of new therapeutic targets and strategies. *European Journal of Pharmacology, 717*, 129–141.

Morasco, B. J., Lovejoy, T. I., Lu, M., Turk, D. C., Lewis, L., & Dobscha, S. K. (2013). The relationship between PTSD and chronic pain: Mediating role of coping strategies and depression. *Pain, 154*, 609–616.

Moriarty, O., McGuire, B. E., & Finn, D. P. (2011). The effect of pain on cognitive function: A review of clinical and preclinical research. *Progress in Neurobiology, 93*, 385–404.

Na, H. S., Choi, S., Kim, J., Park, J., & Shin, H. S. (2008). Attenuated neuropathic pain in Cav3.1 null mice. *Molecules and Cells, 25*, 242–246.

Nahin, R. L. (2015). Estimates of pain prevalence and severity in adults: United States, 2012. *Journal of Pain, 16*, 769–780.

Nahorski, M. S., Chen, Y.-C., & Woods, C. G. (2015). New Mendelian disorders of painlessness. *Trends in Neurosciences, 38*, 712–724.

Nassar, M. A., Levato, A., Stirling, L. C., & Wood, J. N. (2005). Neuropathic pain develops normally in mice lacking both Na(v)1.7 and Na(v)1.8. *Molecular Pain, 1*, 24.

Nassar, M. A., Stirling, L. C., Forlani, G., Baker, M. D., Matthews, E. A., Dickenson, A. H., et al. (2004). Nociceptor-specific gene deletion reveals a major role for Nav1.7 (PN1) in acute and inflammatory pain. *Proceedings of the National Academy of Sciences of the United States of America, 101*, 12706–12711.

Navratilova, E., Xie, J. Y., King, T., & Porreca, F. (2013). Evaluation of reward from pain relief. *Annals of the New York Academy of Sciences, 1282*, 1–11.

Nielsen, C. S., Stubhaug, A., Price, D. D., Vassend, O., Czajkowski, N., Harris, J. R., et al. (2008). Individual differences in pain sensitivity: Genetic and environmental contributions. *Pain, 136*, 21–29.

Nissenbaum, J. (2012). From mouse to humans: Discovery of the CACNG2 pain susceptibility gene. *Clinical Genetics, 82*, 311–320.

Oertel, B. G., & Lötsch, J. (2012). Clinical pharmacology of analgesics assessed with human experimental pain models: Bridging basic and clinical research. *British Journal of Pharmacology, 168*, 534–553.

Orlova, I. A., Alexander, G. M., Qureshi, R. A., Sacan, A., Graziano, A., Barrett, J. E., et al. (2011). MicroRNA modulation in complex regional pain syndrome. *Journal of Translational Medicine, 9*, 195.

Outcalt, S. D., Ang, D. C., Wu, J., Sargent, C., Yu, Z., & Bair, M. J. (2014). Pain experience of Iraq and Afghanistan veterans with comorbid chronic pain and posttraumatic stress. *Journal of Rehabilitation Research and Development, 51*, 559–570.

Percie du Sert, N., & Rice, A. S. C. (2014). Improving the translation of analgesic drugs to the clinic: Animal models of neuropathic pain. *British Journal of Pharmacology, 171*, 2951–2963.

Phifer, J., Skelton, K., Weiss, T., Schwartz, A. C., WIngo, A., Gillespie, C. F., et al. (2011). Pain symptomatology and pain medication use in civilian PTSD. *Pain, 152*, 2233–2240.

Pitman, R. K., Rasmusson, A. M., Koenen, K. C., Shin, L. M., Orr, S. P., Gilbertson, M. W., et al. (2012). Biological studies of post-traumatic stress disorder. *Nature Reviews. Neuroscience, 13*, 769–787.

Qureshi, R. A., Tian, Y., McDonald, M. K., Capasso, K. E., Douglas, S. R., Gao, R., et al. (2015). Circulating microRNA signatures in rodent models of pain. *Molecular Neurobiology*, 1–12. http://dx.doi.org/10.1007/s12035-015-9281-4.

Saegusa, H., Kurihara, T., Zong, S., Kazuno, A., Matsuda, Y., Nonaka, T., et al. (2001). Suppression of inflammatory and neuropathic pain symptoms in mice lacking the N-type Ca^{2+} channel. *The EMBO Journal, 20*, 2349–2356.

Sander, J. D., & Joung, J. K. (2014). CRISPR-Cas systems for editing, regulating and targeting genomes. *Nature Biotechnology, 32*, 347–355.

Seo, S., Grzenda, A., Lomberk, G., Ou, X.-M., Cruciani, R. A., & Urrutia, R. (2013). Epigenetics: A promising paradigm for better understanding and managing pain. *Journal of Pain, 14*, 549–557.

Sharp, T. J., & Harvey, A. G. (2001). Chronic pain and posttraumatic stress disorder: Mutual maintenance? *Clinical Psychology Review, 21*, 857–877.

Sikandar, S., Patel, R., Patel, S., Sikander, S., Bennett, D. L. H., & Dickenson, A. H. (2013). Genes, molecules and patients—Emerging topics to guide clinical pain research. *European Journal of Pharmacology, 716*, 188–202.

Silva, M., Daheron, L., Hurley, H., Bure, K., Barker, R., Carr, A. J., et al. (2015). Generating iPSCs: Translating cell reprogramming science into scalable and robust biomanufacturing strategies. *Cell Stem Cell, 16*, 13–17.

Solle, M., Labasi, J., Perregaux, D. G., Stam, E., Petrushova, N., Koller, B. H., et al. (2001). Altered cytokine production in mice lacking P2X(7) receptors. *Journal of Biological Chemistry, 276*, 125–132.

Stam, R. (2007). PTSD and stress sensitisation: A tale of brain and body. Part 1: Human studies. *Neuroscience and Biobehavioral Reviews, 31*, 530–557.

Suzuki, T., Amata, M., Sakaue, G., Nishimura, S., Inoue, T., Shibata, M., et al. (2007). Experimental neuropathy in mice is associated with delayed behavioral changes related to anxiety and depression. *Anesthesia and Analgesia, 104*, 1570–1577.

Teuns, G. B., Geys, H. M., Geuens, S. M., Stinissen, P., & Meert, T. F. (2014). Abuse liability assessment in preclinical drug development: Predictivity of a translational approach for abuse liability testing using methylphenidate in four standardized preclinical study models. *Journal of Pharmacological and Toxicological Methods, 70*, 295–309.

Uebelacker, L. A., Weisberg, R. B., Herman, D. S., Bailey, G. L., Pinkston-Camp, M. M., & Stein, M. D. (2015). Chronic pain in HIV-infected patients: Relationship to depression, substance use, and mental health and pain treatment. *Pain Medicine, 16*, 1870–1881.

von Frey, M. (1896). Untersuchungen über die Sinnesfunctionen der menschlichen haut. Erste abhandlung: druckempfindung und schmerz (Reproduced in German and English). In H. O. Handwerker & K. Brune (Eds.), *Deutschprachige Klassiker der Schmerzforchung. Classical German Contributions to Pain Research*. Heidelberg: Gesellschaft zum Studium des Schemerzes für Deutschland, Österreich und die Schweiz.

Von Schack, D., Agostino, M. J., Murray, B. S., Li, Y., Reddy, P. S., Chen, J., et al. (2011). Dynamic changes in microRNA expression profile reveal multiple regulatory mechanism in the spinal nerve ligation model of neuropathic pain. *PLoS One, 6*(3), e17670.

Wade, C. L., & Fairbanks, C. A. (2014). The self-administration of analgesic drugs in experimentally induced chronic pain. *Current Topics in Behavioral Neurosciences, 20*, 217–232.

Wade, C. L., Krumenacher, P., Kitto, K. F., Peterson, C. D., Wilcox, G. L., et al. (2013). Effect of chronic pain on fentanyl self-administration in mice. *PLoS One, 8*(11), e79239.

Woolf, C. J. (2010). Overcoming obstacles to developing new analgesics. *Nature Medicine, 16*, 1241–1247.

Yaksh, T. L., Woller, S. A., Ramachandran, R., & Sorkin, L. S. (2015). The search for novel analgesics: Targets and mechanisms. *F1000Prime Reports, 7*, 56.

Yalcin, I., Barthas, F., & Barrot, M. (2014). Emotional consequences of neuropathic pain: Insight from preclinical studies. *Neuroscience and Biobehavioral Reviews, 47*, 154–164.

Young, G. T., Gutteridge, A., Fox, H. D. E., Wilbrey, A. L., Cao, L., Cho, L. T., et al. (2014). Characterizing human stem cell-derived sensory neurons at the single-cell level reveals their ion channel expression and utility in pain research. *Molecular Therapy, 22*, 1530–1543.

Zhang, Y., Simpson-Durand, C. D., & Standifer, K. M. (2015). Nociceptin/orphanin FQ peptide receptor antagonist JTC-801 reverses pain and anxiety symptoms in a rat model of post-traumatic stress disorder. *British Journal of Pharmacology, 172*, 571–582.

CHAPTER TWO

MicroRNA-Based Biomarkers in Pain

Sujay Ramanathan, Seena K. Ajit[1]
Department of Pharmacology and Physiology, Drexel University College of Medicine, Philadelphia, Pennsylvania, USA
[1]Corresponding author: e-mail address: seena.ajit@drexelmed.edu

Contents

Abstract

Biomarkers are measurable characteristics reflective of the physiological or diseased state and a crucial feature in rendering personalized medicine more precise. Dysregulated expression of circulating microRNAs (miRNAs) in bodily fluids is being explored as noninvasive clinical biomarker for a variety of disorders including chronic pain. High-precision qPCR-based signal amplification of these miRNAs enables the detection of small changes making them ideal biomarker candidates. Presence of circulating miRNAs in exosomes, small vesicles that mediate intercellular communication, opens up novel avenues for target intervention and biomarker discovery. miRNA signatures specific to different pain conditions, and their reversal on treatment in patients and animal models can be beneficial in patient stratification, prognosis, and in bridging preclinical and clinical results. Identification of multiple miRNAs as opposed to reliance on one specific molecule as a biomarker could improve treatment efficacies in an extremely heterogeneous pain patient population. Additionally, owing to the stability of miRNAs, retrospective studies could be performed using banked samples

Advances in Pharmacology, Volume 75
ISSN 1054-3589
http://dx.doi.org/10.1016/bs.apha.2015.12.001

from completed clinical trials. Irrespective of the phase and outcome, these studies can provide insights on molecular underpinnings influencing treatment outcome, or specific therapeutic intervention. Identification of miRNAs altered in chronic pain states will have a significant impact on the identification of right leads, targets, doses, and patients. Effective implementation of miRNA-based biomarkers would provide treatment guidance for clinicians, better clinical trial designs for pharmaceutical companies, all leading to individualized care and better treatment outcome for chronic pain patients.

ABBREVIATIONS

CFA complete Freund's adjuvant
CT cycle threshold
miRNA microRNA
NMDA *N*-methyl-D-aspartate
PBMCs peripheral blood mononuclear cells
TLDA TaqMan low density array
TLR Toll-like receptors
UTR untranslated region

1. INTRODUCTION

Chronic pain affects millions of people worldwide impacting the quality of life and posing an enormous burden on healthcare systems (Gereau IV et al., 2014). Chronic pain includes neuropathic pain resulting from injury and malfunction of the nervous system, lower back pain, migraines, osteoarthritis, etc. Traditionally, physiologic and behavioral responses are used to assess pain in animals and people (Peterson & Servinsky, 2007). Pain scoring and assessment in humans are subjective and necessitates the development of objective measures to assess pain (Chizh, Greenspan, Casey, Nemenov, & Treede, 2008). Development of new analgesics is stymied by high failure rates of drugs targeted to treat neuropathic pain. Thus, there is an urgent need to develop biomarkers that may potentially reduce failures in drug discovery (Kola & Landis, 2004; Woodcock, Witter, & Dionne, 2007).

Much of the focus in biomarker discovery in the pain field has been on secreted inflammatory mediators (Marchi, Vellucci, Mameli, Rita Piredda, & Finco, 2009). Unlike cancer biology, where researchers have access to tissue samples, CNS disorders including pain are dependent on biological markers that can be identified from bodily fluids, predominantly blood. Small non-protein coding endogenous ~22 nucleotide RNA molecules called microRNAs (miRNAs) have attracted considerable attention in recent years both as potential biomarkers as well as for their utility in dissecting the molecular changes underlying various diseases. miRNAs play important roles in the regulation of gene expression and function by binding predominantly to the 3′-untranslated region (3′UTR) of target mRNAs that, in turn, causes cleavage or repression of translation of these mRNAs. Each miRNA species regulates multiple genes, and most mRNA targets contain multiple miRNA binding sites within their 3′UTR, rendering a complex regulatory network (Bartel, 2009). Owing to their aberrant expression in a variety of human pathologies, miRNAs are often employed in the pursuit of biomarker identification and to discover and validate novel therapeutic targets (Erson & Petty, 2008).

The first reports of the presence of stable miRNAs in blood were published in 2008 (Chen et al., 2008; Gilad et al., 2008; Mitchell et al., 2008). These reports were followed by a number of studies, predominantly in cancer biology, demonstrating the utility of miRNAs as biomarkers of the disease state and progression (De Guire et al., 2013). It is now well established that miRNAs are present in the serum and plasma of humans and other mammals. This finding opens up the feasibility of using miRNAs as biomarkers of disease. Though the stability of miRNAs in serum was the initial concern, it has now been demonstrated that these circulating miRNAs are protected from plasma RNase activity and are, in fact quite stable (Chen et al., 2008).

2. MECHANISM OF ACTION AND miRNA BIOGENESIS

The modulation of eukaryotic gene expression is regulated at various levels which include the basic genetic mechanisms, like initiation of transcription, transcriptional processing, posttranslational modification, and extends to epigenetic mechanisms. In addition to DNA methylation and histone modification-mediated epigenetic modifications that influence access to DNA and thus protein expression (Jirtle & Skinner, 2007; Vaissiere, Sawan, & Herceg, 2008), RNA-mediated gene silencing is another mechanism that is crucial in posttranscriptional gene silencing (Bartel, 2009). miRNAs comprise a group of short noncoding single-stranded RNA molecules and potentiate epigenetic regulation of a significant proportion of the genome at the posttranscriptional level. miRNA binds to the 8–10 nucleotide long, conserved "seed sequence" present within the UTRs of a target mRNA and thereupon exerts its effect. Numerous studies suggest the involvement of miRNAs in key biological processes such as development, immune system, and cellular homeostasis, and their altered expression and regulation is observed in various pathological conditions such as autoimmune diseases, neurological and vascular diseases, infection, and cancer (Croce, 2009). In humans, genes coding for miRNA are known to be present on all chromosomes, with the exception of the Y chromosome and about 50% of them are located within the intergenic regions and possess their own regulatory elements (Corcoran et al., 2009; Lagos-Quintana, Rauhut, Lendeckel, & Tuschl, 2001).

The biogenesis of a miRNA is initiated in the nucleus with the transcription from its corresponding gene by either RNA polymerase II or RNA polymerase III, giving rise to a long (2–4 kb) primary transcript known as pri-miRNA, which is then poly-adenylated (Cai, Hagedorn, & Cullen, 2004). The pri-miRNA is then processed into an imperfectly base paired stem loop structure of about 70–100 nucleotides known as precursor miRNA (pre-miRNA) by a microprocessor complex consisting of specific double-stranded ribonucleases called Drosha, Pasha, and accessory proteins (Denli, Tops, Plasterk, Ketting, & Hannon, 2004; Lee et al., 2003). A RanGTPase and exportin 5-dependent mechanism aids the translocation of this pre-miRNA to the cytoplasm where it is cleaved into a short (about 22 bp long), imperfectly paired, double-stranded mature miRNA–miRNA* duplex by another double-stranded endonuclease, known as Dicer and accessory protein TRBP (Chendrimada et al., 2005; Yi, Qin, Macara, & Cullen, 2003). Further processing by an argonaute protein, Ago2, allows one of the complementary strands of the duplex, known as the guide-strand to be incorporated into the miRNA-induced silencing complex (RISC), while the miRNA* strand, also known as passenger strand, is often degraded. This asymmetric incorporation into the RISC is supposedly determined by which miRNA strand 5′-end is less tightly paired (Khvorova, Reynolds, & Jayasena, 2003). A Drosha-independent machinery identified in mammals, include the biogenesis of mirtons, spliced from the introns of mRNA coding genes and exported to the cytoplasm and processed by Dicer (Okamura, Hagen, Duan, Tyler, & Lai, 2007; Ruby et al., 2007) (Fig. 1).

The RISC-bound miRNA possesses complementary sequence to the regions within the 3′UTR of the target mRNAs and is the effector complex regulating their posttranscriptional expression by various mechanisms such as mRNA cleavage, mRNA destabilization, and inhibition of translation

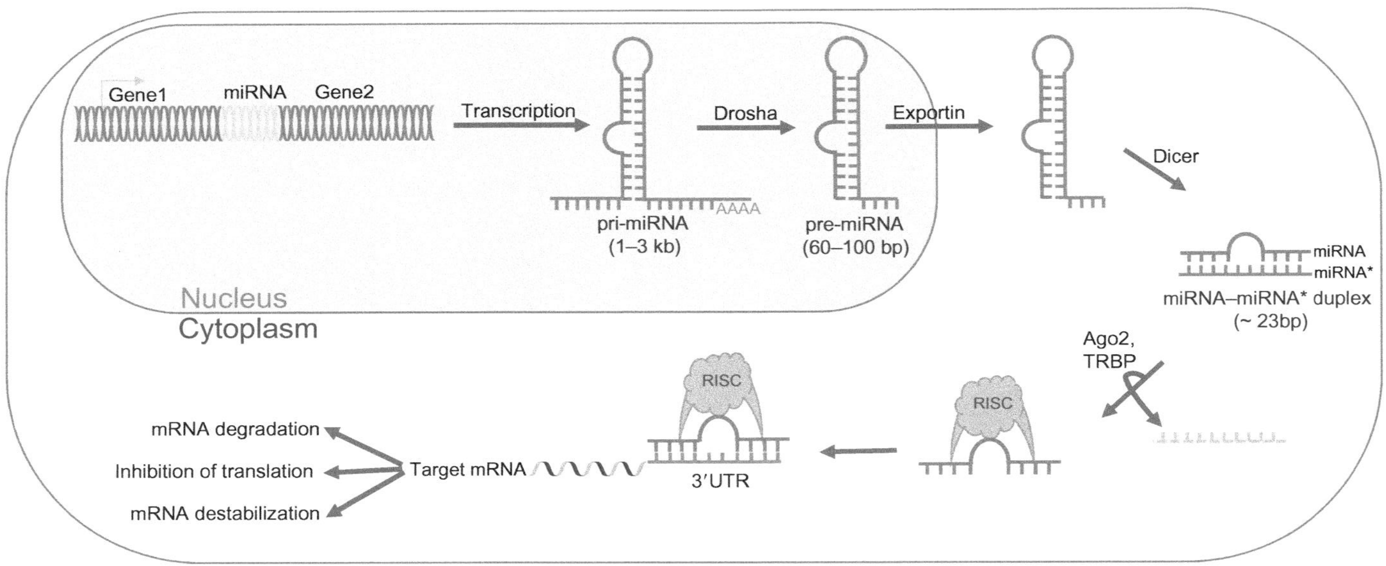

Figure 1 Biogenesis of miRNA and its mode of action. A vast majority of miRNAs are intergenic, and are transcribed by RNA polymerase II, into a long stem looped pri-miRNA transcript in the nucleus. The pri-miRNA is processed by a microprocessing machinery consisting of endonucleases like Drosha, to form a 60–100-bp long pre-miRNA. This is exported into the cytoplasm by exportin and other accessory proteins. In the cytoplasm, further processing by Dicer and auxiliary proteins generate the mature double-stranded miRNA–miRNA* duplex. An asymmetric and selective process governed by the Ago2 and TRBP proteins incorporate the guide strand into the RISC complex, while the passenger strand is usually degraded. The active miRNA–RISC complex regulates target gene expression by its binding to the 3′UTR of target mRNAs, which could either lead to degradation or destabilization of target mRNA, or inhibit protein translation.

(Elramah et al., 2014). While the mechanism of mRNA cleavage requires perfect base pairing (observed in metazoans), the latter two mechanisms involve imperfect base pairing and are more common in mammals. The location of miRNA binding sites (seed region) on the target mRNA plays a key role in their regulation, with the most effective seed regions occurring at the 3′UTRs, and in some cases could also be potentiated by similar regions within the coding region. This could be attributed to higher affinity of the translation complex in comparison to RISC, within the 5′UTR and ORF of the mRNA, thus displacing the silencing complex (Bartel, 2009).

While the composition of the seed region may differ, it always involves a conserved Watson–Crick pairing to the nucleotides at 5′-region of the miRNA, resulting in diverse affinities and inhibition properties. These include canonical sites with a 6- to 8-nt match, noncanonical additional pairing at the 3′-end of the miRNA. Additional factors have been shown to affect miRNA seed efficacy such as AU-rich sites, the position of the seed within the 3′UTR of the target-mRNA (Grimson et al., 2007), with sites at the extremities of the 3′UTR being more accessible than those in the middle because long UTRs may form occlusive interactions, thus greatly reducing miRNA site accessibility.

3. CIRCULATING miRNAs

miRNAs modulate paracrine signaling by their release into circulation in various forms and processes. Often transported either within extracellular vesicles or as RNase resistant complexes through their association with lipoproteins (high density lipoproteins) or RNA binding proteins (Ago2), these miRNA entities collectively, but not limited to, are termed circulating miRNAs (Boon & Vickers, 2013; Grasedieck et al., 2013). Although it is still unclear whether all circulating miRNAs are Ago bound and/or associated in exosomes, miRNAs found in plasma were reportedly resistant to endogenous RNases (Mitchell et al., 2008; Turchinovich, Weiz, Langheinz, & Burwinkel, 2011). The identification of several types of noncoding RNAs in the circulation within extracellular vesicles (El Andaloussi et al., 2013) has generated tremendous interest both from a biomarker perspective and for their therapeutic potential (Alvarez-Erviti et al., 2011). Intercellular communication is predominantly thought to be mediated either through direct cell–cell contact or through the transfer of secreted molecules like peptides, hormones, and cytokines. More recently, a third mode of communication involving extracellular vesicles has been recognized to play an important role in this intercellular information transfer (Kowal, Tkach, & Thery, 2014; Raposo & Stoorvogel, 2013; El Andaloussi et al., 2013). This latter method of transport of biomolecular cargo has gained enormous attention due to the vesicular contents, including but not limited to several species of RNA, proteins, and lipids. It has been recently quite well substantiated that uptake of these vesicles can impart functional consequences in the recipient cells (Raposo & Stoorvogel, 2013).

Exosomes are extracellular vesicles 30–100 nm in size and are derived from the endocytic compartment of the cell. Exosomes are generated by the inward budding of an endosomal membrane that results in the formation of multivesicular bodies (Raiborg, Rusten, & Stenmark, 2003; Stoorvogel, Kleijmeer, Geuze, & Raposo, 2002), which in a specific secretory pathway can fuse with the plasma membrane, releasing the exosomes either to the adjacent cell or into the circulation. Exosomes are released by various cell types, reticulocytes, and platelets and are present in most bodily fluids (Kalra et al., 2012). The protein and lipid composition of exosomes differs from that of other types of extracellular vesicles including apoptotic bodies. In fact, exosomes are enriched in certain proteins and lipids and they are used as markers to differentiate exosomes from other types of extracellular vesicles, organelles, or cellular debris (Gyorgy et al., 2011; Record, Subra, Silvente-Poirot, & Poirot, 2011). Exosomal composition is reflective of the cell secreting them. Changes due to infection, activation, inflammation, or transformation (in tumor cells) will influence and alter the composition of the exosome and thus are the basis for the biological consequences upon its uptake as well as for its biomarker utility. However, not everything that is present in the parent cell is incorporated into the exosomes, suggesting that this well-regulated process is dynamically altered by signaling cues (Stoorvogel, 2012; Villarroya-Beltri, Baixauli, Gutierrez-Vazquez, Sanchez-Madrid, & Mittelbrunn, 2014). An emerging area of research is to use exosomes purified from various sources and disease states to evaluate alterations in gene expression in recipient cells (Fig. 2).

Several methods are currently employed for exosome purification and a recent study compared downstream RNA profiling using exosomes obtained from different isolation methods. They showed that very pure exosomes is a prerequisite to obtain reliable omics data and identify exosome-specific functions and biomarkers (Van Deun et al., 2014). In a recent editorial, the International Society for Extracellular Vesicles has put forth a minimal set of biochemical, biophysical, and functional standards that should be used to attribute any specific biological cargo or functions to EVs (Lötvall et al., 2014).

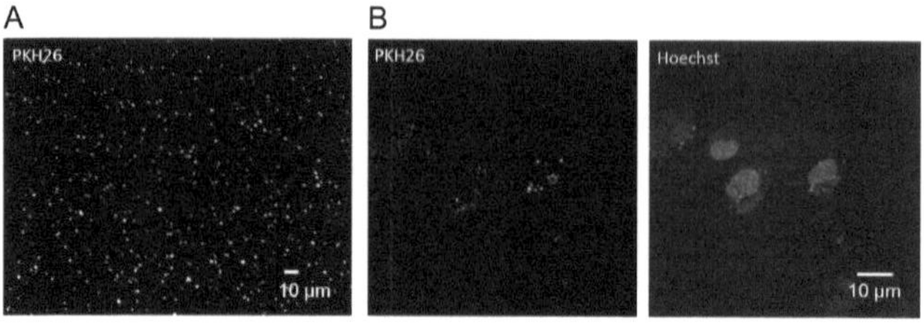

Figure 2 Exosome labeling and uptake. (A) Exosomes isolated from human monocytic THP-1 cell line were labeled with the lipophilic dye, PKH26, used to label cell membranes. The labeled exosomes were imaged (λ_{Em} 535 nm) at 60 × magnification in an Olympus FV 1000 confocal laser scanning microscope. (B) Exosomes isolated from THP-1 cells were labeled with PKH26 dye (red (white in the print version)) and labeled exosomes were added to human umbilical vein endothelial cells and incubated for 1 h. The cells were counterstained with the DNA binding dye Hoechst 33342 (blue (gray in the print version)) the live cells were imaged for exosomal uptake by confocal laser scanning microscope (Magnification: 60 ×).

The precise molecular mechanisms and mediators responsible for determining the exosomal contents are still unknown. Manipulation of the parent cells can influence the packaging of biomolecules, and because exosomes can cross the blood–brain barrier, artificial manipulation of exosomal content, whether loading with nucleic acids or small molecules, is being explored for therapeutic intervention, including in CNS disorders (El Andaloussi et al., 2013). Exosomes derived from antigen-presenting cells have been found to be protective in painful conditions. Dendritic cell-derived exosomes suppress the onset of collagen-induced arthritis in mice and reduce the severity of established arthritis (Kim et al., 2005). Macrophage-derived exosomes also attenuated thermal hyperalgesia associated with complete Freund's adjuvant (CFA)-induced inflammatory pain (McDonald et al., 2014). Thus exosomes derived from antigen presenting cells are capable of eliciting therapeutically relevant immune responses. Preclinical studies exploiting the immunogenicity of dendritic cell-derived exosomes for anticancer therapy are ongoing (Viaud et al., 2010). Release and uptake of exosomes between neurons have been demonstrated *in vitro* (Chivet, Hemming, Pernet-Gallay, Fraboulet, & Sadoul, 2012). Secretion of exosomes in an activity-dependent manner could thus mediate the interneuronal transfer of information, allowing signaling across synapses, necessary for plasticity. Exosomes can carry pathogenic proteins linked to neurodegenerative disorders such as Parkinson, prion, and Alzheimer diseases, suggesting that exosomes might contribute to the spreading of the pathology throughout interconnected cortical areas (Chivet et al., 2012).

Exosomes achieve epigenetic regulation through the transportation of a large number of transcribed mRNA. Analysis of exosomal transcriptome of the naïve or lipopolysaccharide stimulated RAW 264.7 cells by next-generation sequencing revealed protein coding potential of many transcripts; in addition to a high representation of histone H1 subunits within exosomes from unstimulated cells (McDonald et al., 2014) . It has also been shown that extracellular histone H1 is neurotoxic and drives a pro-inflammatory response in microglia (Gilthorpe et al., 2013). This could imply mature miRNAs to modulate inflammation by regulating proinflammatory mRNA or protein levels, while pre-miRNAs mediate a second regulatory wave much later in the recipient cells, thus potentiating a temporal mode of epigenetic regulation. Thus, exosomes provide the benefit of both delivering proteins and miRNA which facilitate direct and immediate action, and translatable transcripts which enable regulation of gene expression during inflammation (McDonald et al., 2014). The mechanisms involved in sorting of different exosomal cargo, exosome release, transport, and finally culminating in uptake by recipient cells is not completely understood (Stoorvogel, 2012; Villarroya-Beltri et al., 2014). However, there is a need to explore novel strategies involving pharmacological interventions capable of either selectively inducing the secretion of a protective exosome pool or inhibit the uptake of pathogenic ones. Exosome biology, in due course of time will open novel avenues in contributing to physiology, pathology, and eventually therapy. From a biomarker perspective, characterization of exosomal content offers a glimpse to biological underpinnings within the body and can be beneficial in elucidating the mechanistic basis of the disease, severity, and stages of disease progression (Ajit, 2015).

4. miRNA PROFILING METHODS

Several methods are available for miRNA detection. The expression profiles of several miRNAs in parallel can be determined by microarray analysis, deep sequencing, or real-time RT-PCR. Northern blotting and *in situ* hybridization can be used to determine the level of individual miRNAs in tissues and cells (van Rooij, 2011). The RT-PCR approach relies on reverse transcription of miRNA to cDNA, followed by qPCR with real-time monitoring of accumulation of reaction products. Two different formats of miRNA profiling, the OpenArray platform, and TaqMan low density array (TLDA) are offered by Applied Biosystems, Foster City, CA. OpenArray platform is commonly used for large-scale miRNA profiling in a high-throughput format (Hudson et al., 2013). These are 3072-well microfluidic OpenArray plates containing nano-liter-scale wells with pre-plated dried TaqMan primers and probes for up to 758 miRNAs and controls. For TLDA microfluidic cards, there is the option of screening 758 miRNAs in two 384-well cards format (Card A and B) or it can be custom designed to examine a small set of miRNAs (for example, miRNAs detected in plasma) in a medium-throughput format. Multiple additional kits and platforms such as those offered by Qiagen (Germantown, MD), Exiqon (Woburn, MA), and nCounter analysis system (Nanostring Technologies, Seattle, WA) can also be employed for qPCR. The advantages of TaqMan miRNA assays include high specificity and sensitivity. Though the platforms mentioned above provide comprehensive coverage of Sanger miRBase v14, the disadvantage of profiling for known miRNAs over sequencing is that we cannot identify novel miRNAs. The methodological challenges in utilizing miRNAs as circulating biomarkers and key procedural aspects of miRNA isolation contributing to variability in miRNA assessment from body fluids have been covered before (Moldovan et al., 2014).

5. DATA ANALYSIS

Several methods are used in data normalization to account for variability. These include mean, quantile, endogenous, and discovered miRNAs. For calculating the mean normalization, the average (CT0) of all miRNAs is subtracted from each CT (cycle threshold) value. Quantile normalization is commonly used in microarray expression analysis and uses the ranking of the raw CT expression values on each plate. Vendors usually recommend endogenous control miRNAs, in which case only these miRNAs are used for calculation of CT0. Alternatively, one can identify endogenous controls appropriate for the current study using various stability criteria. Standard deviation of the CT values across all samples as the stability measure for each miRNA can be determined and the most stable miRNAs can be selected as endogenous controls (Orlova et al., 2011). The mean of these values can then be used as CT0 to calculate the delta CT (ΔCT) values of the target miRNAs on each plate ($\Delta CT = CTtarget - CTreference$ where CTreference is the average CT value of the endogenous controls) (Schmittgen & Livak, 2008). Statistical significance of differential expression can be determined for ΔCT values by performing a two-tailed independent samples *t*-test. Fold change can be determined according to the formula

FC = 2^− ΔΔCT. The ΔΔCT values are calculated by subtracting the ΔCT values of the control individuals from the ΔCT values of the patient samples. Upon the completion of miRNA profiling, hierarchical clustering can be performed and the results can be combined with a heat map of the log-transformed fold changes for the significant miRNAs.

6. miRNAs AS POTENTIAL BIOMARKERS IN PAIN

The first study to demonstrate a role for miRNAs in mediating pain employed a conditional knockout of the miRNA biogenesis enzyme Dicer, within a subset of sensory neurons (Zhao et al., 2010) in mice, and interestingly, these animals had reduced levels of several transcripts associated with nociception and exhibited attenuated inflammatory pain. Several studies have examined alterations in miRNA expression in tissue samples procured from rodent models of inflammatory and neuropathic pain models and have been reviewed (Bali & Kuner, 2014; Elramah et al., 2014; Kress et al., 2013; Kynast, Russe, Geisslinger & Niederberger, 2013; McDonald & Ajit, 2015; Sakai & Suzuki, 2014; Tan, Pao, Cheng, Hung, & Liu, 2013). Several studies indicate roles of miRNAs including miR-103, miR-124a, miR-203, and miR-7a in mediating pain (Favereaux et al., 2011; Kynast, Russe, Moser, Geisslinger & Niederberger, 2013; Sakai et al., 2013; Sun et al., 2012).

One of the first studies investigating circulating miRNAs in a chronic neuropathic pain condition was in whole blood from patients with complex regional pain syndrome (CRPS) (Orlova et al., 2011). CRPS is a chronic neuropathic pain syndrome characterized by pain, inflammation, and aberrant sensory motor and trophic disturbances. The pathophysiology of CRPS is not completely understood, but its complex multifactor pathogenesis includes inflammatory, vascular, sympathetic nervous system, cortical, and spinal mechanisms. This study demonstrated the utility of circulating miRNAs in patient stratification. Of the three different groups that emerged from miRNA profiling, one group comprised 60% of CRPS patients; miRNA profiles from the remaining patients were interspersed among control samples from the other two groups. These findings suggest that clinically relevant patient stratification is possible on the basis of alterations in miRNA expression. Eighteen miRNAs were significantly different in CRPS patients. Analysis of inflammatory markers showed that vascular endothelial growth factor, interleukin-1 receptor antagonist, and monocyte chemotactic protein-1 were significantly elevated in CRPS patients. Several other markers exhibited trends that did not reach significance. Analysis of the patients who were clustered according to their miRNA profile revealed correlations that were not significant in the total patient population, again indicating that miRNA profiles can be useful in grouping patients and in identifying additional biomarkers, the significance of which may be diminished when the patient population is considered overall. This is particularly important in CRPS, a syndrome with differing symptoms (Orlova et al., 2011).

To determine whether exosomal miRNAs reflect the miRNA signature in whole blood of patients with CRPS (Orlova et al., 2011), the same group of researchers analyzed miRNAs in exosomes purified from the serum of six patients with CRPS and six healthy controls (McDonald et al., 2014). A total of 503 miRNAs were detected in at least one human serum-derived exosomal sample and 127 miRNAs were significantly different between CRPS and control-derived exosomes. Sixteen of the 18 miRNAs dysregulated in patients with CRPS from their previous study were detected in human serum-derived exosomes, but only five of these (miR-25-3p, miR-320B, miR-939, miR-126-3p, and RNU48) were significantly altered. Additionally, the exosomal miRNA signature differed in the directionality of changes compared with that of the whole blood. In the exosomal fraction of patient blood, miR-320B, miR-939, miR-126-3p, and RNU48 were significantly upregulated, whereas they were downregulated in whole blood. Thus, hsa-miR-25-3p was the only miRNA exhibiting the same trend in whole blood and exosomes in patients with CRPS (McDonald et al., 2014). Authors suggest that analysis of exosomes from a larger sample of patients is required to determine whether exosomal miRNA could be a useful biomarker or can serve as a secondary strategy for patient stratification. The fact that exosomes can be purified from stored serum samples suggests the feasibility of retrospective analysis of banked samples.

In a study investigating the relationship among pain, psychological characteristics, plasma cytokines, and miRNAs in whole blood from 22 healthy controls, 33 subjects with chronic pelvic pain (vestibulodynia, VBD), and 23 subjects with VBD and irritable bowel syndrome (IBS), the utility of miRNAs in patient stratification and for individual-based diagnosis and treatment was demonstrated (Ciszek et al., 2015). They identified separate pathways for localized versus widespread pain predicted based on miRNA profiles. miRNA dysregulation in VBD is predicted to affect estrogen-relevant pathways and the authors suggest that this may be a contributing factor in localized pain to the pelvis. In patients with both VBD and IBS, miRNA alterations were linked to alterations in muscle, nerve, and glial cell function, thereby contributing to widespread pain. MicroRNA-132 modulates cholinergic signaling and inflammation in human inflammatory bowel disease. Higher levels of miR-132, with a correspondingly lower AChE (acetyl cholinesterase) activity were observed in IBD patients in comparison to healthy controls which support an inflammation-dependent homeostatic role in cholinergic signaling (Maharshak et al., 2013).

Aberrant miRNA expression has been identified in both bodily fluids and tissue biopsy samples from patients with other painful conditions. In patients with bladder pain syndrome, miR-199a-5p has been suggested to play a role in regulation of urothelial permeability (Monastyrskaya et al., 2013), and expression of miR-449b and miR-500 in the bladder smooth muscle cells is increased (Sanchez Freire et al., 2010). miR-146a was upregulated in different cell types and tissues in patients with rheumatoid arthritis, a systemic autoimmune disorder characterized by the inflammation of synovial tissue (Ceribelli, Nahid, Satoh, & Chan, 2011), as well as in osteoarthritis (Li et al., 2011). Altered miRNA expression profiles have been reported for immune disorders such as rheumatoid arthritis (Ammari, Jorgensen, & Apparailly, 2013) and systemic lupus erythematosus (Shen, Liang, Tang, de Vries, & Tak, 2012), painful conditions such as irritable bowel syndrome (Fourie et al., 2014), chronic bladder syndrome (Gheinani, Burkhard, & Monastyrskaya, 2013), visceral pain (Zhang & Banerjee, 2015), migraine (Andersen, Duroux, & Gazerani, 2015; Tafuri et al., 2015), and endometriosis (Ohlsson Teague, Print, & Hull, 2010) when compared with healthy controls.

Profiling of cerebrospinal fluid in 10 women with fibromyalgia and 8 healthy control subjects showed that the expression of nine miRNAs was significantly lower in patients when compared with healthy controls (Bjersing, Lundborg, Bokarewa, & Mannerkorpi, 2013). Two recent studies identified differential expression of eight miRNAs in fibromyalgia patients compared to healthy women. One study was conducted in serum samples (Bjersing, Bokarewa, & Mannerkorpi, 2015) and the second study used peripheral blood mononuclear cells (PBMCs) (Cerdá-Olmedo, Mena-Durán, Monsalve, & Oltra, 2015). The eight miRNAs identified differed between the two reports indicating that the source of miRNAs being investigated is crucial and may result in the identification of different subsets of miRNAs. miRNAs altered in different painful disorders indicates that each disease has a specific miRNA "signature" rendering specificity for miRNA biomarkers. Pain is a very heterogeneous phenomenon and different etiologies and comorbidities likely contribute to the differences in miRNAs altered in these disorders. Currently, miRNA profiling in several neuropathic conditions reported do not provide a strong evidence of any particular miRNA to be exclusively involved in a molecular feedback mechanism to alleviate or aggravate pain due to a paucity in follow-up mechanistic studies. However, a few reports as stated above show the regulation of pro and antiinflammatory miRNAs in the pain-inflammatory axis. We have investigated the role of hsa-miR-939, the miRNA that ranked first and showed a 4.3-fold downregulation ($p = 6.0 \times 10^{-6}$) in CRPS patients (Orlova et al., 2011). Hsa-miR-939 is predicted to target several proinflammatory genes, including interleukin-6 (IL-6), vascular endothelial growth factor A (VEGFA), and tumor necrosis factor-α (TNFα), TNFα-induced protein 1 (TNFAIP1); nuclear factor-κB2 (NFκB2); and nitric oxide synthase 2 (NOS2A). Our unpublished results suggest that hsa-miR-939 can regulate multiple proinflammatory genes and that downregulation of hsa-miR-939 in CRPS patients may increase expression of target genes, including those involved in amplification of an inflammatory pain signal transduction cascade. Studies focusing on individual miRNAs and their target genes, miRNA-based patient stratification coupled to next-generation sequencing analysis for potential miRNA target genes and pathway analysis are all strategies that could be beneficial in elucidating the functional significance of miRNA alterations in observed in various chronic pain conditions.

7. miRNA MODULATION IN RESPONSE TO TREATMENT

Changes are needed on how new analgesics are discovered and developed because of the high rate of failure of drugs targeted to treat neuropathic pain (Kola & Landis, 2004; Woodcock et al., 2007). Studies targeting well-defined patient populations for clinical trials and delineating placebo response will help in developing drugs efficacious in a subset of patients. Circulating miRNAs can potentially be used in patient stratification. This combined with the ability to predict treatment response would be immensely useful in the development of pain therapeutics. Development of experimental paradigms more predictive of trial outcomes (Kola & Landis, 2004; Woodcock et al., 2007) are urgently needed. The ability to predict treatment outcome by a simple qPCR-based blood test could revolutionize both treatment and clinical trials design. Efficacy trials could be conducted in mechanistically defined patient groups. Existing clinical trial samples can be used to conduct proof-of-concept studies to evaluate the feasibility and utility of assessing miRNA signatures. This will be beneficial in assessing the predictive validity of this approach. Assessing miRNA changes before and after treatment will provide insight into miRNA signatures and its alterations in good responders, non-treatment (placebo) responders, and poor responders. Samples from both unsuccessful and successful clinical trials can provide meaningful insights and guidance for future or even ongoing trials. A patient's miRNA signature may differ even prior to treatment initiation and changes in signature may correlate with treatment outcome. Identifying the potential target genes for individual miRNAs could provide insights into the molecular bases of different types of pain and help identify novel targets for pain therapy. If implemented successfully, these studies can potentially reduce future failures by targeting well-defined patient population for clinical trials along with delineating placebo response.

Ketamine, an *N*-methyl-D-aspartate (NMDA) receptor antagonist and widely used anesthetic, is currently being studied in the treatment of depression (aan het Rot et al., 2012) and pain, including CRPS. NMDA receptors are upregulated in CRPS causing the pain, allodynia, and hyperalgesia that hallmark the disease (Costigan, Scholz, & Woolf, 2009). Although controversial for its potential abuses and side effects (psychotomimetic effects), ketamine, when administered intravenously over several days with antipsychotics and antihallucinogenics, has been shown to provide relief to CRPS sufferers (Borsook, 2009) that often lasts for weeks, or even months after treatment (Dahanl et al., 2011; Schwartzman et al., 2009). Patients for whom all other treatments have failed are typically considered for ketamine treatment. Though ketamine can reduce pain, approximately 30% of the patients do not respond to ketamine therapy (Dahan et al., 2011). There is no known clinical symptom or biomarker for predicting response to ketamine.

In a recent proof-of-principle study, intravenous ketamine treatment induced miRNA alterations in CRPS patients were investigated by profiling blood samples before and after treatment (Douglas et al., 2015). The patients were grouped as good and poor responders based on whether they reported pain relief after ketamine therapy. Analysis of circulating miRNAs in CRPS patients undergoing ketamine therapy demonstrated differential expression of miRNAs in responders and poor responders before and after ketamine treatment. Differential expression of several miRNAs between good and poor responders before treatment indicates that miRNA profile can predict treatment response. The miRNA changes were not identical between responders and nonresponders, indicating that ketamine elicited response differed between the two groups (Douglas et al., 2015). This study also investigated the mechanistic basis of miRNA alterations and provided molecular evidence suggesting that downregulation of hsa-miR-548d-5p in poor responders can influence the expression of its target mRNA UDP-glucuronosyltransferase UGT1A1. Authors propose that higher UDP-GT activity can lead to higher levels of inactive glucuronide conjugates and thereby can minimize the therapeutic efficacy of ketamine in poor responders (Douglas et al., 2015). This is an example of how potential biomarker discovery can be extended to mechanistic studies that can generate insight on disease. Thus differences in miRNA signatures can provide molecular insights distinguishing responders from poor responders prior to treatment.

8. MODULATION OF CIRCULATING miRNAs IN RODENT MODELS OF PAIN

Animal models have been crucial in understanding the mechanisms and maintenance of chronic pain and have an important role in facilitating translational research (Gregory et al., 2013; Mogil, Davis, & Derbyshire, 2010). In conjunction with human studies, these models can be instrumental in elucidating the role of miRNAs in pain states. As mentioned above, recent reviews have cataloged the studies linking miRNAs to various pain conditions (Bali & Kuner, 2014; Elramah et al., 2014; Kress et al., 2013; Kynast, Russe, Geisslinger, et al., 2013; Sakai & Suzuki, 2014; Tan et al., 2013). Profiling studies have identified tissue-specific dysregulated expression of miRNAs in dorsal root ganglia (DRG) and spinal cord (SC) after peripheral inflammatory stimulus (Bai, Ambalavanar, Wei, & Dessem, 2007; Kusuda et al., 2011), nerve injury (Aldrich, Frakes, Kasuya, Hammond, & Kitamoto, 2009; Bali, Hackenberg, Lubin, Kuner, & Devor, 2014; Kusuda et al., 2011; Sakai et al., 2013; Strickland et al., 2011; von Schack et al., 2011; Yu et al., 2011), and cancer pain (Bali et al., 2013). Additionally, differential regulation of individual miRNAs has been observed in specific regions of the brain in acute and chronic pain models (Arai et al., 2013; Imai et al., 2011; Poh, Yeo, & Ong, 2011). The few studies that link specific miRNA changes to a pain condition suggest that temporal and spatial regulation of intracellular miRNA expression occurs at specific time points that correspond to early or late phases of pain conditions (Bali & Kuner, 2014; Kynast, Russe, Geisslinger, et al., 2013; Sakai & Suzuki, 2014). miRNAs altered in animal models could be beneficial in elucidating the pathophysiology of pain; miRNA changes specific to certain models representing a pain condition could provide insights unique to the model being studied. While several recent studies have successfully established negative correlation between miRNAs and target mRNA levels (Chen et al., 2014; Im et al., 2012; Ni et al., 2013; Sengupta et al., 2013; Sun et al., 2012), a few have provided evidence for the role of specific miRNAs in impacting nociceptive behavior using rodent models (Favereaux et al., 2011; Kynast et al., 2013b; Sakai et al., 2013; Willemen et al., 2012). miRNA-induced attenuation or augmentation of pain phenotype has also been demonstrated in rodent models of inflammatory, neuropathic, and cancer pain (Bali et al., 2013; Favereaux et al., 2011; Kynast et al., 2013b; Pan et al., 2014; Sakai et al., 2013; Willemen et al., 2012).

Circulating miRNAs can act extracellularly by directly interacting with cell-surface receptors. It was demonstrated that miR-21, miR-29a, and let-7b can act as agonists of Toll-like receptors (TLR) 7 and 8 and thereby influence downstream signaling pathway in target cells (Fabbri, Paone, Calore, Galli, & Croce, 2013). Secreted miRNAs represent a new class of pain mediators; extracellular let-7b is required and sufficient for inducing inflammatory pain via the activation of TLR7 and TRPA1. Let-7b is highly enriched in DRG and endogenous let-7b can be released from DRG neurons in an activity-dependent manner (Park et al., 2014). This study suggests that miRNAs could potentially act in an autocrine fashion on nociceptors, or mediate novel signaling mechanisms.

Profiling using blood obtained from multiple rodent models of pain, including spinal nerve ligation, spared nerve injury surgical models of neuropathic pain, and the administration of CFA as a model of inflammatory pain showed differential expression of circulating miRNAs (Qureshi et al., 2015). Circulating miRNAs differed between rats and mice indicating that there are species specific differences (Qureshi et al., 2015). This study also investigated the temporal regulation of miRNA alterations in CFA model. Thus, 13 miRNAs were differentially expressed in the blood of mice 3 days after CFA-injection mice versus controls, while 31 miRNAs were significant in the blood 10 days after CFA-injection. There were only three common differentially expressed miRNAs in the blood after 3 and 10 days. The magnitude of downregulation increased for mir-384-5p, and mir-190b after 10 days compared to changes observed after 3 days. An increase in number of miRNAs altered 10 days after CFA-injection suggests that chronic inflammation can induce significant dysregulation of miRNAs. Thus, different rodent models of pain have unique miRNA expression signatures in blood.

9. PHARMACOLOGICAL MODULATION OF CIRCULATING miRNAs IN MICE

Celecoxib is a selective COX2 inhibitor and extensively used to treat inflammatory pain including rheumatoid arthritis, osteoarthritis, headache, and musculoskeletal pain. Induction of COX-2 accounts largely for the high prostanoid production at the site of inflammation (Chen, Yang, & Grosser, 2013). To study whether celecoxib administration can induce miRNA modulation, the drug was administered for 7 days in a CFA model of inflammatory pain. Comparison of four experimental conditions including saline, celecoxib, CFA, and CFA–celecoxib co-administration showed that several miRNAs dysregulated by CFA were restored to baseline levels after the administration of celecoxib (Qureshi et al., 2015). This study suggests that reversal of miRNA expression to physiological levels may be important for therapeutic effect of celecoxib. miRNA target prediction and pathway enrichment for rodent models of pain showed that Wnt signaling pathway was consistently enriched across all experimental conditions (Qureshi et al., 2015). WNT family of secreted signaling molecules has an important role in both healthy and diseased states (Rosso & Inestrosa, 2013). Binding of WNT ligands to Frizzled receptors can activate the canonical or β-catenin-dependent pathway, the noncanonical planar cell polarity pathway, and the Wnt/Ca^{2+} pathway. Wnt signaling pathways are regulated by nociceptive input and their activation can mediate the development of acute and chronic pain (Shi et al., 2012; Simonetti et al., 2014; Zhang et al., 2013). Exosomes have a role in Wnt secretion and transport and their signaling activities have been functionally implicated in the development of *Drosophila* and in fibroblast-promoted cancer metastasis (Zhang & Wrana, 2014).

10. CONCLUSION

The journey of miRNAs to the diagnostic lab is still long and needs improved approaches at multiple levels (Angelini & Emanueli, 2015). The investigation of circulating miRNA as novel biomarkers for physiological and pathological conditions, owing to its noninvasive nature, can be both beneficial and cost effective. The selective sorting and excretion of miRNAs via lipoproteins or microvesicles, functioning as a mode of intercellular communication, is a fairly recent idea of crucial importance in relation to the potential of miRNA as biomarkers (Stoorvogel, 2015). The advent of new and improved procedures for the purification and quantification of circulating miRNAs, especially quantitative RT-PCR, have paved way to enable the detection of low abundance miRNAs. Lack of reliable normalizers that can be used as universal standards is to be expected considering the dynamic nature of the composition of circulating RNAs. It is still necessary to standardize the profiling platforms, methodologies, including sample collection, storage, data normalization, and statistical analysis, as well as the clinical parameters, before an miRNA can be developed into a reliable biomarker that can be used routinely. It has been suggested that miRNA clusters may render more specificity than an individual miRNAs (Angelini & Emanueli, 2015). To capture biological variability, a central database cataloging the levels of miRNAs in both the healthy male and female populations, stratified by ethnicity, age, and geography, would serve as a useful reference and would greatly reduce the challenges associated with data reproducibility. Most of the studies published to date were performed on limited cohort size. The array of fluids and samples to profile just from blood include serum, plasma, PBMC, whole blood, and exosomes. As mentioned earlier the results differ depending on the source (whole blood vs. exosomes for CRPS (McDonald et al., 2014; Orlova et al., 2011), serum vs. PBMC for fibromyalgia (Bjersing et al., 2015; Cerdá-Olmedo et al., 2015)). Data collection from selected patient populations along with controls can serve as a starting reference and can be tracked temporally to capture the effects of chronic pain, medical interventions and/or life style changes in these individuals. Identification of patients likely to experience pain relief without side effects, and predicting the risk of drug abuse prior to initiating therapy, though highly desired, is a huge unmet need. Combining cytokine and chemokine data with miRNAs will undoubtedly be beneficial in determining treatment options and for better understanding of the disease. Although pain is the common denominator in a variety of disorders, the underlying neurobiological mechanisms leading to pain can differ. Thus it is reasonable to expect an overlap of miRNA populations altered in different pathologies associated with pain, but every disorder, including different kinds of pain itself, may have its own unique miRNA signature (Fig. 3).

A number of studies investigating circulating miRNAs demonstrate their feasibility as potential biomarkers. Though the mechanisms that determine the loading of exosomes and the means by which they reach the recipient cells at distant locations though the circulation are not completely known,

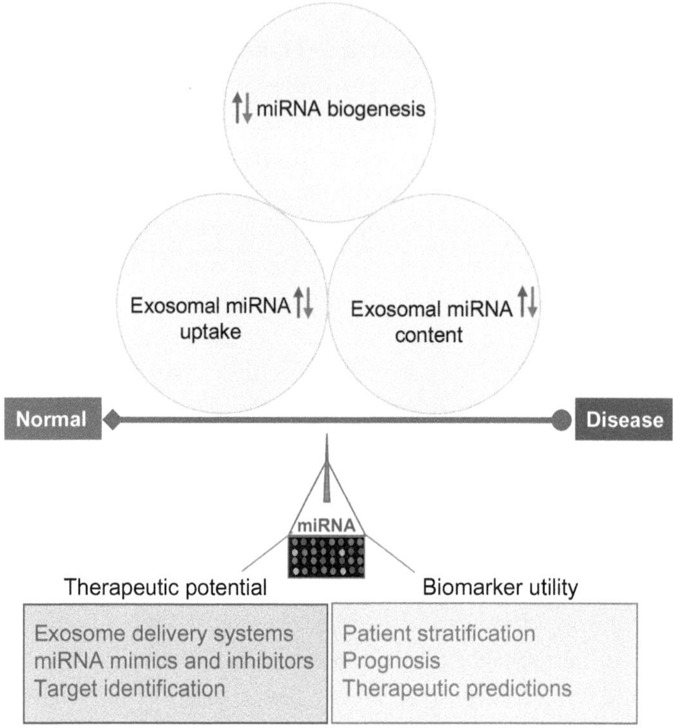

Figure 3 miRNAs as biomarkers. Expression profiling and analysis of circulating and tissue-specific miRNAs could help assess disease variants contributed by perturbations at various stages of miRNA biogenesis, transport, and/or uptake mechanisms. Designation of miRNAs known to affect target gene expression in recipient cells could help in developing biomarker assays and therapeutic intervention strategies.

exosome biology is another aspect of circulating miRNAs that will undoubtedly open novel avenues in understanding normal physiology, disease mechanisms, and therapeutic intervention strategies. Accurate and precise diagnostic tests that are specific and sensitive enough to categorize patients with potential benefit from targeted therapies will be crucial for the success of personalized medicine. Clinical trials should be conducted on selected patient populations possessing molecular markers associated with specific drug targets. Ultimately, novel products and approaches successfully incorporated into clinical practice would evaluate our progress in making personalized medicine a reality (Hamburg & Collins, 2010).

CONFLICT OF INTEREST

The authors have no conflicts of interest to declare.

ACKNOWLEDGMENTS

We gratefully acknowledge the funding from Rita Allen Foundation, National Institute of Health (1R21NS082991-01), PhRMA Foundation, Pennsylvania Department of Health Commonwealth Universal Research Enhancement (CURE), and Drexel University Clinical and Translational Research Institute to S. A.

REFERENCES

aan het Rot, M., Zarate, C. A., Jr., Charney, D. S., & Mathew, S. J. (2012). Ketamine for depression: Where do we go from here? *Biological Psychiatry, 72*(7), 537–547. http://dx.doi.org/10.1016/j.biopsych.2012.05.003.

Ajit, S. K. (2015). Chapter 14—Epigenetics and personalized pain management. In T. O. Tollefsbol (Ed.), *Personalized epigenetics* (pp. 389–427). Boston: Academic Press.

Aldrich, B. T., Frakes, E. P., Kasuya, J., Hammond, D. L., & Kitamoto, T. (2009). Changes in expression of sensory organ-specific microRNAs in rat dorsal root ganglia in association with mechanical hypersensitivity induced by spinal nerve ligation. *Neuroscience, 164*(2), 711–723. http://dx.doi.org/10.1016/j.neuroscience.2009.08.033. S0306-4522(09)01391-8 [pii].

Alvarez-Erviti, L., Seow, Y., Yin, H., Betts, C., Lakhal, S., & Wood, M. J. A. (2011). Delivery of siRNA to the mouse brain by systemic injection of targeted exosomes. *Nature Biotechnology, 29*(4), 341–345. http://www.nature.com/nbt/journal/v29/n4/abs/nbt.1807.html#supplementary-information.

Ammari, M., Jorgensen, C., & Apparailly, F. (2013). Impact of microRNAs on the understanding and treatment of rheumatoid arthritis. *Current Opinion in Rheumatology, 25*(2), 225–233. http://dx.doi.org/10.1097/BOR.0b013e32835d8385.

Andersen, H., Duroux, M., & Gazerani, P. (2015). Serum microRNA signatures in migraineurs during attacks and in pain-free periods. *Molecular Neurobiology, 1–7*. http://dx.doi.org/10.1007/s12035-015-9106-5.

Angelini, T. G., & Emanueli, C. (2015). MicroRNAs as clinical biomarkers? *Frontiers in Genetics, 6*, 240. http://dx.doi.org/10.3389/fgene.2015.00240. eCollection 2015. PMID:26236333.

Arai, M., Genda, Y., Ishikawa, M., Shunsuke, T., Okabe, T., & Sakamoto, A. (2013). The miRNA and mRNA changes in rat hippocampi after chronic constriction injury. *Pain Medicine, 14*(5), 720–729. http://dx.doi.org/10.1111/pme.12066.

Bai, G., Ambalavanar, R., Wei, D., & Dessem, D. (2007). Downregulation of selective microRNAs in trigeminal ganglion neurons following inflammatory muscle pain. *Molecular Pain, 3*(15). http://dx.doi.org/10.1186/1744-8069-3-15. 1744-8069-3-15 [pii].

Bali, K., Hackenberg, M., Lubin, A., Kuner, R., & Devor, M. (2014). Sources of individual variability: miRNAs that predispose to neuropathic pain identified using genome-wide sequencing. *Molecular Pain, 10*(1), 22.

Bali, K. K., & Kuner, R. (2014). Noncoding RNAs: Key molecules in understanding and treating pain. *Trends in Molecular Medicine, 20*(8), 437–448. http://dx.doi.org/10.1016/j.molmed.2014.05.006.

Bali, K. K., Selvaraj, D., Satagopam, V. P., Lu, J., Schneider, R., & Kuner, R. (2013). Genome-wide identification and functional analyses of microRNA signatures associated with cancer pain. *EMBO Molecular Medicine, 5*(11), 1740–1758. http://dx.doi.org/10.1002/emmm.201302797.

Bartel, D. P. (2009). MicroRNAs: Target recognition and regulatory functions. *Cell, 136*(2), 215–233. http://dx.doi.org/10.1016/j.cell.2009.01.002. S0092-8674(09)00008-7 [pii].

Bjersing, J., Bokarewa, M., & Mannerkorpi, K. (2015). Profile of circulating microRNAs in fibromyalgia and their relation to symptom severity: An exploratory study. *Rheumatology International, 35*(4), 635–642. http://dx.doi.org/10.1007/s00296-014-3139-3.

Bjersing, J. L., Lundborg, C., Bokarewa, M. I., & Mannerkorpi, K. (2013). Profile of cerebrospinal microRNAs in fibromyalgia. *PLoS One*. *8*(10). http://dx.doi.org/10.1371/journal.pone.0078762. e78762.

Boon, R. A., & Vickers, K. C. (2013). Intercellular transport of microRNAs. *Arteriosclerosis, Thrombosis, and Vascular Biology*, *33*(2), 186–192. http://dx.doi.org/10.1161/ATVBAHA.112.300139.

Borsook, D. (2009). Ketamine and chronic pain—Going the distance. *Pain*, *145*(3), 271–272. http://dx.doi.org/10.1016/j.pain.2009.05.021.

Cai, X., Hagedorn, C. H., & Cullen, B. R. (2004). Human microRNAs are processed from capped, polyadenylated transcripts that can also function as mRNAs. *RNA*, *10*(12), 1957–1966. http://dx.doi.org/10.1261/rna.7135204.

Cerdá-Olmedo, G., Mena-Durán, A. V., Monsalve, V., & Oltra, E. (2015). Identification of a microRNA signature for the diagnosis of fibromyalgia. *PLoS One*, *10*(3), e0121903. http://dx.doi.org/10.1371/journal.pone.0121903.

Ceribelli, A., Nahid, M. A., Satoh, M., & Chan, E. K. L. (2011). MicroRNAs in rheumatoid arthritis. *FEBS Letters*, *585*(23), 3667–3674. http://dx.doi.org/10.1016/j.febslet.2011.05.020.

Chen, H.-P., Zhou, W., Kang, L.-M., Yan, H., Zhang, L., Xu, B.-H., et al. (2014). Intrathecal miR-96 inhibits Nav1.3 expression and alleviates neuropathic pain in rat following chronic construction injury. *Neurochemical Research*, *39*(1), 76–83. http://dx.doi.org/10.1007/s11064-013-1192-z.

Chen, L., Yang, G., & Grosser, T. (2013). Prostanoids and inflammatory pain. *Prostaglandins & Other Lipid Mediators*, *104*, 58–66. http://dx.doi.org/10.1016/j.prostaglandins.2012.08.006.

Chen, X., Ba, Y., Ma, L., Cai, X., Yin, Y., Wang, K., et al. (2008). Characterization of microRNAs in serum: A novel class of biomarkers for diagnosis of cancer and other diseases. *Cell Research*, *18*(10), 997–1006. http://dx.doi.org/10.1038/cr.2008.282. cr2008282 [pii].

Chendrimada, T. P., Gregory, R. I., Kumaraswamy, E., Norman, J., Cooch, N., Nishikura, K., et al. (2005). TRBP recruits the dicer complex to Ago2 for microRNA processing and gene silencing. *Nature*, *436*(7051), 740–744. http://dx.doi.org/10.1038/nature03868.

Chivet, M., Hemming, F., Pernet-Gallay, K., Fraboulet, S., & Sadoul, R. (2012). Emerging role of neuronal exosomes in the central nervous system. *Frontiers in Physiology*, *3*, 145. http://dx.doi.org/10.3389/fphys.2012.00145.

Chizh, B. A., Greenspan, J. D., Casey, K. L., Nemenov, M. I., & Treede, R. D. (2008). Identifying biological markers of activity in human nociceptive pathways to facilitate analgesic drug development. *Pain*, *140*(2), 249–253. http://dx.doi.org/10.1016/j.pain.2008.09.024. S0304-3959(08)00559-9 [pii].

Ciszek, B. P., Khan, A. A., Dang, H., Slade, G. D., Smith, S., Bair, E., et al. (2015). MicroRNA expression profiles differentiate chronic pain condition subtypes. *Translational Research*, *166*(6). http://dx.doi.org/10.1016/j.trsl.2015.06.008. 706–720.e711.

Corcoran, D. L., Pandit, K. V., Gordon, B., Bhattacharjee, A., Kaminski, N., & Benos, P. V. (2009). Features of mammalian microRNA promoters emerge from polymerase II chromatin immunoprecipitation data. *PLoS One*, *4*(4), e5279. http://dx.doi.org/10.1371/journal.pone.0005279.

Costigan, M., Scholz, J., & Woolf, C. J. (2009). Neuropathic pain: A maladaptive response of the nervous system to damage. *Annual Review of Neuroscience*, *32*, 1–32.

Croce, C. M. (2009). Causes and consequences of microRNA dysregulation in cancer. *Nature Reviews. Genetics*, *10*(10), 704–714. http://dx.doi.org/10.1038/nrg2634.

Dahan, A., Olofsen, E., Sigtermans, M., Noppers, I., Niesters, M., Aarts, L., et al. (2011). Population pharmacokinetic-pharmacodynamic modeling of ketamine-induced pain relief of chronic pain. *European Journal of Pain, 15*(3), 258–267. http://dx.doi.org/10.1016/j.ejpain.2010.06.016.

Dahanl, A., Olofsenl, E., Sigtermans, M., Noppers, I., Niesters, M., Aarts, L., et al. (2011). Population pharmacokinetic—Pharmacodynamic modeling of ketamine-induced pain relief of chronic pain. *European Journal of Pain, 15*(3), 258–267.

De Guire, V., Robitaille, R., Tetreault, N., Guerin, R., Menard, C., Bambace, N., et al. (2013). Circulating miRNAs as sensitive and specific biomarkers for the diagnosis and monitoring of human diseases: Promises and challenges. *Clinical Biochemistry, 46*(10–11), 846–860. http://dx.doi.org/10.1016/j.clinbiochem.2013.03.015.

Denli, A. M., Tops, B. B., Plasterk, R. H., Ketting, R. F., & Hannon, G. J. (2004). Processing of primary microRNAs by the microprocessor complex. *Nature, 432*(7014), 231–235. http://dx.doi.org/10.1038/nature03049.

Douglas, S. R., Shenoda, B. B., Qureshi, R. A., Sacan, A., Alexander, G. M., Perreault, M., et al. (2015). Analgesic response to intravenous ketamine is linked to a circulating microRNA signature in female complex regional pain syndrome patients. *Journal of Pain, 16*(9), 814–824. http://dx.doi.org/10.1016/j.jpain.2015.05.008.

El Andaloussi, S., Mäger, I., Breakefield, X. O., & Wood, M. J. (2013). Extracellular vesicles: Biology and emerging therapeutic opportunities. *Nature Reviews. Drug Discovery, 12*(5), 347–357. http://dx.doi.org/10.1038/nrd3978.

Elramah, S., Landry, M., & Favereaux, A. (2014). MicroRNAs regulate neuronal plasticity and are involved in pain mechanisms. *Frontiers in Cellular Neuroscience, 8*, 31. http://dx.doi.org/10.3389/fncel.2014.00031.

Erson, A. E., & Petty, E. M. (2008). MicroRNAs in development and disease. *Clinical Genetics, 74*(4), 296–306. http://dx.doi.org/10.1111/j.1399-0004.2008.01076.x. CGE1076 [pii].

Fabbri, M., Paone, A., Calore, F., Galli, R., & Croce, C. M. (2013). A new role for microRNAs, as ligands of toll-like receptors. *RNA Biology, 10*(2), 169–174.

Favereaux, A., Thoumine, O., Bouali-Benazzouz, R., Roques, V., Papon, M. A., Salam, S. A., et al. (2011). Bidirectional integrative regulation of Cav1.2 calcium channel by microRNA miR-103: Role in pain. *EMBO Journal, 30*(18), 3830–3841. http://dx.doi.org/10.1038/emboj.2011.249. emboj2011249.

Fourie, N. H., Peace, R. M., Abey, S. K., Sherwin, L. B., Rahim-Williams, B., Smyser, P. A., et al. (2014). Elevated circulating miR-150 and miR-342-3p in patients with irritable bowel syndrome. *Experimental and Molecular Pathology, 96*(3), 422–425. http://dx.doi.org/10.1016/j.yexmp.2014.04.009.

Gereau IV, R. W., Sluka, K. A., Maixner, W., Savage, S. R., Price, T. J., Murinson, B. B., et al. (2014). A pain research agenda for the 21st century. *Journal of Pain, 15*, 1203–1214. http://dx.doi.org/10.1016/j.jpain.2014.09.004.

Gheinani, A., Burkhard, F., & Monastyrskaya, K. (2013). Deciphering microRNA code in pain and inflammation: Lessons from bladder pain syndrome. *Cellular and Molecular Life Sciences, 70*(20), 3773–3789. http://dx.doi.org/10.1007/s00018-013-1275-7.

Gilad, S., Meiri, E., Yogev, Y., Benjamin, S., Lebanony, D., Yerushalmi, N., et al. (2008). Serum microRNAs are promising novel biomarkers. *PLoS One, 3*(9), e3148. http://dx.doi.org/10.1371/journal.pone.0003148.

Gilthorpe, J. D., Oozeer, F., Nash, J., Calvo, M., Bennett, D. L. H., Lumsden, A., et al. (2013). Extracellular histone H1 is neurotoxic and drives a pro-inflammatory response in microglia. *F1000, Research, 2*(148), 1–11. http://dx.doi.org/10.12688/f1000research.2-148.v1. eCollection 2013.

Grasedieck, S., Sorrentino, A., Langer, C., Buske, C., D$\sqrt{\partial}$hner, H., Mertens, D., et al. (2013). Circulating microRNAs in hematological diseases: Principles, challenges, and perspectives. *Blood, 121*(25), 4977–4984.

Gregory, N. S., Harris, A. L., Robinson, C. R., Dougherty, P. M., Fuchs, P. N., & Sluka, K. A. (2013). An overview of animal models of pain: Disease models and outcome measures. *Journal of Pain, 14*(11), 1255–1269. http://dx.doi.org/10.1016/j.jpain.2013.06.008.

Grimson, A., Farh, K. K., Johnston, W. K., Garrett-Engele, P., Lim, L. P., & Bartel, D. P. (2007). MicroRNA targeting specificity in mammals: Determinants beyond seed pairing. *Molecular Cell, 27*(1), 91–105. http://dx.doi.org/10.1016/j.molcel.2007.06.017.

Gyorgy, B., Szabo, T. G., Pasztoi, M., Pal, Z., Misjak, P., Aradi, B., et al. (2011). Membrane vesicles, current state-of-the-art: Emerging role of extracellular vesicles. *Cellular and Molecular Life Sciences, 68*(16), 2667–2688. http://dx.doi.org/10.1007/s00018-011-0689-3.

Hamburg, M. A., & Collins, F. S. (2010). The path to personalized medicine. *New England Journal of Medicine, 363*(4), 301–304. http://dx.doi.org/10.1056/NEJMp1006304.

Hudson, J., Duncavage, E., Tamburrino, A., Salerno, P., Xi, L., Raffeld, M., et al. (2013). Overexpression of miR-10a and miR-375 and downregulation of YAP1 in medullary thyroid carcinoma. *Experimental and Molecular Pathology, 95*(1), 62–67. http://dx.doi.org/10.1016/j.yexmp.2013.05.001.

Im, Y. B., Jee, M. K., Choi, J. I., Cho, H. T., Kwon, O. H., & Kang, S. K. (2012). Molecular targeting of NOX4 for neuropathic pain after traumatic injury of the spinal cord. *Cell Death & Disease, 3*, e426. http://www.nature.com/cddis/journal/v3/n11/suppinfo/cddis2012168s1.html.

Imai, S., Saeki, M., Yanase, M., Horiuchi, H., Abe, M., Narita, M., et al. (2011). Change in microRNAs associated with neuronal adaptive responses in the nucleus accumbens under neuropathic pain. *Journal of Neuroscience, 31*(43), 15294–15299. http://dx.doi.org/10.1523/jneurosci.0921-11.2011.

Jirtle, R. L., & Skinner, M. K. (2007). Environmental epigenomics and disease susceptibility. *Nature Reviews. Genetics, 8*(4), 253–262. http://dx.doi.org/10.1038/nrg2045.nrg2045 [pii].

Kalra, H., Simpson, R. J., Ji, H., Aikawa, E., Altevogt, P., Askenase, P., et al. (2012). Vesiclepedia: A compendium for extracellular vesicles with continuous community annotation. *PLoS Biology, 10*(12). http://dx.doi.org/10.1371/journal.pbio.1001450.e1001450.

Khvorova, A., Reynolds, A., & Jayasena, S. D. (2003). Functional siRNAs and miRNAs exhibit strand bias. *Cell, 115*(2), 209–216.

Kim, S. H., Lechman, E. R., Bianco, N., Menon, R., Keravala, A., Nash, J., et al. (2005). Exosomes derived from IL-10-treated dendritic cells can suppress inflammation and collagen-induced arthritis. *Journal of Immunology, 174*(10), 6440–6448.

Kola, I., & Landis, J. (2004). Can the pharmaceutical industry reduce attrition rates? *Nature Reviews. Drug Discovery, 3*(8), 711–715. http://dx.doi.org/10.1038/nrd1470nrd1470.

Kowal, J., Tkach, M., & Thery, C. (2014). Biogenesis and secretion of exosomes. *Current Opinion in Cell Biology, 29*, 116–125. http://dx.doi.org/10.1016/j.ceb.2014.05.004.

Kress, M., Hüttenhofer, A., Landry, M., Kuner, R., Favereaux, A., Greenberg, D. S., et al. (2013). MicroRNAs in nociceptive circuits as predictors of future clinical applications. *Frontiers in Molecular Neuroscience, 6*, 33.

Kusuda, R., Cadetti, F., Ravanelli, M. I., Sousa, T. A., Zanon, S., De Lucca, F. L., et al. (2011). Differential expression of microRNAs in mouse pain models. *Molecular Pain, 7*, 17. http://dx.doi.org/10.1186/1744-8069-7-1. 1744-8069-7-17 [pii].

Kynast, K. L., Russe, O. Q., Geisslinger, G., & Niederberger, E. (2013a). Novel findings in pain processing pathways: Implications for miRNAs as future therapeutic targets. *Expert Review of Neurotherapeutics, 13*(5), 515–525. http://dx.doi.org/10.1586/ern.13.34.

Kynast, K. L., Russe, O. Q., Moser, C. V., Geisslinger, G., & Niederberger, E. (2013b). Modulation of central nervous system-specific microRNA-124a alters the inflammatory response in the formalin test in mice. *Pain*, *154*(3), 368–376. http://dx.doi.org/10.1016/j.pain.2012.11.010.

Lagos-Quintana, M., Rauhut, R., Lendeckel, W., & Tuschl, T. (2001). Identification of novel genes coding for small expressed RNAs. *Science*, *294*(5543), 853–858. http://dx.doi.org/10.1126/science.1064921.

Lee, Y., Ahn, C., Han, J., Choi, H., Kim, J., Yim, J., et al. (2003). The nuclear RNase III Drosha initiates microRNA processing. *Nature*, *425*(6956), 415–419. http://dx.doi.org/10.1038/nature01957.

Li, X., Gibson, G., Kim, J. S., Kroin, J., Xu, S., van Wijnen, A. J., et al. (2011). MicroRNA-146a is linked to pain-related pathophysiology of osteoarthritis. *Gene*, *480*(1–2), 34–41. http://dx.doi.org/10.1016/j.gene.2011.03.003. S0378-1119(11)00093-X [pii].

Lötvall, J., Hill, A. F., Hochberg, F., Buzás, E. I., Di Vizio, D., Gardiner, C., et al. (2014). Minimal experimental requirements for definition of extracellular vesicles and their functions: A position statement from the International Society for Extracellular Vesicles. *Journal of Extracellular Vesicles*, *3*, 26913. http://dx.doi.org/10.3402/jev.v3.26913. eCollection 2014. PMID:25536934.

Maharshak, N., Shenhar-Tsarfaty, S., Aroyo, N., Orpaz, N., Guberman, I., Canaani, J., et al. (2013). MicroRNA-132 modulates cholinergic signaling and inflammation in human inflammatory bowel disease. *Inflammatory Bowel Diseases*, *19*(7), 1346–1353. http://dx.doi.org/10.1097/MIB.0b013e318281f47d.

Marchi, A., Vellucci, R., Mameli, S., Rita Piredda, A., & Finco, G. (2009). Pain biomarkers. *Clinical Drug Investigation*, *29*(Suppl. 1), 41–46. http://dx.doi.org/10.2165/0044011-200929001-00006.

McDonald, M. K., & Ajit, S. K. (2015). Chapter eight—MicroRNA biology and pain. In J. P. Theodore & D. Gregory (Eds.), *Progress in molecular biology and translational science: Vol. 131* (pp. 215–249). Cambridge, MA: Academic Press.

McDonald, M. K., Tian, Y., Qureshi, R. A., Gormley, M., Ertel, A., Gao, R., et al. (2014). Functional significance of macrophage-derived exosomes in inflammation and pain. *PAIN*, *155*(8), 1527–1539. http://dx.doi.org/10.1016/j.pain.2014.04.029.

Mitchell, P. S., Parkin, R. K., Kroh, E. M., Fritz, B. R., Wyman, S. K., Pogosova-Agadjanyan, E. L., et al. (2008). Circulating microRNAs as stable blood-based markers for cancer detection. *Proceedings of the National Academy of Sciences of the United States of America*, *105*(30), 10513–10518. http://dx.doi.org/10.1073/pnas.0804549105. 0804549105 [pii].

Mogil, J. S., Davis, K. D., & Derbyshire, S. W. (2010). The necessity of animal models in pain research. *Pain*, *151*(1), 12–17. http://dx.doi.org/10.1016/j.pain.2010.07.015. S0304-3959(10)00437-9 [pii].

Moldovan, L., Batte, K. E., Trgovcich, J., Wisler, J., Marsh, C. B., & Piper, M. (2014). Methodological challenges in utilizing miRNAs as circulating biomarkers. *Journal of Cellular and Molecular Medicine*, *18*(3), 371–390. http://dx.doi.org/10.1111/jcmm.12236.

Monastyrskaya, K., Sánchez-Freire, V., Hashemi Gheinani, A., Klumpp, D. J., Babiychuk, E. B., Draeger, A., et al. (2013). miR-199a-5p regulates urothelial permeability and may play a role in bladder pain syndrome. *American Journal of Pathology*, *182*(2), 431–448. http://dx.doi.org/10.1016/j.ajpath.2012.10.020.

Ni, J., Gao, Y., Gong, S., Guo, S., Hisamitsu, T., & Jiang, X. (2013). Regulation of mu-opioid type 1 receptors by microRNA134 in dorsal root ganglion neurons following peripheral inflammation. *European Journal of Pain*, *17*(3), 313–323. http://dx.doi.org/10.1002/j.1532-2149.2012.00197.x.

Ohlsson Teague, E. M. C., Print, C. G., & Hull, M. L. (2010). The role of microRNAs in endometriosis and associated reproductive conditions. *Human Reproduction Update*, *16*(2), 142–165. http://dx.doi.org/10.1093/humupd/dmp034.

Okamura, K., Hagen, J. W., Duan, H., Tyler, D. M., & Lai, E. C. (2007). The mirtron pathway generates microRNA-class regulatory RNAs in Drosophila. *Cell*, *130*(1), 89–100. http://dx.doi.org/10.1016/j.cell.2007.06.028.

Orlova, I. A., Alexander, G. M., Qureshi, R. A., Sacan, A., Graziano, A., Barrett, J. E., et al. (2011). MicroRNA modulation in complex regional pain syndrome. *Journal of Translational Medicine*, *9*(1), 195. http://dx.doi.org/10.1186/1479-5876-9-195. 1479-5876-9-195 [pii].

Pan, Z., Zhu, L.-J., Li, Y.-Q., Hao, L.-Y., Yin, C., Yang, J.-X., et al. (2014). Epigenetic modification of spinal miR-219 expression regulates chronic inflammation pain by targeting CaMKIIγ. *Journal of Neuroscience*, *34*(29), 9476–9483. http://dx.doi.org/10.1523/jneurosci.5346-13.2014.

Park, C. K., Xu, Z. Z., Berta, T., Han, Q., Chen, G., Liu, X. J., et al. (2014). Extracellular microRNAs activate nociceptor neurons to elicit pain via TLR7 and TRPA1. *Neuron*, *82*(1), 47–54. http://dx.doi.org/10.1016/j.neuron.2014.02.011.

Peterson, N. C., & Servinsky, M. D. (2007). Development of molecular and cellular biomarkers of pain. *Comparative Medicine*, *57*(6), 554–562.

Poh, K. W., Yeo, J. F., & Ong, W. Y. (2011). MicroRNA changes in the mouse prefrontal cortex after inflammatory pain. *European Journal of Pain*. *15*(8), http://dx.doi.org/10.1016/j.ejpain.2011.02.002. S1090-3801(11)00035-8 [pii], 801 e801-812.

Qureshi, R., Tian, Y., McDonald, M., Capasso, K., Douglas, S., Gao, R., et al. (2015). Circulating microRNA signatures in rodent models of pain. *Molecular Neurobiology*, *1–12*. http://dx.doi.org/10.1007/s12035-015-9281-4.

Raiborg, C., Rusten, T. E., & Stenmark, H. (2003). Protein sorting into multivesicular endosomes. *Current Opinion in Cell Biology*, *15*(4), 446–455. S0955067403000802 [pii].

Raposo, G., & Stoorvogel, W. (2013). Extracellular vesicles: Exosomes, microvesicles, and friends. *Journal of Cell Biology*, *200*(4), 373–383. http://dx.doi.org/10.1083/jcb.201211138.

Record, M., Subra, C., Silvente-Poirot, S., & Poirot, M. (2011). Exosomes as intercellular signalosomes and pharmacological effectors. *Biochemical Pharmacology*, *81*(10), 1171–1182. http://dx.doi.org/10.1016/j.bcp.2011.02.011. S0006-2952(11)00115-8 [pii].

Rosso, S. B., & Inestrosa, N. C. (2013). WNT signaling in neuronal maturation and synaptogenesis. *Frontiers in Cellular Neuroscience*, 7, 103. http://dx.doi.org/10.3389/fncel.2013.00103.

Ruby, J. G., Stark, A., Johnston, W. K., Kellis, M., Bartel, D. P., & Lai, E. C. (2007). Evolution, biogenesis, expression, and target predictions of a substantially expanded set of Drosophila microRNAs. *Genome Research*, *17*(12), 1850–1864. http://dx.doi.org/10.1101/gr.6597907.

Sakai, A., Saitow, F., Miyake, N., Miyake, K., Shimada, T., & Suzuki, H. (2013). miR-7a alleviates the maintenance of neuropathic pain through regulation of neuronal excitability. *Brain*, *136*(Pt. 9), 2738–2750. http://dx.doi.org/10.1093/brain/awt191.

Sakai, A., & Suzuki, H. (2014). Emerging roles of microRNAs in chronic pain. *Neurochemistry International*, 77, 58–67. http://dx.doi.org/10.1016/j.neuint.2014.05.010.

Sanchez Freire, V., Burkhard, F. C., Kessler, T. M., Kuhn, A., Draeger, A., & Monastyrskaya, K. (2010). MicroRNAs may mediate the down-regulation of neurokinin-1 receptor in chronic bladder pain syndrome. *American Journal of Pathology*, *176*(1), 288–303. http://dx.doi.org/10.2353/ajpath.2010.090552.

Schmittgen, T. D., & Livak, K. J. (2008). Analyzing real-time PCR data by the comparative C(T) method. *Nature Protocols*, *3*(6), 1101–1108.

Schwartzman, R. J., Alexander, G. M., Grothusen, J. R., Paylor, T., Reichenberger, E., & Perreault, M. (2009). Outpatient intravenous ketamine for the treatment of complex regional pain syndrome: A double-blind placebo controlled study. *Pain*, *147*(1), 107–115.

Sengupta, J. N., Pochiraju, S., Kannampalli, P., Bruckert, M., Addya, S., Yadav, P., et al. (2013). MicroRNA-mediated GABAAα-1 receptor subunit down-regulation in adult spinal cord following neonatal cystitis-induced chronic visceral pain in rats. *PAIN*, *154*(1), 59–70. http://dx.doi.org/10.1016/j.pain.2012.09.002.

Shen, N., Liang, D., Tang, Y., de Vries, N., & Tak, P. P. (2012). MicroRNAs—Novel regulators of systemic lupus erythematosus pathogenesis. *Nature Reviews. Rheumatology*, *8*(12), 701–709. http://dx.doi.org/10.1038/nrrheum.2012.142.

Shi, Y., Yuan, S., Li, B., Wang, J., Carlton, S., Chung, K., et al. (2012). Regulation of Wnt signaling by nociceptive input in animal models. *Molecular Pain*, *8*(1), 47.

Simonetti, M., Agarwal, N., Stösser, S., Bali, Kiran K., Karaulanov, E., Kamble, R., et al. (2014). Wnt-Fzd signaling sensitizes peripheral sensory neurons via distinct noncanonical pathways. *Neuron*, *83*(1), 104–121. http://dx.doi.org/10.1016/j.neuron.2014.05.037.

Stoorvogel, W. (2012). Functional transfer of microRNA by exosomes. *Blood*, *119*(3), 646–648. http://dx.doi.org/10.1182/blood-2011-11-389478.

Stoorvogel, W. (2015). Resolving sorting mechanisms into exosomes. *Cell Research*, *25*(5), 531–532. http://dx.doi.org/10.1038/cr.2015.39.

Stoorvogel, W., Kleijmeer, M. J., Geuze, H. J., & Raposo, G. (2002). The biogenesis and functions of exosomes. *Traffic*, *3*(5), 321–330. tra030502 [pii].

Strickland, I. T., Richards, L., Holmes, F. E., Wynick, D., Uney, J. B., & Wong, L.-F. (2011). Axotomy-induced miR-21 promotes axon growth in adult dorsal root ganglion neurons. *PLoS One*, *6*(8), e23423.

Sun, Y., Li, X. Q., Sahbaie, P., Shi, X. Y., Li, W. W., Liang, D. Y., et al. (2012). miR-203 regulates nociceptive sensitization after incision by controlling phospholipase A2 activating protein expression. *Anesthesiology*, *117*(3), 626–638. http://dx.doi.org/10.1097/ALN.0b013e31826571aa.

Tafuri, E., Santovito, D., de Nardis, V., Marcantonio, P., Paganelli, C., Affaitati, G., et al. (2015). MicroRNA profiling in migraine without aura: Pilot study. *Annals of Medicine*, *47*(6), 468–473. http://dx.doi.org/10.3109/07853890.2015.1071871.

Tan, P.-H., Pao, Y.-Y., Cheng, J.-K., Hung, K.-C., & Liu, C.-C. (2013). MicroRNA-based therapy in pain medicine: Current progress and future prospects. *Acta Anaesthesiologica Taiwanica*, *51*(4), 171–176. http://dx.doi.org/10.1016/j.aat.2013.11.001.

Turchinovich, A., Weiz, L., Langheinz, A., & Burwinkel, B. (2011). Characterization of extracellular circulating microRNA. *Nucleic Acids Research*, *39*(16), 7223–7233. http://dx.doi.org/10.1093/nar/gkr254. gkr254 [pii].

Vaissiere, T., Sawan, C., & Herceg, Z. (2008). Epigenetic interplay between histone modifications and DNA methylation in gene silencing. *Mutation Research*, *659*(1–2), 40–48. http://dx.doi.org/10.1016/j.mrrev.2008.02.004. S1383-5742(08)00032-X [pii].

Van Deun, J., Mestdagh, P., Sormunen, R., Cocquyt, V., Vermaelen, K., Vandesompele, J., et al. (2014). The impact of disparate isolation methods for extracellular vesicles on downstream RNA profiling. *Journal of Extracellular Vesicles*, *3*. http://dx.doi.org/10.3402/jev.v3.24858. 10.3402/jev.v3403.24858. eCollection 2014.

van Rooij, E. (2011). The art of microRNA research. *Circulation Research*, *108*(2), 219–234. http://dx.doi.org/10.1161/circresaha.110.227496.

Viaud, S., Thery, C., Ploix, S., Tursz, T., Lapierre, V., Lantz, O., et al. (2010). Dendritic cell-derived exosomes for cancer immunotherapy: What's next? *Cancer Research*, *70*(4), 1281–1285. http://dx.doi.org/10.1158/0008-5472.can-09-3276.

Villarroya-Beltri, C., Baixauli, F., Gutierrez-Vazquez, C., Sanchez-Madrid, F., & Mittelbrunn, M. (2014). Sorting it out: Regulation of exosome loading. *Seminars in Cancer Biology*, *28*, 3–13. http://dx.doi.org/10.1016/j.semcancer.2014.04.009.

von Schack, D., Agostino, M. J., Murray, B. S., Li, Y., Reddy, P. S., Chen, J., et al. (2011). Dynamic changes in the microRNA expression profile reveal multiple regulatory mechanisms in the spinal nerve ligation model of neuropathic pain. *PLoS One*, *6*(3), e17670. http://dx.doi.org/10.1371/journal.pone.0017670.

Willemen, H., Huo, X.-J., Mao-Ying, Q.-L., Zijlstra, J., Heijnen, C., & Kavelaars, A. (2012). MicroRNA-124 as a novel treatment for persistent hyperalgesia. *Journal of Neuroinflammation*, *9*(1), 143.

Woodcock, J., Witter, J., & Dionne, R. A. (2007). Stimulating the development of mechanism-based, individualized pain therapies. *Nature Reviews. Drug Discovery*, *6*(9), 703–710. http://dx.doi.org/10.1038/nrd2335. nrd2335 [pii].

Yi, R., Qin, Y., Macara, I. G., & Cullen, B. R. (2003). Exportin-5 mediates the nuclear export of pre-microRNAs and short hairpin RNAs. *Genes & Development*, *17*(24), 3011–3016. http://dx.doi.org/10.1101/gad.1158803.

Yu, B., Zhou, S., Wang, Y., Ding, G., Ding, F., & Gu, X. (2011). Profile of microRNAs following rat sciatic nerve injury by deep sequencing: Implication for mechanisms of nerve regeneration. *PLoS One*, *6*(9), e24612. http://dx.doi.org/10.1371/journal.pone.0024612.

Zhang, J., & Banerjee, B. (2015). Role of microRNA in visceral pain. *Journal of Neurogastroenterology and Motility*, *21*(2), 159–171. http://dx.doi.org/10.5056/jnm15027.

Zhang, L., & Wrana, J. L. (2014). The emerging role of exosomes in Wnt secretion and transport. *Current Opinion in Genetics & Development*, *27*, 14–19. http://dx.doi.org/10.1016/j.gde.2014.03.006.

Zhang, Y. K., Huang, Z. J., Liu, S., Liu, Y. P., Song, A. A., & Song, X. J. (2013). WNT signaling underlies the pathogenesis of neuropathic pain in rodents. *Journal of Clinical Investigation*, *123*(5), 2268–2286. http://dx.doi.org/10.1172/JCI65364.

Zhao, J., Lee, M. C., Momin, A., Cendan, C. M., Shepherd, S. T., Baker, M. D., et al. (2010). Small RNAs control sodium channel expression, nociceptor excitability, and pain thresholds. *Journal of Neuroscience*, *30*(32), 10860–10871. http://dx.doi.org/10.1523/JNEUROSCI.1980-10.2010. 30/32/10860 [pii].

CHAPTER THREE

Modulation of Chronic Pain by Metabotropic Glutamate Receptors

Santina Chiechio[1]
Department of Drug Sciences, University of Catania, Catania, Italy
[1]Corresponding author: e-mail address: chiechio@unict.it

Contents

Abstract

Metabotropic glutamate receptors (mGluRs) belong to class C G-protein-coupled receptors. They are expressed throughout the nervous system on both neurons and glial cells. In the central nervous system (CNS), mGluRs are mainly located in the proximity of the synaptic cleft where they regulate glutamatergic transmission in addition to a number of other neurotransmitters. To date, eight subtypes of mGluRs (mGluR1–mGluR8) have been cloned and classified into three groups on the basis of sequence similarities, and pharmacological and biochemical properties. Consequently, group I mGluRs includes mGluR1 and mGluR5, group II mGluRs includes mGluR2 and mGluR3, and group III mGluRs consists of mGluR4, mGluR6, mGluR7, and mGluR8. With the exception of mGluR6, whose localization is restricted within the retina, all mGluRs are ubiquitously expressed throughout the peripheral and CNS with some subtype specificity in different anatomical regions. mGluRs participate in many physiological processes and play important roles in a number of neurological conditions including anxiety, depression, schizophrenia, and neurodegenerative disorders. mGluRs also participate in the physiological transmission of pain stimuli as well as to mechanisms involved in the establishment of chronic pain. Therefore, these receptors are attractive targets for therapeutic intervention in several neurological disorders including chronic

Advances in Pharmacology, Volume 75
ISSN 1054-3589
http://dx.doi.org/10.1016/bs.apha.2015.11.001

pain. Thus, understanding the physiological function and role of each mGluR subtype in the development of chronic pain will provide a better insight into the potential use of subtype-selective drugs currently being developed as orthosteric or allosteric ligands.

ABBREVIATIONS

AMPA α-amino-3-hydroxy-5-methyl-isoxazole-4-propionate
cAMP cyclic adenosine monophosphate
CNS central nervous system
CPCRs G-protein-coupled receptors
DH dorsal horn
DRG dorsal root ganglion
ERK extracellular signal-related kinase
iGluRs ionotropic glutamate receptors
IP_3 inositol 1,4,5-trisphosphate
mGluRs metabotropic glutamate receptors
NAM negative allosteric modulator
NMDA *N*-methyl-D-aspartate
PAG periaqueductal gray matter
PAM positive allosteric modulator
PLC phospholipase C
RVM rostral ventromedial medulla

1. INTRODUCTION

Pain is usually classified as either nociceptive, inflammatory, or neuropathic, according to its origin, symptoms, and underlying mechanisms (Costigan, Scholz, & Woolfet, 2009). Although this classification is very useful from a didactic point of view, it does not reflect the complexity of pain disorders in clinical conditions. In chronic pain patients, the presence of more than one component extremely complicates the assessment and management of pain (Baron & Binder, 2004). In this chapter, recent literature describing the role of glutamate transmission via metabotropic glutamate receptor (mGluR) subtypes in the pathophysiology of chronic pain is reviewed.

Glutamate is the main excitatory amino acid in the central nervous system (CNS) and is involved in brain function and pathology. As neurotransmitter, glutamate activates two different types of receptors: ionotropic glutamate receptors (iGluRs) and mGluRs. According to their response to different agonists, iGluRs have been further subdivided into three distinct types: *N*-methyl-D-aspartate (NMDA), α-amino-3-hydroxy-5-methyl-isoxazole-4-propionate (AMPA), and kainate (KA) receptors (Hollmann & Heinemann, 1994; Monaghan, Bridges, & Cotman, 1989). iGluRs are directly coupled to a membrane ion channel and mediate fast excitatory synaptic transmission. On the contrary, mGluRs are cell membrane receptors belonging to the class C of the G-protein-coupled receptor (GPCR) superfamily that modulate rather than mediate neuronal excitability and neurotransmitter release via G-protein-dependent and non-G-protein-dependent signaling pathways (Anwyl, 1999).

By activating iGluRs and/or mGluRs, glutamate participates not only in the physiological transmission of nociceptive information but also in the development of peripheral and central mechanisms of pain hypersensitivity (Latremoliere & Woolf, 2009). Glutamate plays a primary role in the increased synaptic efficacy occurring after injury, a mechanism that has been referred to activity-dependent central sensitization (Woolf, 1983). As for the hippocampal long-term potentiation (LTP) of the synaptic strength (Ji, Kohno, Moore, & Woolf, 2003) which is a key mechanism for memory consolidation (Nicoll, 2003), glutamate-induced plasticity is a fundamental step for the development of the so-called "memory of pain" that is the basis for the establishment of chronic pain symptoms such as hyperalgesia, allodynia, and spontaneous pain (Woolf, 1983). Both NMDA and AMPA receptors, together with a number of metabotropic receptors, can trigger central sensitization through an increase in intracellular calcium levels that activate intracellular pathways strengthening the excitatory synapse (Latremoliere & Woolf, 2009). The blockade of NMDA receptors consistently resulting in the prevention of hyperexcitability of nociceptive neurons suggests the potential use of NMDA antagonist in the treatment of pain hypersensitivity (Woolf & Thompson, 1991). However, besides the selective antagonists of the NMDA receptor NR2B subunit (Boyce et al., 1999), the direct blockade of glutamate transmission by iGluRs antagonists is known to have detrimental effects on learning and memory processes (Chizh, 2007; Nakazato, Kato, & Watanabe, 2005; Wei et al., 2001; Zhang, Chen, & Pan, 2009); therefore, an NMDA antagonist-based therapy for chronic pain is unlikely to be developed. Consequently, understanding the function, expression, and role of mGluRs in pain modulation and their involvement in the induction and maintenance of central sensitization may help to find a practicable alternative to reduce hypersensitivity in chronic pain conditions.

2. CLASSIFICATION OF mGluRs

mGluRs belong to the class C of GPCRs (Schiöth & Fredriksson, 2005). There are eight types of mGluRs (mGluR1–8) that can be divided into three different groups according to their sequence similarity, pharmacology and intracellular signal transduction pathways (Fig. 1; Conn & Pin, 1997; Pin & Duvoisin, 1995). Group I include mGluR1 and mGluR5; group II include mGluR2 and mGluR3; and group III is formed by mGluR4, mGluR6, mGluR7, and mGluR8. Moreover, virtually all mGluR genes have been described to undergo alternative splicing to generate splice variants (reviewed by Yin & Niswender, 2014). Group I mGluRs are predominantly, but not exclusively, localized at postsynaptic level where they regulate neuronal excitability. By coupling to $G_{\alpha q/11}$ proteins and activating phospholipase

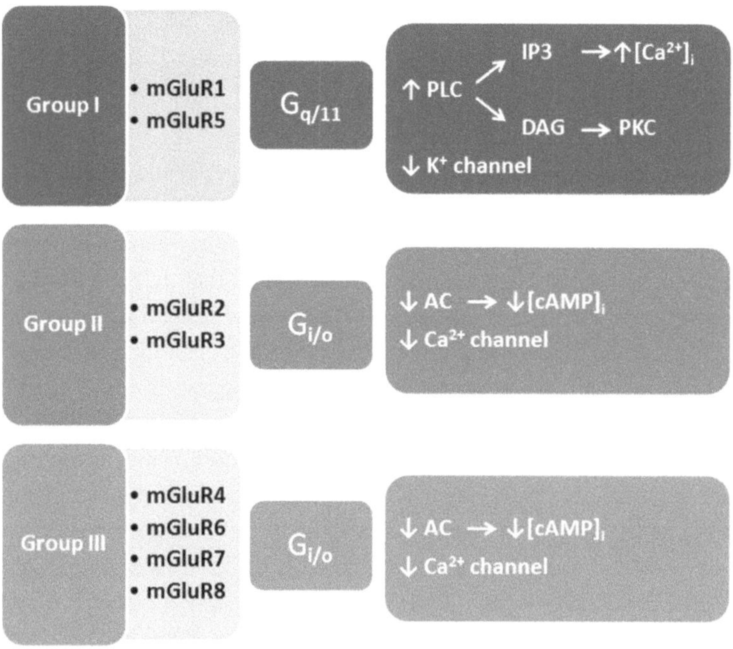

Figure 1 mGluR receptor families, subtypes, and transduction pathways. mGluRs are classified into three families: group I, II, and III. Stimulation of group I mGluRs activates phospholipase C (PLC) and induces phosphoinositide hydrolysis with formation of inositol 1,4,5-triphosphate (IP_3) and diacylglycerol (DAG), whereas activation of group I and group III mGluRs induces a decrease of the intracellular levels of cyclic adenosine monophosphate (cAMP) by a negative coupling to adenylyl cyclase (AC).

C (PLC), group I mGluRs primarily stimulate phosphoinositide hydrolysis leading to the formation of two second messengers: inositol 1,4,5-trisphosphate (IP_3) and diacylglycerol (DAG) that initiate a cascade of intracellular events starting from the IP_3-induced calcium mobilization from intracellular stores. In addition, a number of intracellular signaling molecules such as protein kinase A (PKA), protein kinase C (PKC), mitogen-activated protein kinase (MAPK), extracellular signal-related kinase (ERK), and cAMP response element binding protein (CREB) are activated. Conversely, group II and group III mGluRs are negatively coupled to adenylyl cyclase through $G_{\alpha i/o}$ proteins and are often localized on presynaptic terminals. Thus, activation of group II and III mGluRs results in a decreased formation of intracellular cyclic adenosine monophosphate (cAMP) (Conn & Pin, 1997; Niswender & Conn, 2010; Schoepp, Jane, & Monn, 1999). These receptors primarily act as autoreceptors providing negative feedback for the release of glutamate and other neurotransmitters (Alagarsamy, Sorensen, & Conn, 2001; Conn & Pin, 1997). The different pattern of intracellular signal pathways among mGluRs accounts for the substantial differences in the effect mediated by group I mGluRs that trigger excitatory responses, and group II and III mGluRs that mostly mediate inhibitory effects. mGluRs can also modulate ion channel currents via $G_{\beta\gamma}$ subunits (Conn & Pin, 1997) and numerous other receptors via G-protein-dependent and -independent pathways (reviewed by Yin & Niswender, 2014).

As other GPGRs, mGluRs are characterized by a seven-transmembrane domain (7TMD) structure; however, a distinguishing feature of mGluRs is the very long extracellular amino terminal domain containing the Venus-flytrap (VFT) and a cysteine-rich domains (CRD). The VFT domain, highly conserved among all eight mGluRs, contains the ligand bind site for glutamate and orthosteric ligands, while the CRD is crucial to transferring the signal to the transmembrane domain (Hu, Hauache, & Spiegel, 2000; Muto, Tsuchiya, Morikawa, & Jingami, 2007; Wellendorph & Bräuner-Osborne, 2009). Furthermore, mGluRs form, at least *in vitro*, homo- and/or heterodimers by interacting via their VFT domains through a disulfide linkage (Romano, Yang, & O'Malley, 1996) with other mGluRs (Doumazane et al., 2011; Kniazeff, Prézeau, Rondard, Pin, & Goudet, 2011; Pin, Galvez, & Prézeau, 2003). The existence of heterodimers formed by mGluR5 and μ-opioid receptors (Schröder et al., 2009), calcium sensing receptors (Gama, Wilt, & Breitwieser, 2001), or with serotonin 5-HT2A receptors (González-Maeso et al., 2008), as well as a functional interaction with adenosine A2A (Ferré et al., 2002; Rodrigues, Alfaro, Rebola,

Oliveira, & Cunha, 2005) and dopamine D2 receptors (Cabello et al., 2009), has been also described. Recently, the existence of mGluR2/mGluR4 heterodimers at corticostriatal synapses in rodents has been postulated using biochemical and pharmacological approaches (Yin et al., 2014). The ability of mGluRs to form heterodimers has been used to develop bivalent ligands with increased analgesic efficacy, such as compounds endowed with μ-opioid agonist and mGluR5 antagonist pharmacophores that produce potent antinociception in models of inflammatory and chronic cancer pain in mice (Akgün et al., 2013; Smeester, Lunzer, Akgün, Beitz, & Portoghese, 2014).

3. ORTHOSTERIC LIGANDS AND ALLOSTERIC MODULATORS OF mGluRs

During the last decades, a number of synthetic compounds have been developed with the ability to modulate glutamatergic transmission by either activating or inhibiting specific mGluR groups or subtypes. Among these several compounds, orthosteric ligands and allosteric modulators have been employed to investigate the specific role of mGluRs in pain modulation (Chiechio & Nicoletti, 2012; Montana & Gereau, 2011). Since the majority of allosteric modulators bind to a site within the 7TMD, which, among all mGluR subtypes, is less conserved than the FTV domain, a subtype selectivity is more likely to be achieved (Gregory, Noetzel, & Niswender, 2013). Thus, besides classical agonists or antagonists at mGluRs, a number of subtype-selective positive (PAM), negative (NAM) allosteric modulators have been developed to potentiate or reduce the physiological activation of specific mGluRs by endogenous glutamate and many of these have been used to understand the specific role of mGluR subtypes function in pain conditions (Dolan, Gunn, Crossan, & Nolan, 2011; Goudet et al., 2008; Hao et al., 2013; Ji & Neugebauer, 2014; Kiritoshi et al., 2013; Palazzo et al., 2013, 2015; Rossi et al., 2014; Salt, Jones, Copeland, & Sillito, 2014; Wang, Jiang, Yang, & Li, 2011). Table 1 reports a list of the most employed ligands in pain studies. In addition, a number of new compounds with mGluR1 antagonist properties (Cho et al., 2015; Kim et al., 2014; Nam et al., 2015) or negative allosteric modulators (Ai, Wood, & Welsh, 2015) have been recently developed for their potential use in neuropathic pain conditions.

Table 1 Orthosteric and Allosteric mGluR Receptor Ligands Employed in Pain Studies

Group/ Subtype	Activity	Other Effects	References
Group I ligands			
Quisqualic acid	Agonist	Selectivity for mGluR1 and mGlur5	Ohashi et al. (2002)
		Activity at AMPA receptors	Watkins, Krogsgaard-Larsen, and Honoré (1990)
(*S*)-3,5-DHPG	Agonist	More selective for mGluR5 over mGluR1	Schoepp et al. (1999)
(*S*)-4CPG	Antagonist	Activity at mGluR2	Schoepp et al. (1999)
(*S*)-4C3HPG	Antagonist	Activity at mGluR2	Schoepp et al. (1999)
(*S*)-MCPG	Antagonist	Activity at mGluR2	Schoepp et al. (1999)
mGluR1 selective			
AIDA	Antagonist		Lavreysen et al. (2003)
LY367385	Antagonist		Kingston, Burnett, Mayne, and Lodge (1995)
Ro67-4853	PAM		Knoflach et al. (2001)
CPCCOEt	NAM		Litschig et al. (1999)
JNJ16259685	NAM		Lavreysen et al. (2004)
YM-298198	NAM		Kohara et al. (2005)
FTIDC	NAM		Suzuki, Kimura, et al. (2007) and Suzuki, Tsukamoto, et al. (2007)
mGluR5 selective			
CHPG	Agonist	High selectivity at mGluR5 over mGluR1	Doherty, Palmer, Henley, Collingridge, and Jane (1997)
SIB-1757	NAM		Varney et al. (1999)
Fenobam	NAM		Porter et al. (2005)
MPEP	NAM	mGluR4 PAM	Gasparini et al. (1999)
MTEP	NAM		Cosford et al. (2003)

Continued

Table 1 Orthosteric and Allosteric mGluR Receptor Ligands Employed in Pain Studies—cont'd

Group/ Subtype	Activity	Other Effects	References
Group II ligands			
DCG IV	Agonists	Potent agonist at mGluR2 and mGluR3	Schweitzer et al. (2000)
		NMDA receptor agonist activity	Ishida, Saitoh, Shimamoto, Ohfune, and Shinozaki (1993)
		Antagonist activity at group I and group III	
		mGluRs at high concentrations	Brabet et al. (1998)
2*R*,4*R*-APDC	Agonist		Schoepp et al. (1999)
LY379268	Agonist	Activate mGluR4, mGluR6 and mGluR8 at high concentrations	
			Monn et al. (1999)
LY341495	Antagonist	Little antagonism on group I and III mGluRs	Johnson et al. (1999)
			Jane, Thomas, Tse, and Watkins (1996)
LY354740	Agonist		Bond, Monn, and Lodge (1997)
EGLU	Antagonist	Little antagonism on group I and III mGluRs	Jane et al. (1996)
mGluR2 selective			
LY487379	PAM		Schaffhauser et al. (2003)
mGluR3 selective			
NAAG	Agonist		Schweitzer et al. (2000)
Group III ligands			
L-AP4	Agonist	Activate mGluR4, mGluR6 and mGluR8 with similar potencies	
			Schoepp et al. (1999)

Table 1 Orthosteric and Allosteric mGluR Receptor Ligands Employed in Pain Studies—cont'd

Group/ Subtype	Activity	Other Effects	References
L-SOP	Agonist	Activate mGluR7 at higher concentrations	Wright, Arnold, Wheeler, Ornstein, and Schoepp (2000)
CPPG	Antagonist		Jane et al. (1996)
mGluR4 selective			
LSP4-2022	Agonist	300-fold selectivity for mGluR4 over mGluR8	Goudet et al. (2012)
PHCCC	PAM	Activity on mGluR6	Beqollari and Kammermeier (2008)
VU0155041	PAM		Niswender et al. (2008)
mGluR7 selective			
AMN082	PAM		Mitsukawa et al. (2005)
MMPIP	NAM		Suzuki, Kimura, et al. (2007) and Suzuki, Tsukamoto, et al. (2007)
XAP044	NAM		Gee et al. (2014)
mGluR8 selective			
(*S*)-3,4-DCPG	Agonist	100-fold selectivity for mGluR8 over mGluR4	Thomas et al. (2001)
AZ12216052	PAM		Duvoisin et al. (2010)

NAM, negative allosteric modulator; PAM, positive allosteric modulator; (*S*)-3,5-DHPG, (*S*)-3,-5-dihydroxyphenylglycine; (*S*)-4CPG, (*S*)-4-carboxyphenylglycine; (*S*)-4C3HPG, (*S*)-4-carboxy-3-hydroxyphenylglycine; (*S*)-MCPG, (*S*)-α-methyl-4-carboxyphenylglycine; AIDA, (*RS*)-1-aminoindan-1,5-dicarboxylic acid; LY367385, (*S*)-(+)-*a*-amino-4-carboxy-2-methylbenzeneacetic acid; Ro67-4853, (9*H*-xanthen-9-ylcarbonyl)-carbamic acid butyl ester; CPCCOEt, 7-(hydroxyimino)cyclopropa[*b*]chromen-1*a*-carboxylate ethyl ester; JNJ16259685, 3-4-dihydro-2*H*-pyrano[2,3-b]quinolin-7-yl-(*cis*-4-methoxycyclohexyl)-methanone; YM-298198, 6-amino-*N*-cyclohexyl-*N*,3-dimethylthiazolo[3,2-*a*]benzimidazole-2-carboxamide; FTIDC, 4-[1-(2-fluoropyridin-3-yl)-5-methyl-1*H*-1,2,3-triazol-4-yl]-*N*-isopropyl-*N*-methyl-3,6-dihydropyridine-1(2*H*)-carboxamide; CHPG, (*RS*)-2-chloro-5--hydroxyphenylglycine; SIB-1757, 6-methyl-2-(phenylazo)-3-pyridinol; Fenobam, *N*-(3-chlorophenyl)-*N*′-(4,5-dihydro-1-methyl-4-oxo-1*H*-imidazol-2-yl)urea; MPEP, 2-methyl-6-(phenylethynyl)pyridine; MTEP, 3-[(2-methyl-1,3-thiazol-4-yl)ethynyl]pyridine; DCG IV, (2*S*,2′*R*,3′*R*)-2-(2′,3′-dicarboxycyclopropyl)glycine; 2*R*,4*R*-APDC, (2*R*,4*R*)-4-aminopyrrolidine-2,4-dicarboxylate; LY379268, (1*R*,4*R*,5*S*,6*R*)-4-amino-2-oxabicyclo[3.1.0]hexane-4,6-dicarboxylic acid; LY341495, (2*S*)-2-amino-2-[(1*S*,2*S*)-2-carboxycycloprop-1-yl]-3-(xanth-9-yl) propanoic acid; LY354740, (1*S*,2*S*,5*R*,6*S*)-2-aminobicyclo[3.1.0]hexane-2,6-dicarboxylic acid; EGLU, (2*S*)-α-ethylglutamic acid; LY487379, 2,2,2-trifluoro-*N*-[4-(2-methoxyphenoxy)phenyl]-*N*-(3-pyridinylmethyl)ethanesulfonamide; NAAG, *N*-acetyl-L-aspartyl-L-glutamic acid; L-AP4, L-(+)-2-amino-4-phosphonobutyric acid; L-SOP, L-serine-*O*-phosphate; CPPG, (*RS*)-*a*-cyclopropyl-4-phosphonophenylglycine; LSP4-2022, (2*S*)-2-amino-4-({[4-(carboxymethoxy)phenyl](hydroxy)methyl}(hydroxy)phosphoryl)butanoic acid; PHCCC, *N*-phenyl-7-(hydroxyimino)cyclopropa[*b*]chromen-1*a*-carboxamide; VU0155041, *cis*-2-[[(3,5-dichlorophenyl)amino]carbonyl] cyclohexanecarboxylic acid; AMN082, *N*,*N*/-bis(diphenylmethyl)-1,2-ethanediamine; MMPIP, 6-(4-methoxyphenyl)-5-methyl-3-(4-pyridinyl)-isoxazolo[4,5-*c*]pyridin-4(5*H*)-one hydrochloride; XAP044, 7-hydroxy-3-(4-iodophenoxy)-4*H*-1-benzopyran-4-one, (*S*)-3,4-DCPG, (*S*)-3,4-dicarboxyphenylglycine; AZ12216052, 2-[[(4-bromophenyl)methyl]thio]-*N*-[4-(1-methylpropyl)phenyl] acetamide.

4. mGluR SUBTYPES IN PAIN

The assessment and management of chronic pain syndromes can be extremely complicated by the coexistence of mixed pain forms (Baron & Binder, 2004). By counteracting both nociceptive and persistent forms of pain, mGluRs are excellent candidates for chronic pain treatment. mGluRs are able to reduce pain hypersensitivity acting at different levels, from the periphery to brain regions involved in the perception and modulation of pain. With the exception of the mGluR6 subtype, whose localization is restricted to dendrites of ON bipolar cells in the retina (Vardi, Duvoisin, Wu, & Sterling, 2000), all mGluRs are ubiquitously expressed throughout the nervous system in both neurons and glial cells, with some selectivity for each subtype in specific brain regions (Fig. 2; Ferraguti & Shigemoto, 2006). Within the pain neuraxis, mGluRs modulate the perception of physiological pain and participate in the development of peripheral and central sensitization in chronic pain conditions (Chiechio & Nicoletti, 2012; Goudet et al., 2009; Varney & Gereau, 2002). In neurons, mGluRs are located both pre- and postsynaptically. In particular, group I mGluRs are mainly located at postsynaptic level where they positively modulate neuronal excitability, while group II and III mGluRs are predominately located at presynaptic level where they negatively regulate neurotransmitter release. In addition, several mGluR subtypes are also expressed in glial cells, such as astrocytes, where they have a crucial role in modulating neuronal excitability and pain hypersensitivity (Boye Larsen et al., 2014; Byrnes et al., 2009; Osikowicz, Mika, & Przewlocka, 2013; Saab, Wang, Gu, Garner, & Al-Chaer, 2006; Weisshaar et al., 2010).

A number of studies have been addressed to elucidate the precise role and contribution of each subtype on pain modulation. Although specific mGluR subtypes can have both pronociceptive and antinociceptive effects depending on the anatomical site of activation, it is generally agreed that while group I mGluRs mediate hyperalgesia, group II and III mGluRs are able to reduce hyperalgesia in animal models of inflammatory and neuropathic pain.

5. ROLE OF GROUP I mGluRs IN PAIN MODULATION

Pharmacological interventions for pain relief are usually aimed at inhibiting group I mGluRs and/or potentiating group II and III mGluR

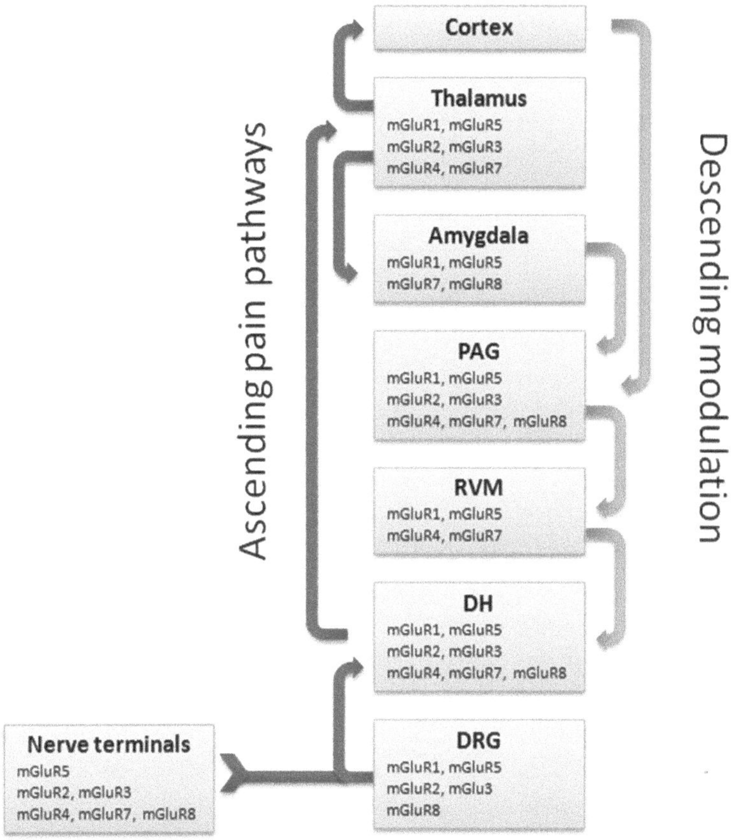

Figure 2 mGluRs in the pain pathways. Schematic representation of mGluR expression in peripheral, spinal, and supraspinal structures involved in pain transmission and modulation. Besides the mGluR6 subtype, all mGluR subtypes are expressed all along the pain neuraxis where they modulate pain sensitivity. Ascending and descending pain pathways are indicated. PAG: periaqueductal gray; RVM: rostral ventromedial medulla; DRG: dorsal root ganglion.

signaling. Glutamate released from primary afferent neurons is a key event for persistent activation of spinal neurons leading to hypersensitivity in chronic pain states. Among group I mGluRs, the mGluR5 subtype, together with NMDA receptors, gives an important contribution in nociceptive processing and in the development of central sensitization by activating a variety of intracellular pathways (Dolan, Kelly, Monteiro, & Nolan, 2003; Ren et al., 2012). Pharmacological studies have shown an implication of both mGluR1 and mGluR5 in the physiological modulation of pain and in the development of chronic pain states. In particular, the administration of group I mGluRs agonists induces spontaneous pain and increases inflammatory and neuropathic pain that can be blocked by antibodies raised against the C-terminals of mGluR1 and mGluR5 (Fundytus, Fisher, Dray, Henry, & Coderre, 1998; Karim, Wang, & Gereau, 2001). More recent studies have shown that mGluR5 antagonists are effective in animal models of inflammatory, neuropathic, and visceral pain (Crock, Stemler, et al., 2012; Lindström et al., 2008; Montana et al., 2009, 2011). Strikingly, drugs that block or negatively modulate mGluR5 are not only effective in chronic pain but also have positive reinforcing effects only in the context of neuropathic pain, as demonstrated in a model of analgesic conditioned place preference (Lax, George, Ignatz, & Kolber, 2014). This interesting finding makes the mGluR5 an attractive candidate in chronic pain conditions. Thus, although both mGluR1 and mGluR5 antagonists or NAMs are both effective in chronic pain models, the mGluR5 seems to be a better target for chronic pain treatment. However, it is important to point out that although group I mGluR-mediated signaling is a key event in peripheral and central sensitization of pain (Bhave, Karim, Carlton, & Gereau, 2001), group I mGluRs can mediate both pro- and antinociceptive effects, depending on the site of activation. While activation of group I mGluRs in peripheral sensory afferents in the dorsal horn (DH) of the spinal cord has been shown to facilitate nociception, group I mGluRs can differently modulate pain sensitivity with different mechanisms at supraspinal levels (Chiechio & Nicoletti, 2012).

In the periphery, group I mGluR-mediated hyperalgesia is elicited through a number of mechanisms that often require the cooperation of different receptors, ion channels and intracellular pathways. For example, in the peripheral terminal of sensory neurons, group I mGluRs increase pain sensitivity by enhancing the transient receptor potential vanilloid 1 (TRPV1) function (Hu, Bhave, & Gereau, 2002). Also, a biphasic modulation of the TRPV1 function by mGluR5 has been shown in peripheral sensory neurons (Masuoka et al., 2015). Interestingly, mGluR5-mediated sensitization of TRPV1 function seems to require the intervention of the scaffolding protein A-kinase anchoring protein 79/150 (AKAP150) (Szteyn et al., 2015). A functional interaction between group I mGluRs and TRPV1 receptors via AKAP150 has also been shown in trigeminal sensory neurons responsible for mechanical hyperalgesia in muscle tissues (Chung, Lee, Joseph, Saloman, & Ro, 2015). In the DH of the spinal cord, mGluR1 and mGluR5 also play a pronociceptive role by activating the ERK signaling (Karim et al., 2001) that in turn inhibits Kv4.2-containing potassium channels resulting in increased DH neuronal excitability (Hu, Alter, Carrasquillo, Qiu, & Gereau, 2007; Hu & Gereau, 2011).

At the supraspinal level, stimulation of group I mGluRs has both pronociceptive and antinociceptive effects. In the amygdala, group I mGluRs mediate hyperalgesic effects in inflammatory models of persistent pain (Kolber et al., 2010; Neugebauer, 2015) and mGluR5 are involved in the modulation of visceral pain (Crock, Kolber, et al., 2012). Moreover, mGluR1 seems to be involved in the crosstalk among the basolateral amygdala and the prefrontal cortex in inflammatory pain in rats (Ji & Neugebauer, 2011; Luongo et al., 2013). Interestingly, within the periaqueductal gray matter (PAG), activation of all groups of mGluRs, including group I mediate antinociceptive effects presumably by the activation of the descending antinociceptive pathways via the inhibition of the GABAergic transmission (Drew & Vaughan, 2004; Maione et al., 2000). In addition, in the PAG, mGluR5 seems to participate in the analgesic effects mediated by cannabinoids (de Novellis et al., 2005; Palazzo et al., 2001). Group I mGluRs are also highly expressed in the prefrontal cortex, a region involved in decision-making functions and behavioral control which has been shown to be impaired in patients suffering from chronic pain (Apkarian et al., 2004) and in animal models of inflammatory and neuropathic pain (Ji et al., 2010; Metz, Yau, Centeno, Apkarian, & Martina, 2009; Pais-Vieira, Mendes-Pinto, Lima, & Galhardo, 2009). mGluR5 located in the prefrontal cortex also influences amygdala neuronal hyperactivity and pain behavior in models of arthritis pain (Ji & Neugebauer, 2014).

Group I mGluRs also play an important role in nociceptive processing in the thalamus, which is an important center for the integration of pain stimuli coming from the spinal cord, through the spinothalamic tract, and from the descending projection from the somatosensory cortex via the corticothalamic projections (Sherman, 2012). The thalamic circuitry nociceptive responses are largely mediated by glutamate via both NMDA receptors (Bordi & Quartaroli, 2000; Eaton & Salt, 1990; Kolhekar, Murphy, & Gebhart, 1997) and group I mGluRs (Eaton et al., 1993; Salt & Binns, 2000; Salt & Turner, 1998) where the postsynaptic mGluR1 subtype seems to play a prominent role in the modulation of nociceptive processing (Salt et al., 2014).

6. ROLE OF GROUP II mGluRs IN PAIN MODULATION

The role of group II mGluRs has been extensively investigated for their ability to reduce hyperalgesia in animal models of persistent pain (Fisher & Coderre, 1996; Fisher, Lefebvre, & Coderre, 2002; Sharpe, Kingston, Lodge, Monn, & Headley, 2000; Simmons, Webster, Kalra, & Iyengar, 2002). mGluR2 and mGluR3 are generally located presynaptically on sensory nerve terminals. In the synapse, these receptors function as presynaptic auto- or heteroreceptors, regulate neurotransmitter release, and mainly respond to glutamate released from astrocytes (Kalivas, 2009). When systemically injected, group II mGluR agonists depress pain transmission by acting at different levels of pain neuraxis, including nociceptors, DH neurons, and supraspinal regions involved in pain modulation, such as the amygdala and PAG (Chiechio & Nicoletti, 2012). In periphery, group II mGluRs attenuate hyperalgesia following inflammation. This has been shown after local administration of a group II agonist, APDC, in the knee joint in a model of inflammatory pain such as the carrageenan-induced arthritis (Lee, Park, Cho, Kim, & Han, 2013). In peripheral terminals of sensory neurons, group II mGluRs regulate TRPV1 channels (Carlton, Du, & Zhou, 2009; Carlton, Zhou, Govea, & Du, 2011, Yang & Gereau, 2002) and TTX-resistant sodium channels (Yang & Gereau, 2004). An important contribution to pain control mediated by group II mGluRs occurs in the DH of the spinal cord where they depress synaptic transmission between primary afferent fibers and DH neurons (Gerber, Zhong, Youn, & Randic, 2000). Analgesia is also mediated by group II mGluRs at the supraspinal level, including the amygdala (Li & Neugebauer, 2006), the PAG (Drew & Vaughan, 2004; Maione et al., 2000), and the medial prefrontal cortex (Kiritoshi & Neugebauer, 2015). As for group I mGluRs, group II mGluRs are also highly expressed in the prefrontal cortex where they inhibit glutamatergic excitatory transmission and modulate arthritis pain-related synaptic transmission (Kiritoshi & Neugebauer, 2015). Among group II mGluRs, mGluR2 seems to play a more prominent role in the control of pain transmission, at least in inflammatory pain (Zammataro et al., 2011). The expression of mGluR2 has been shown to be regulated by several epigenetic drugs, such as L-acetylcarnitine, or several histone deacetylase or acetyltransferase inhibitors in different regions such as dorsal root ganglion (DRG) and DH (Chiechio et al., 2002; Chiechio, Copani, De Petris, et al., 2006; Chiechio, Copani, Nicoletti, & Gereau, 2006; Chiechio, Copani,

Gereau, & Nicoletti, 2007; Chiechio et al., 2009; Chiechio et al., 2010; Onofrj et al., 2013; Zammataro, Sortino, Parenti, Gereau, & Chiechio, 2014). Interestingly, changes of the mGluR2 expression level in the DRG and spinal cord have been shown to modify the analgesic potency of group II mGluR agonists (Zammataro et al., 2014). Accordingly, drug-induced mGluR2 overexpression could be an effective strategy for the control of inflammatory and neuropathic pain. Accordingly, *N*-acetyl-cysteine, a drug that induces analgesia in models of inflammatory and neuropathic pain (Bernabucci et al., 2012) by enhancing the endogenous activation of mGluR2 and mGluR3 via the glutamate/cystine antiporter, has been show to inhibit nociceptive transmission in humans (Truini et al., 2015), suggesting that group II mGluRs are excellent candidates for novel analgesic drugs.

7. ROLE OF GROUP III mGluRs IN PAIN MODULATION

mGluR subtypes belonging to group III are also expressed throughout the pain neuraxis from peripheral nerves to the CNS. In particular, the expression of mGluR8 has been shown in unmyelinated fibers of digital nerves where they negatively modulate the activity of TRPV1 receptors on nociceptors via the inhibition of adenylyl cyclase (Govea, Zhou, & Carlton, 2012). Consistently, the intraplantar injection of the group III mGluRs agonist, L-AP4, is able to attenuate the hyperalgesia induced by the TRPV1 agonist, capsaicin (Carlton et al., 2011; Govea et al., 2012).

Similarly to group II, peripheral group III mGluRs are also involved in the control of hyperalgesia following inflammation. Local administration of the group III mGluRs agonist, L-AP4, in the knee joint is able to reduce hyperalgesia in the carrageenan-induced arthritic pain model (Lee et al., 2013). In the DH of the spinal cord, activation of spinal group III mGluRs has been shown to decrease the firing of projection second order neurons by controlling the excess of glutamatergic transmission in inflammatory and neuropathic pain (Chen & Pan, 2005; Fisher et al., 2002; Zhang et al., 2009).

Among group III mGluRs, the presence of the mGluR4 subtype has been shown in the inner laminae II of the DH on both presynaptic terminals of C-fibers and spinal neuron terminals (Azkue et al., 2001; Ohishi, Akazawa, Shigemoto, Nakanishi, & Mizuno, 1995). In the DH, stimulation of mGluR4 inhibits the development of inflammatory and neuropathic pain by reducing glutamatergic transmission (Vilar et al., 2013). The control of pain hypersensitivity mediated by mGluR4 seem particularly interesting since intrathecal injection of selective mGluR4 agonists or PAMs are able to reduce hypersensitivity in animal models of inflammatory and neuropathic pain without affecting normal nociception in models of acute pain in naive animals (Goudet et al., 2008; Vilar et al., 2013; Wang et al., 2011).

Another group III mGluR, the mGluR7 subtype, has also been found in presynaptic terminals of sensory neurons in laminae I and II of the DH (Li et al., 1997; Ohishi, Nomura, et al., 1995). However, mGluR7 does not seem to play a prominent role in chronic pain since intrathecal administration of mGluR7 PAMs does not reduce hyperalgesia in neuropathic pain (Wang et al., 2011).

Group III mGluRs are extensively expressed at supraspinal region S involved in pain. However, in regions such as the amygdala, PAG, and rostral ventromedial medulla (RVM), mGluR7 and mGluR8 often elicit opposite effects. Indeed, although systemic activation of mGluR7 and mGluR8 is effective in reducing inflammatory and neuropathic pain (Marabese, de Novellis, et al., 2007; Osikowicz, Mika, Makuch, & Przewlocka, 2008), local stimulation of mGluR7 within the PAG and amygdala increases pain, while the mGluR7 blockade reduces inflammatory and neuropathic pain. On the other hand, stimulation of mGluR8 in the PAG, dorsal striatum, amygdala, and RVM reduces inflammatory and neuropathic pain (Marabese, de Novellis, et al., 2007; Marabese, Rossi, et al., 2007; Palazzo, Fu, Ji, Maione, & Neugebauer, 2008; Palazzo et al., 2013, 2011, 2015; Rossi et al., 2014). Altogether, results obtained with group III mGluR ligands suggest that these receptors are interesting therapeutic targets to alleviate pain hypersensitivity in chronic pain conditions. This is particularly relevant for the mGluR4 subtype because its activation in the spinal cord does not interfere with the physiological perception of pain while counteracts chronic pain.

8. CONCLUSION

The treatment of chronic pain can be extremely complicated due to the coexistence of mixed pain forms that often occur in patients. Over the past decades, the role of mGluRs has been investigated in different forms of pain. The increasing availability of novel subtype-selective pharmacological ligands acting at mGluRs has helped to clarify the precise role of each mGluR subtype in pain processing and in mechanisms of nociceptive sensitization suggesting that these receptors can serve as promising targets for the treatment of chronic pain. Thus, different approaches involving mGluRs are possible to relieve pain. As a general concept, an effective control of pain hypersensitivity can be achieved by either blocking group I mGluRs or stimulating group II and group III mGluRs. This can possibly be obtained by using orthosteric ligands that can either directly activate or block specific mGluR subtypes or allosteric ligands that positively (PAM) or negatively (NAM) modulate mGluR function. Moreover, an epigenetic approach leading to an increased expression of mGluR2 has shown promising effects in chronic pain models.

CONFLICT OF INTEREST

No conflicts of interest to declare.

REFERENCES

Ai, N., Wood, R. D., & Welsh, W. J. (2015). Identification of nitazoxanide as a group I metabotropic glutamate receptor negative modulator for the treatment of neuropathic pain: An in silico drug repositioning study. *Pharmaceutical Research*, *32*(8), 2798–2807.

Akgün, E., Javed, M. I., Lunzer, M. M., Smeester, B. A., Beitz, A. J., & Portoghese, P. S. (2013). Ligands that interact with putative MOR-mGluR5 heteromer in mice with inflammatory pain produce potent antinociception. *Proceedings of the National Academy of Sciences of the United States of America*, *110*, 11595–11599.

Alagarsamy, S., Sorensen, S. D., & Conn, P. J. (2001). Coordinate regulation of metabotropic glutamate receptors. *Current Opinion in Neurobiology*, *11*(3), 357–362.

Anwyl, R. (1999). Metabotropic glutamate receptors: Electrophysiological properties and role in plasticity. *Brain Research Reviews*, *29*(1), 83–120.

Apkarian, A. V., Sosa, Y., Krauss, B. R., Thomas, P. S., Fredrickson, B. E., Levy, R. E., et al. (2004). Chronic pain patients are impaired on an emotional decision-making task. *Pain*, *108*(1–2), 129–136.

Azkue, J. J., Murga, M., Fernández-Capetillo, O., Mateos, J. M., Elezgarai, I., Benítez, R., et al. (2001). Immunoreactivity for the group III metabotropic glutamate receptor subtype mGluR4a in the superficial laminae of the rat spinal dorsal horn. *The Journal of Comparative Neurology*, *430*(4), 448–457.

Baron, R., & Binder, A. (2004). How neuropathic is sciatica? The mixed pain concept. *Orthopade*, *33*(5), 568–575.

Beqollari, D., & Kammermeier, P. J. (2008). The mGlu(4) receptor allosteric modulator N-phenyl-7-(hydroxyimino)cyclopropa[b]chromen-1a-carboxamide acts as a direct agonist at mGlu(6) receptors. *European Journal of Pharmacology*, *589*(1–3), 49–52.

Bernabucci, M., Notartomaso, S., Zappulla, C., Fazio, F., Cannella, M., Motolese, M., et al. (2012). N-Acetyl-cysteine causes analgesia by reinforcing the endogenous activation of type-2 metabotropic glutamate receptors. *Molecular Pain*, *8*, 77.

Bhave, G., Karim, F., Carlton, S. M., & Gereau, R. W., IV. (2001). Peripheral group I metabotropic glutamate receptors modulate nociception in mice. *Nature Neuroscience*, *4*(4), 417–423.

Bond, A., Monn, J. A., & Lodge, D. (1997). A novel orally active group 2 metabotropic glutamate receptor agonist: LY354740. *Neuroreport*, *8*(6), 1463–1466.

Bordi, F., & Quartaroli, M. (2000). Modulation of nociceptive transmission by NMDA/glycine site receptor in the ventroposterolateral nucleus of the thalamus. *Pain*, *84*(2–3), 213–224.

Boyce, S., Wyatt, A., Webb, J. K., O'Donnell, R., Mason, G., Rigby, M., et al. (1999). Selective NMDA NR2B antagonists induce antinociception without motor dysfunction: Correlation with restricted localisation of NR2B subunit in dorsal horn. *Neuropharmacology*, *38*(5), 611–623.

Boye Larsen, D., Ingemann Kristensen, G., Panchalingam, V., Laursen, J. C., Nørgaard Poulsen, J., Skallerup Andersen, M., et al. (2014). Investigating the expression of metabotropic glutamate receptors in trigeminal ganglion neurons and satellite glial cells: Implications for craniofacial pain. *Journal of Receptor and Signal Transduction Research*, *34*(4), 261–269.

Brabet, I., Parmentier, M. L., DeColle, C., Bockaert, J., Acher, F., & Pin, J. P. (1998). Comparative effect of L-CCG-I, DCG-IV and gamma-carboxy-L-glutamate on all cloned metabotropic glutamate receptor subtypes. *Neuropharmacology*, *37*(8), 1043–1051.

Byrnes, K. R., Stoica, B., Loane, D. J., Riccio, A., Davis, M. I., & Faden, A. I. (2009). Metabotropic glutamate receptor 5 activation inhibits microglial associated inflammation and neurotoxicity. *Glia*, *57*(5), 550–560.

Cabello, N., Gandía, J., Bertarelli, D. C., Watanabe, M., Lluís, C., Franco, R., et al. (2009). Metabotropic glutamate type 5, dopamine D2 and adenosine A2a receptors form higher-order oligomers in living cells. *Journal of Neurochemistry*, *109*(5), 1497–1507.

Carlton, S. M., Du, J., & Zhou, S. (2009). Group II metabotropic glutamate receptor activation on peripheral nociceptors modulates TRPV1 function. *Brain Research*, *1248*, 86–95.

Carlton, S. M., Zhou, S., Govea, R., & Du, J. (2011). Group II/III metabotropic glutamate receptors exert endogenous activity-dependent modulation of TRPV1 receptors on peripheral nociceptors. *The Journal of Neuroscience*, *31*(36), 12727–12737.

Chen, S. R., & Pan, H. L. (2005). Distinct roles of group III metabotropic glutamate receptors in control of nociception and dorsal horn neurons in normal and nerve-injured Rats. *The Journal of Pharmacology and Experimental Therapeutics*, *312*(1), 120–126.

Chiechio, S., Caricasole, A., Barletta, E., Storto, M., Catania, M. V., Copani, A., et al. (2002). L-Acetylcarnitine induces analgesia by selectively up-regulating mGlu2 metabotropic glutamate receptors. *Molecular Pharmacology*, *61*(5), 989–996.

Chiechio, S., Copani, A., De Petris, L., Morales, M. E., Nicoletti, F., & Gereau, R. W., IV. (2006a). Transcriptional regulation of metabotropic glutamate receptor 2/3 expression by the NF-kappaB pathway in primary dorsal root ganglia neurons: A possible mechanism for the analgesic effect of L-acetylcarnitine. *Molecular Pain*, *9*, 2–20.

Chiechio, S., Copani, A., Gereau, R. W., IV, & Nicoletti, F. (2007). Acetyl-L-carnitine in neuropathic pain: Experimental data. *CNS Drugs*, *21*(1), 31–38.

Chiechio, S., Copani, A., Nicoletti, F., & Gereau, R. W., IV (2006b). L-acetylcarnitine: A proposed therapeutic agent for painful peripheral neuropathies. *Current Neuropharmacology*, *4*(3), 233–237.

Chiechio, S., Copani, A., Zammataro, M., Battaglia, G., Gereau, R. W., IV, & Nicoletti, F. (2010). Transcriptional regulation of type-2 metabotropic glutamate receptors: An epigenetic path to novel treatments for chronic pain. *Trends in Pharmacological Sciences*, *31*(4), 153–160.

Chiechio, S., & Nicoletti, F. (2012). Metabotropic glutamate receptors and the control of chronic pain. *Current Opinion in Pharmacology*, *12*(1), 28–34.

Chiechio, S., Zammataro, M., Morales, M. E., Busceti, C. L., Drago, F., Gereau, R. W., IV, et al. (2009). Epigenetic modulation of mGlu2 receptors by histone deacetylase inhibitors in the treatment of inflammatory pain. *Molecular Pharmacology*, *75*(5), 1014–1020.

Chizh, B. A. (2007). Low dose ketamine: A therapeutic and research tool to explore N-methyl-D-aspartate (NMDA) receptor-mediated plasticity in pain pathways. *Journal of Psychopharmacology*, *21*(3), 259–271.

Cho, G. H., Kim, T., Son, W. S., Seo, S. H., Min, S. J., Cho, Y. S., et al. (2015). Synthesis and biological evaluation of aryl isoxazole derivatives as metabotropic glutamate receptor 1 antagonists: A potential treatment for neuropathic pain. *Bioorganic & Medicinal Chemistry Letters*, *25*(6), 1324–1328.

Chung, M. K., Lee, J., Joseph, J., Saloman, J., & Ro, J. Y. (2015). Peripheral group I metabotropic glutamate receptor activation leads to muscle mechanical hyperalgesia through TRPV1 phosphorylation in the rat. *The Journal of Pain*, *16*(1), 67–76.

Conn, P. J., & Pin, J. P. (1997). Pharmacology and functions of metabotropic glutamate receptors. *Annual Review of Pharmacology and Toxicology*, *37*, 205–237.

Cosford, N. D., Tehrani, L., Roppe, J., Schweiger, E., Smith, N. D., et al. (2003). 3-[(2-Methyl-1,3-thiazol-4-yl)ethynyl]-pyridine: A potent and highly selective metabotropic glutamate subtype 5 receptor antagonist with anxiolytic activity. *Journal of Medicinal Chemistry*, *46*(2), 204–206.

Costigan, M., Scholz, J., & Woolf, C. J. (2009). Neuropathic pain: A maladaptive response of the nervous system to damage. *The Annual Review of Neuroscience*, *32*, 1–32.

Crock, L. W., Kolber, B. J., Morgan, C. D., Sadler, K. E., Vogt, S. K., Bruchas, M. R., et al. (2012). Central amygdala metabotropic glutamate receptor 5 in the modulation of visceral pain. *The Journal of Neuroscience*, *32*(41), 14217–14226.

Crock, L. W., Stemler, K. M., Song, D. G., Abbosh, P., Vogt, S. K., Qiu, C. S., et al. (2012). Metabotropic glutamate receptor 5 (mGluR5) regulates bladder nociception. *Molecular Pain*, *26*(8), 20.

de Novellis, V., Mariani, L., Palazzo, E., Vita, D., Marabese, I., Scafuro, M., et al. (2005). Periaqueductal grey CB1 cannabinoid and metabotropic glutamate subtype 5 receptors modulate changes in rostral ventromedial medulla neuronal activities induced by subcutaneous formalin in the rat. *Neuroscience*, *134*(1), 269–281.

Doherty, A. J., Palmer, M. J., Henley, J. M., Collingridge, G. L., & Jane, D. E. (1997). (RS)-2-chloro-5-hydroxyphenylglycine (CHPG) activates mGlu5, but no mGlu1, receptors expressed in CHO cells and potentiates NMDA responses in the hippocampus. *Neuropharmacology*, *36*(2), 265–267.

Dolan, S., Gunn, M. D., Crossan, C., & Nolan, A. M. (2011). Activation of metabotropic glutamate receptor 7 in spinal cord inhibits pain and hyperalgesia in a novel formalin model in sheep. *Behavioural Pharmacology*, *22*(5–6), 582–588.

Dolan, S., Kelly, J. G., Monteiro, A. M., & Nolan, A. M. (2003). Up-regulation of metabotropic glutamate receptor subtypes 3 and 5 in spinal cord in a clinical model of persistent inflammation and hyperalgesia. *Pain*, *106*(3), 501–512.

Doumazane, E., Scholler, P., Zwier, J. M., Trinquet, E., Rondard, P., & Pin, J. P. (2011). A new approach to analyze cell surface protein complexes reveals specific heterodimeric metabotropic glutamate receptors. *FASEB Journal*, *25*(1), 66–77.

Drew, G. M., & Vaughan, C. W. (2004). Multiple metabotropic glutamate receptor subtypes modulate GABAergic neurotransmission in rat periaqueductal grey neurons in vitro. *Neuropharmacology*, *46*(7), 927–934.

Duvoisin, R. M., Pfankuch, T., Wilson, J. M., Grabell, J., Chhajlani, V., Brown, D. G., et al. (2010). Acute pharmacological modulation of mGluR8 reduces measures of anxiety. *Behavioural Brain Research*, *212*(2), 168–173.

Eaton, S. A., Birse, E. F., Wharton, B., Sunter, D. C., Udvarhelyi, P. M., Watkins, J. C., et al. (1993). Mediation of thalamic sensory responses in vivo by ACPD-activated excitatory amino acid receptors. *The European Journal of Neuroscience*, *5*(2), 186–189.

Eaton, S. A., & Salt, T. E. (1990). Thalamic NMDA receptors and nociceptive sensory synaptic transmission. *Neuroscience Letters*, *110*(3), 297–302.

Ferraguti, F., & Shigemoto, R. (2006). Metabotropic glutamate receptors. *Cell and Tissue Research*, *326*(2), 483–504.

Ferré, S., Karcz-Kubicha, M., Hope, B. T., Popoli, P., Burgueño, J., Gutiérrez, M. A., et al. (2002). Synergistic interaction between adenosine A2A and glutamate mGlu5 receptors: Implications for striatal neuronal function. *Proceedings of the National Academy of Sciences of the United States of America*, *99*(18), 11940–11945.

Fisher, K., & Coderre, T. J. (1996). The contribution of metabotropic glutamate receptors (mGluRs) to formalin-induced Nociception. *Pain*, *68*, 255–263.

Fisher, K., Lefebvre, C., & Coderre, T. J. (2002). Antinociceptive effects following intrathecal pretreatment with selective metabotropic glutamate receptor compounds in a rat model of neuropathic pain. *Pharmacology, Biochemistry, and Behavior*, *73*(2), 411–418.

Fundytus, M. E., Fisher, K., Dray, A., Henry, J. L., & Coderre, T. J. (1998). In vivo antinociceptive activity of anti-rat mGluR1 and mGluR5 antibodies in rats. *Neuroreport*, *9*(4), 731–735.

Gama, L., Wilt, S. G., & Breitwieser, G. E. (2001). Heterodimerization of calcium sensing receptors with metabotropic glutamate receptors in neurons. *The Journal of Biological Chemistry*, *276*(42), 39053–39059.

Gasparini, F., Lingenhöhl, K., Stoehr, N., Flor, P. J., Heinrich, M., Vranesic, I., et al. (1999). 2-Methyl-6-(phenylethynyl)-pyridine (MPEP), a potent, selective and systemically active mGlu5 receptor antagonist. *Neuropharmacology*, *38*(10), 1493–1503.

Gee, C. E., Peterlik, D., Neuhäuser, C., Bouhelal, R., Kaupmann, K., Laue, G., et al. (2014). Blocking metabotropic glutamate receptor subtype 7 (mGlu7) via the Venus flytrap domain (VFTD) inhibits amygdala plasticity, stress, and anxiety-related behavior. *The Journal of Biological Chemistry*, *289*(16), 10975–10987.

Gerber, G., Zhong, J., Youn, D., & Randic, M. (2000). Group II and group III metabotropic glutamate receptor agonists depress synaptic transmission in the rat spinal cord dorsal horn. *Neuroscience*, *100*, 393–406.

González-Maeso, J., Ang, R. L., Yuen, T., Chan, P., Weisstaub, N. V., López-Giménez, J. F., et al. (2008). Identification of a serotonin/glutamate receptor complex implicated in psychosis. *Nature*, *452*(7183), 93–97.

Goudet, C., Chapuy, E., Alloui, A., Acher, F., Pin, J. P., & Eschalier, A. (2008). Group III metabotropic glutamate receptors inhibit hyperalgesia in animal models of inflammation and neuropathic pain. *Pain*, *137*(1), 112–124.

Goudet, C., Magnagh, V., Landry, M., Nagy, F., Gereau, R. W., IV, & Pin, J. P. (2009). Metabotropic receptors for glutamate and GABA in pain. *Brain Research Reviews*, *60*(1), 43–56.

Goudet, C., Vilar, B., Courtiol, T., Deltheil, T., Bessiron, T., Brabet, I., et al. (2012). A novel selective metabotropic glutamate receptor 4 agonist reveals new possibilities for developing subtype selective ligands with therapeutic potential. *FASEB Journal*, *26*(4), 1682–1693.

Govea, R. M., Zhou, S., & Carlton, S. M. (2012). Group III metabotropic glutamate receptors and transient receptor potential vanilloid 1 co-localize and interact on nociceptors. *Neuroscience*, *217*, 130–139.

Gregory, K. J., Noetzel, M. J., & Niswender, C. M. (2013). Pharmacology of metabotropic glutamate receptor allosteric modulators: Structural basis and therapeutic potential for CNS disorders. *Progress in Molecular Biology and Translational Science*, *115*, 61–121.

Hao, J., Dehlinger, V., Fivush, A. M., Rudyk, H. C., Britton, T. C., Hollinshead, S. P., et al. (2013). Discovery of (1R,2R)-N-(4-(6-isopropylpyridine-2-yl)-3-(2-methyl-2H-indazol-5-yl)isothiazol-5-yl)-2-methylcyclopropanecarboxamide, a potent and orally efficacious mGlu5 receptor negative allosteric modulator. *Bioorganic & Medicinal Chemistry Letters*, *23*(5), 1249–1252.

Hollmann, M., & Heinemann, S. (1994). Cloned glutamate receptors. *Annual Review of Neuroscience*, *17*, 31–108.

Hu, H. J., Alter, B. J., Carrasquillo, Y., Qiu, C. S., & Gereau, R. W., IV. (2007). Metabotropic glutamate receptor 5 modulates nociceptive plasticity via extracellular signal-regulated kinase-Kv4.2 signaling in spinal cord dorsal horn neurons. *The Journal of Neuroscience*, *27*(48), 13181–13191.

Hu, H. J., Bhave, G., & Gereau, R. W., IV. (2002). Prostaglandin and protein kinase A-dependent modulation of vanilloid receptor function by metabotropic glutamate receptor 5: Potential mechanism for thermal hyperalgesia. *The Journal of Neuroscience*, *22*(17), 7444–7452.

Hu, H. J., & Gereau, R. W., IV. (2011). Metabotropic glutamate receptor 5 regulates excitability and Kv4.2-containing K^+ channels primarily in excitatory neurons of the spinal dorsal horn. *Journal of Neurophysiology*, *105*(6), 3010–3021.

Hu, J., Hauache, O., & Spiegel, A. M. (2000). Human Ca2+ receptor cysteine-rich domain. Analysis of function of mutant and chimeric receptors. *The Journal of Biological Chemistry*, *275*(21), 16382–16389.

Ishida, M., Saitoh, T., Shimamoto, K., Ohfune, Y., & Shinozaki, H. (1993). A novel metabotropic glutamate receptor agonist: Marked depression of monosynaptic excitation in the newborn rat isolated spinal cord. *British Journal of Pharmacology*, *109*(4), 1169–1177.

Jane, D. E., Thomas, N. K., Tse, H. W., & Watkins, J. C. (1996). Potent antagonists at the L-AP4- and (1S,3S)-ACPD-sensitive presynaptic metabotropic glutamate receptors in the neonatal rat spinal cord. *Neuropharmacology*, *35*(8), 1029–1035.

Ji, R. R., Kohno, T., Moore, K. A., & Woolf, C. J. (2003). Central sensitization and LTP: Do pain and memory share similar mechanisms? *Trends in Neurosciences*, *26*(12), 696–705.

Ji, G., & Neugebauer, V. (2011). Pain-related deactivation of medial prefrontal cortical neurons involves mGluR1 and GABA(A) receptors. *Journal of Neurophysiology*, *106*(5), 2642–2652.

Ji, G., & Neugebauer, V. (2014). CB1 augments mGluR5 function in medial prefrontal cortical neurons to inhibit amygdala hyperactivity in an arthritis pain model. *The European Journal of Neuroscience*, *39*(3), 455–466.

Ji, G., Sun, H., Fu, Y., Li, Z., Pais-Vieira, M., Galhardo, V., et al. (2010). Cognitive impairment in pain through amygdala-driven prefrontal cortical deactivation. *The Journal of Neuroscience*, *30*(15), 5451–5464.

Johnson, B. G., Wright, R. A., Arnold, M. B., Wheeler, W. J., Ornstein, P. L., & Schoepp, D. D. (1999). [3H]-LY341495 as a novel antagonist radioligand for group II metabotropic glutamate (mGlu) receptors: Characterization of binding to membranes of mGlu receptor subtype expressing cells. *Neuropharmacology*, *38*(10), 1519–1529.

Kalivas, P. (2009). The glutamate homeostatic hypothesis of addiction. *Nature Reviews. Neuroscience*, *10*, 561–572.

Karim, F., Wang, C. C., & Gereau, R. W., IV. (2001). Metabotropic glutamate receptor subtypes 1 and 5 are activators of extracellular signal-regulated kinase signaling required for inflammatory pain in mice. *The Journal of Neuroscience*, *21*(11), 3771–3779.

Kim, Y., Kim, J., Kim, S., Ki, Y., Seo, S. H., Tae, J., et al. (2014). Novel thienopyrimidinones as mGluR1 antagonists. *European Journal of Medicinal Chemistry*, *85*, 629–637.

Kingston, A. E., Burnett, J. P., Mayne, N. G., & Lodge, D. (1995). Pharmacological analysis of 4-carboxyphenylglycine derivatives: Comparison of effects on mGluR1 alpha and mGluR5a subtypes. *Neuropharmacology*, *34*(8), 887–894.

Kiritoshi, T., & Neugebauer, V. (2015). Group II mGluRs modulate baseline and arthritis pain-related synaptic transmission in the rat medial prefrontal cortex. *Neuropharmacology*, *95*, 388–394.

Kiritoshi, T., Sun, H., Ren, W., Stauffer, S. R., Lindsley, C. W., Conn, P. J., et al. (2013). Modulation of pyramidal cell output in the medial prefrontal cortex by mGluR5 interacting with CB1. *Neuropharmacology*, *66*, 170–178.

Kniazeff, J., Prézeau, L., Rondard, P., Pin, J. P., & Goudet, C. (2011). Dimers and beyond: The functional puzzles of class C GPCRs. *Pharmacology & Therapeutics*, *130*(1), 9–25.

Knoflach, F., Mutel, V., Jolidon, S., Kew, J. N., Malherbe, P., Vieira, E., et al. (2001). Positive allosteric modulators of metabotropic glutamate 1 receptor: Characterization, mechanism of action, and binding site. *Proceedings of the National Academy of Sciences of the United States of America*, *98*(23), 13402–13407.

Kohara, A., Toya, T., Tamura, S., Watabiki, T., Nagakura, Y., Shitaka, Y., et al. (2005). Radioligand binding properties and pharmacological characterization of 6-amino-N-cyclohexyl-N,3-dimethylthiazolo[3,2-a]benzimidazole-2-carboxamide (YM-298198), a high-affinity, selective, and noncompetitive antagonist of metabotropic glutamate receptor type 1. *The Journal of Pharmacology and Experimental Therapeutics*, *315*(1), 163–169.

Kolber, B. J., Montana, M. C., Carrasquillo, Y., Xu, J., Heinemann, S. F., Muglia, L. J., et al. (2010). Activation of metabotropic glutamate receptor 5 in the amygdala modulates pain-like behavior. *The Journal of Neuroscience*, *30*(24), 8203–8213.

Kolhekar, R., Murphy, S., & Gebhart, G. F. (1997). Thalamic NMDA receptors modulate inflammation-produced hyperalgesia in the rat. *Pain*, *71*(1), 31–40.

Latremoliere, A., & Woolf, C. J. (2009). Central sensitization: A generator of pain hypersensitivity by central neural plasticity. *The Journal of Pain*, *10*(9), 895–926.

Lavreysen, H., Janssen, C., Bischoff, F., Langlois, X., Leysen, J. E., & Lesage, A. S. (2003). [3H]R214127: A novel high-affinity radioligand for the mGlu1 receptor reveals a common binding site shared by multiple allosteric antagonists. *Molecular Pharmacology*, *63*, 1082–1093.

Lavreysen, H., Wouters, R., Bischoff, F., NóbregaPereira, S., Langlois, X., Blokland, S., et al. (2004). JNJ16259685, a highly potent, selective and systemically active mGlu1 receptor antagonist. *Neuropharmacology*, *47*(7), 961–972.

Lax, N. C., George, D. C., Ignatz, C., & Kolber, B. J. (2014). The mGluR5 antagonist fenobam induces analgesic conditioned place preference in mice with spared nerve injury. *PLoS One*, *9*(7), e103524.

Lee, K. S., Park, E. H., Cho, H. Y., Kim, Y. I., & Han, H. C. (2013). Peripheral group II and III metabotropic glutamate receptors in the knee joint attenuate carrageenan-induced nociceptive behavior in rats. *Neuroscience Letters*, *542*, 21–25.

Li, W., & Neugebauer, V. (2006). Differential changes of group II and group III mGluR function in central amygdala neurons in a model of arthritic pain. *Journal of Neurophysiology*, *96*, 1803–1815.

Li, H., Ohishi, H., Kinoshita, A., Shigemoto, R., Nomura, S., & Mizuno, N. (1997). Localization of a metabotropic glutamate receptor, mGluR7, in axon terminals of presumed nociceptive, primary afferent fibers in the superficial layers of the spinal dorsal horn: An electron microscope study in the rat. *Neuroscience Letters*, *223*(3), 153–156.

Lindström, E., Brusberg, M., Hughes, P. A., Martin, C. M., Brierley, S. M., Phillis, B. D., et al. (2008). Involvement of metabotropic glutamate 5 receptor in visceral pain. *Pain*, *137*(2), 295–305.

Litschig, S., Gasparini, F., Rueegg, D., Stoehr, N., Flor, P. J., Vranesic, I., et al. (1999). CPCCOEt, a noncompetitive metabotropic glutamate receptor 1 antagonist, inhibits receptor signaling without affecting glutamate binding. *Molecular Pharmacology*, *55*, 453–461.

Luongo, L., de Novellis, V., Gatta, L., Palazzo, E., Vita, D., Guida, F., et al. (2013). Role of metabotropic glutamate receptor 1 in the basolateral amygdala-driven prefrontal cortical deactivation in inflammatory pain in the rat. *Neuropharmacology*, *66*, 317–329.

Maione, S., Oliva, P., Marabese, I., Palazzo, E., Rossi, F., Berrino, L., et al. (2000). Periaqueductal gray matter metabotropic glutamate receptors modulate formalin-induced nociception. *Pain*, *85*(1–2), 183–189.

Marabese, I., de Novellis, V., Palazzo, E., Scafuro, M. A., Vita, D., Rossi, F., et al. (2007). Effects of (S)-3,4-DCPG, an mGlu8 receptor agonist, on inflammatory and neuropathic pain in mice. *Neuropharmacology*, *52*, 253–262.

Marabese, I., Rossi, F., Palazzo, E., de Novellis, V., Starowicz, K., Cristino, L., et al. (2007). Periaqueductal gray metabotropic glutamate receptor subtype 7 and 8 mediate opposite effects on amino acid release, rostral ventromedial medulla cell activities, and thermal nociception. *Journal of Neurophysiology*, *98*, 43–53.

Masuoka, T., Nakamura, T., Kudo, M., Yoshida, J., Takaoka, Y., Kato, N., et al. (2015). Biphasic modulation by mGlu5 receptors of TRPV1-mediated intracellular calcium elevation in sensory neurons contributes to heat sensitivity. *British Journal of Pharmacology*, *172*(4), 1020–1033.

Metz, A. E., Yau, H. J., Centeno, M. V., Apkarian, A. V., & Martina, M. (2009). Morphological and functional reorganization of rat medial prefrontal cortex in neuropathic pain. *Proceedings of the National Academy of Sciences of the United States of America*, *106*(7), 2423–2428.

Mitsukawa, K., Yamamoto, R., Ofner, S., Nozulak, J., Pescott, O., Lukic, S., et al. (2005). A selective metabotropic glutamate receptor 7 agonist: Activation of receptor signaling via an allosteric site modulates stress parameters in vivo. *Proceedings of the National Academy of Sciences of the United States of America*, *102*, 18712–18717.

Monaghan, D. T., Bridges, R. J., & Cotman, C. W. (1989). The excitatory amino acid receptors: Their classes, pharmacology, and distinct properties in the function of the central nervous system. *Annual Review of Pharmacology and Toxicology*, *29*, 365–402.

Monn, J. A., Valli, M. J., Massey, S. M., Hansen, M. M., Kress, T. J., Wepsiec, J. P., et al. (1999). Synthesis, pharmacological characterization, and molecular modeling of hetero bicyclic amino acids related to (+)-2-aminobicyclo[3.1.0] hexane-2,6-dicarboxylic acid (LY354740): Identification of two new potent, selective, and systemically active agonists for group II metabotropic glutamate receptors. *Journal of Medicinal Chemistry*, *42*(6), 1027–1040.

Montana, M. C., Cavallone, L. F., Stubbert, K. K., Stefanescu, A. D., Kharasch, E. D., & Gereau, R. W., IV. (2009). The metabotropic glutamate receptor subtype 5 antagonist fenobam is analgesic and has improved in vivo selectivity compared with the prototypical antagonist 2-methyl-6-(phenylethynyl)-pyridine. *The Journal of Pharmacology and Experimental Therapeutics*, *330*(3), 834–843.

Montana, M. C., Conrardy, B. A., Cavallone, L. F., Kolber, B. J., Rao, L. K., Greco, S. C., et al. (2011). Metabotropic glutamate receptor 5 antagonism with fenobam: Examination of analgesic tolerance and side effect profile in mice. *Anesthesiology*, *115*(6), 1239–1250.

Montana, M. C., & Gereau, R. W. (2011). Metabotropic glutamate receptors as targets for analgesia: Antagonism, activation, and allosteric modulation. *Current Pharmaceutical Biotechnology*, *12*(10), 1681–1688.

Muto, T., Tsuchiya, D., Morikawa, K., & Jingami, H. (2007). Structures of the extracellular regions of the group II/III metabotropic glutamate receptors. *Proceedings of the National Academy of Sciences of the United States of America*, *104*(10), 3759–3764.

Nakazato, E., Kato, A., & Watanabe, S. (2005). Brain but not spinal NR2B receptor is responsible for the anti-allodynic effect of an NR2B subunit-selective antagonist CP-101,606 in a rat chronic constriction injury model. *Pharmacology*, *73*(1), 8–14.

Nam, M., Kim, T., Kwak, J., Seo, S. H., Ko, M. K., Lim, E. J., et al. (2015). Discovery and biological evaluation of tetrahydrothieno[2,3-c]pyridine derivatives as selective metabotropic glutamate receptor 1 antagonists for the potential treatment of neuropathic pain. *European Journal of Medicinal Chemistry*, *97*, 245–258.

Neugebauer, V. (2015). Amygdala pain mechanisms. *Handbook of Experimental Pharmacology*, *227*, 261–284.

Nicoll, R. A. (2003). Expression mechanisms underlying long-term potentiation: A postsynaptic view. *Philosophical Transactions of the Royal Society of London*, *358*(1432), 721–726.

Niswender, C. M., & Conn, P. J. (2010). Metabotropic glutamate receptors: Physiology, pharmacology, and disease. *Annual Review of Pharmacology and Toxicology*, *50*, 295–322.

Niswender, C. M., Johnson, K. A., Weaver, C. D., Jones, C. K., Xiang, Z., Luo, Q., et al. (2008). Discovery, characterization, and antiparkinsonian effect of novel positive allosteric modulators of metabotropic glutamate receptor 4. *Molecular Pharmacology*, *74*(5), 1345–1358.

Ohashi, H., Maruyama, T., Higashi-Matsumoto, H., Nomoto, T., Nishimura, S., & Takeuchi, Y. (2002). A novel binding assay for metabotropic glutamate receptors using [3H]L-quisqualic acid and recombinant receptors. *Zeitschrift für Naturforschung C*, *57*(3–4), 348–355.

Ohishi, H., Akazawa, C., Shigemoto, R., Nakanishi, S., & Mizuno, N. (1995). Distributions of the mRNAs for L-2-amino-4-phosphonobutyrate-sensitive metabotropic glutamate receptors, mGluR4 and mGluR7, in the rat brain. *The Journal of Comparative Neurology*, *360*(4), 555–570.

Ohishi, H., Nomura, S., Ding, Y. Q., Shigemoto, R., Wada, E., Kinoshita, A., et al. (1995). Presynaptic localization of a metabotropic glutamate receptor, mGluR7, in the primary afferent neurons: An immunohistochemical study in the rat. *Neuroscience Letters*, *202*(1–2), 85–88.

Onofrj, M., Ciccocioppo, F., Varanese, S., di Muzio, A., Calvani, M., Chiechio, S., et al. (2013). Acetyl-L-carnitine: From a biological curiosity to a drug for the peripheral nervous system and beyond. *Expert Review of Neurotherapeutics*, *13*(8), 925–936.

Osikowicz, M., Mika, J., Makuch, W., & Przewlocka, B. (2008). Glutamate receptor ligands attenuate allodynia and hyperalgesia and potentiate morphine effects in a mouse model of neuropathic pain. *Pain*, *139*, 117–126.

Osikowicz, M., Mika, J., & Przewlocka, B. (2013). The glutamatergic system as a target for neuropathic pain relief. *Experimental Physiology*, *98*(2), 372–384.

Pais-Vieira, M., Mendes-Pinto, M. M., Lima, D., & Galhardo, V. (2009). Cognitive impairment of prefrontal-dependent decision-making in rats after the onset of chronic pain. *Neuroscience*, *161*(3), 671–679.

Palazzo, E., Fu, Y., Ji, G., Maione, S., & Neugebauer, V. (2008). Group III mGluR7 and mGluR8 in the amygdala differentially modulate nocifensive and affective pain behaviors. *Neuropharmacology*, *55*, 537–545.

Palazzo, E., Marabese, I., de Novellis, V., Oliva, P., Rossi, F., Berrino, L., et al. (2001). Metabotropic and NMDA glutamate receptors participate in the cannabinoid-induced antinociception. *Neuropharmacology*, *40*(3), 319–326.

Palazzo, E., Marabese, I., Luongo, L., Boccella, S., Bellini, G., Giordano, M. E., et al. (2013). Effects of a metabotropic glutamate receptor subtype 7 negative allosteric modulator in the periaqueductal grey on pain responses and rostral ventromedial medulla cell activity in rat. *Molecular Pain*, *9*, 44.

Palazzo, E., Marabese, I., Soukupova, M., Luongo, L., Boccella, S., Giordano, C., et al. (2011). Metabotropic glutamate receptor subtype 8 in the amygdala modulates thermal threshold, neurotransmitter release, and rostral ventromedial medulla cell activity in inflammatory pain. *The Journal of Neuroscience*, *31*, 4687–4697.

Palazzo, E., Romano, R., Luongo, L., Boccella, S., De Gregorio, D., Giordano, M. E., et al. (2015). MMPIP, an mGluR7-selective negative allosteric modulator, alleviates pain and normalizes affective and cognitive behavior in neuropathic mice. *Pain*, *156*(6), 1060–1073.

Pin, J. P., & Duvoisin, R. (1995). The metabotropic glutamate receptors: Structure and functions. *Neuropharmacology*, *34*(1), 1–26.

Pin, J. P., Galvez, T., & Prézeau, L. (2003). Evolution, structure, and activation mechanism of family 3/C G-protein-coupled receptors. *Pharmacology & Therapeutics*, *98*(3), 325–354.

Porter, R. H., Jaeschke, G., Spooren, W., Ballard, T. M., Büttelmann, B., Kolczewski, S., et al. (2005). Fenobam: A clinically validated nonbenzodiazepine anxiolytic is a potent, selective, and noncompetitive mGlu5 receptor antagonist with inverse agonist activity. *The Journal of Pharmacology and Experimental Therapeutics*, *315*(2), 711–721.

Ren, B. X., Gu, X. P., Zheng, Y. G., Liu, C. L., Wang, D., Sun, Y. E., et al. (2012). Intrathecal injection of metabotropic glutamate receptor subtype 3 and 5 agonist/antagonist attenuates bone cancer pain by inhibition of spinal astrocyte activation in a mouse model. *Anesthesiology*, *116*(1), 122–132.

Rodrigues, R. J., Alfaro, T. M., Rebola, N., Oliveira, C. R., & Cunha, R. A. (2005). Co-localization and functional interaction between adenosine A(2A) and metabotropic group 5 receptors in glutamatergic nerve terminals of the rat striatum. *Journal of Neurochemistry*, *92*(3), 433–441.

Romano, C., Yang, W. L., & O'Malley, K. L. (1996). Metabotropic glutamate receptor 5 is a disulfide-linked dimer. *The Journal of Biological Chemistry*, *271*(45), 28612–28616.

Rossi, F., Marabese, I., De Chiaro, M., Boccella, S., Luongo, L., Guida, F., et al. (2014). Dorsal striatum metabotropic glutamate receptor 8 affects nocifensive responses and rostral ventromedial medulla cell activity in neuropathic pain conditions. *Journal of Neurophysiology*, *111*(11), 2196–2209.

Saab, C. Y., Wang, J., Gu, C., Garner, K. N., & Al-Chaer, E. D. (2006). Microglia: A newly discovered role in visceral hypersensitivity? *Neuron Glia Biology*, *2*(4), 271–277.

Salt, T. E., & Binns, K. E. (2000). Contributions of mGlu1 and mGlu5 receptors to interactions with N-methyl-D-aspartate receptor-mediated responses and nociceptive sensory responses of rat thalamic neurons. *Neuroscience*, *100*(2), 375–380.

Salt, T. E., Jones, H. E., Copeland, C. S., & Sillito, A. M. (2014). Function of mGlu1 receptors in the modulation of nociceptive processing in the thalamus. *Neuropharmacology*, *79*, 405–411.

Salt, T. E., & Turner, J. P. (1998). Reduction of sensory and metabotropic glutamate receptor responses in the thalamus by the novel metabotropic glutamate receptor-1-selective antagonist S-2-methyl-4-carboxy-phenylglycine. *Neuroscience*, *85*(3), 655–658.

Schaffhauser, H., Rowe, B. A., Morales, S., Chavez-Noriega, L. E., Yin, R., Jachec, C., et al. (2003). Pharmacological characterization and identification of amino acids involved in the positive modulation of metabotropic glutamate receptor subtype 2. *Molecular Pharmacology*, *64*, 798–810.

Schiöth, H. B., & Fredriksson, R. (2005). The GRAFS classification system of G-protein coupled receptors in comparative perspective. *General and Comparative Endocrinology*, *142*(1–2), 94–101.

Schoepp, D. D., Jane, D. E., & Monn, J. A. (1999). Pharmacological agents acting at subtypes of metabotropic glutamate receptors. *Neuropharmacology*, *38*(10), 1431–1476.

Schröder, H., Wu, D. F., Seifert, A., Rankovic, M., Schulz, S., Höllt, V., et al. (2009). Allosteric modulation of metabotropic glutamate receptor 5 affects phosphorylation, internalization, and desensitization of the micro-opioid receptor. *Neuropharmacology*, *56*(4), 768–778.

Schweitzer, C., Kratzeisen, C., Adam, G., Lundstrom, K., Malherbe, P., Ohresser, S., et al. (2000). Characterization of [(3)H]-LY354740 binding to rat mGlu2 and mGlu3 receptors expressed in CHO cells using semliki forest virus vectors. *Neuropharmacology*, *39*, 1700–1706.

Sharpe, E. F., Kingston, A. E., Lodge, D., Monn, J. A., & Headley, P. M. (2000). Systemic pre-treatment with a group II mGlu agonist, LY379268, reduces hyperalgesia in vivo. *British Journal of Pharmacology*, *135*, 1255–1262.

Sherman, S. M. (2012). Thalamocortical interactions. *Current Opinion in Neurobiology*, *22*(4), 575–579.
Simmons, R. M., Webster, A. A., Kalra, A. B., & Iyengar, S. (2002). Group II mGluR receptor agonists are effective in persistent and neuropathic pain models in rats. *Pharmacology, Biochemistry, and Behavior*, *73*, 419–427.
Smeester, B. A., Lunzer, M. M., Akgün, E., Beitz, A. J., & Portoghese, P. S. (2014). Targeting putative mu opioid/metabotropic glutamate receptor-5 heteromers produces potent antinociception in a chronic murine bone cancer model. *European Journal of Pharmacology*, *743*, 48–52.
Suzuki, G. T., Kimura, A., Satow, N., Kaneko, J., Fukuda, H., Hikichi, N., et al. (2007). Pharmacological characterization of a new, orally active and potent allosteric metabotropic glutamate receptor 1 antagonist, 4-[1-(2-fluoropyridin-3-yl)-5-methyl-1H-1,2,3-triazol-4-yl]-N-isopropyl-N-methyl-3,6-dihydropyridine-1(2H)-carboxamide (FTIDC). *The Journal of Pharmacology and Experimental Therapeutics*, *321*(3), 1144–1153.
Suzuki, G., Tsukamoto, N., Fushiki, H., Kawagishi, A., Nakamura, M., Kurihara, H., et al. (2007). In vitro pharmacological characterization of novel isoxazolopyridone derivatives as allosteric metabotropic glutamate receptor 7 antagonists. *The Journal of Pharmacology and Experimental Therapeutics*, *323*(1), 147–156.
Szteyn, K., Rowan, M. P., Gomez, R., Du, J., Carlton, S. M., & Jeske, N. A. (2015). A-Kinase anchoring protein 79/150 coordinates metabotropic glutamate receptor sensitization of peripheral sensory neurons. *Pain*, *156*, 2364–2372.
Thomas, N. K., Wright, R. A., Howson, P. A., Kingston, A. E., Schoepp, D. D., & Jane, D. E. (2001). (S)-3,4-DCPG, a potent and selective mGlu8a receptor agonist, activates metabotropic glutamate receptors on primary afferent terminals in the neonatal rat spinal cord. *Neuropharmacology*, *40*(3), 311–318.
Truini, A., Piroso, S., Pasquale, E., Notartomaso, S., Di Stefano, G., Lattanzi, R., et al. (2015). N-acetyl-cysteine, a drug that enhances the endogenous activation of group-II metabotropic glutamate receptors, inhibits nociceptive transmission in humans. *Molecular Pain*, *11*, 14.
Vardi, N., Duvoisin, R., Wu, G., & Sterling, P. (2000). Localization of mGluR6 to dendrites of ON bipolar cells in primate retina. *The Journal of Comparative Neurology*, *423*(3), 402–412.
Varney, M. A., Cosford, N. D., Jachec, C., Rao, S. P., Sacaan, A., Lin, F. F., et al. (1999). SIB-1757 and SIB-1893: Selective, noncompetitive antagonists of metabotropic glutamate receptor type 5. *The Journal of Pharmacology and Experimental Therapeutics*, *290*(1), 170–181.
Varney, M. A., & Gereau, R. W., IV (2002). Metabotropic glutamate receptor involvement in models of acute and persistent pain: Prospects for the development of novel analgesics. *Current Drug Targets. CNS and Neurological Disorders*, *1*(3), 283–296.
Vilar, B., Busserolles, J., Ling, B., Laffray, S., Ulmann, L., Malhaire, F., et al. (2013). Alleviating pain hypersensitivity through activation of type 4 metabotropic glutamate receptor. *The Journal of Neuroscience*, *33*(48), 18951–18965.
Wang, H., Jiang, W., Yang, R., & Li, Y. (2011). Spinal metabotropic glutamate receptor 4 is involved in neuropathic pain. *Neuroreport*, *22*(5), 244–248.
Watkins, J. C., Krogsgaard-Larsen, P., & Honoré, T. (1990). Structure-activity relationships in the development of excitatory amino acid receptor agonists and competitive antagonists. *Trends in Pharmacological Sciences*, *11*(1), 25–33.
Wei, F., Wang, G. D., Kerchner, G. A., Kim, S. J., Xu, H. M., Chen, Z. F., et al. (2001). Genetic enhancement of inflammatory pain by forebrain NR2B overexpression. *Nature Neuroscience*, *4*(2), 164–169.
Weisshaar, C. L., Dong, L., Bowman, A. S., Perez, F. M., Guarino, B. B., Sweitzer, S. M., et al. (2010). Metabotropic glutamate receptor-5 and protein kinase C-epsilon increase in

dorsal root ganglion neurons and spinal glial activation in an adolescent rat model of painful neck injury. *Journal of Neurotrauma, 27*(12), 2261–2271.

Wellendorph, P., & Bräuner-Osborne, H. (2009). Molecular basis for amino acid sensing by family C G-protein-coupled receptors. *British Journal of Pharmacology, 156*(6), 869–884.

Woolf, C. J. (1983). Evidence for a central component of post-injury pain hypersensitivity. *Nature, 306*(5944), 686–688.

Woolf, C. J., & Thompson, S. W. (1991). The induction and maintenance of central sensitization is dependent on N-methyl-D-aspartic acid receptor activation; implications for the treatment of post-injury pain hypersensitivity states. *Pain, 44*(3), 293–299.

Wright, R. A., Arnold, M. B., Wheeler, W. J., Ornstein, P. L., & Schoepp, D. D. (2000). Binding of [3H](2S,1'S,2'S)-2-(9-xanthylmethyl)-2-(2'-carboxycyclopropyl) glycine ([3H]LY341495) to cell membranes expressing recombinant human group III metabotropic glutamate receptor subtypes. *Naunyn-Schmiedeberg's Archives of Pharmacology, 362*(6), 546–554.

Yang, D., & Gereau, R. W., IV. (2002). Peripheral group II metabotropic glutamate receptors (mGluR2/3) regulate prostaglandin E2-mediated sensitization of capsaicin responses and thermal nociception. *The Journal of Neuroscience, 22*, 6388–6393.

Yang, D., & Gereau, R. W., IV. (2004). Group II metabotropic glutamate receptors inhibit cAMP-dependent protein kinase-mediated enhancement of tetrodotoxin-resistant sodium currents in mouse dorsal root ganglion neurons. *Neuroscience Letters, 357*, 159–162.

Yin, S., & Niswender, C. M. (2014). Progress toward advanced understanding of metabotropic glutamate receptors: Structure, signaling and therapeutic indications. *Cellular Signalling, 26*(10), 2284–2297.

Yin, S., Noetzel, M. J., Johnson, K. A., Zamorano, R., Jalan-Sakrikar, N., Gregory, K. J., et al. (2014). Selective actions of novel allosteric modulators reveal functional heteromers of metabotropic glutamate receptors in the CNS. *The Journal of Neuroscience, 34*(1), 79–94.

Zammataro, M., Chiechio, S., Montana, M. C., Traficante, A., Copani, A., & Nicoletti, F. (2011). mGlu2 metabotropic glutamate receptors restrain inflammatory pain and mediate the analgesic activity of dual mGlu2/mGlu3 receptor agonists. *Molecular Pain, 7*, 6.

Zammataro, M., Sortino, M. A., Parenti, C., Gereau, R. W., IV, & Chiechio, S. (2014). HDAC and HAT inhibitors differently affect analgesia mediated by group II metabotropic glutamate receptors. *Molecular Pain, 18*(10), 68.

Zhang, H. M., Chen, S. R., & Pan, H. L. (2009). Effects of activation of group III metabotropic glutamate receptors on spinal synaptic transmission in a rat model of neuropathic pain. *Neuroscience, 158*(2), 875–884.

CHAPTER FOUR

Purinergic Mechanisms and Pain

Geoffrey Burnstock[1]
Autonomic Neuroscience Centre, Royal Free and University College Medical School, London, United Kingdom
Department of Pharmacology and Therapeutics, The University of Melbourne, Melbourne, Australia
[1]Corresponding author: e-mail address: g.burnstock@ucl.ac.uk

Contents

Abstract

There is a brief introductory summary of purinergic signaling involving ATP storage, release, and ectoenzymatic breakdown, and the current classification of receptor subtypes for purines and pyrimidines. The review then describes purinergic mechanosensory transduction involved in visceral, cutaneous, and musculoskeletal nociception and on the roles played by receptor subtypes in neuropathic and inflammatory pain. Multiple purinoceptor subtypes are involved in pain pathways both as an initiator and modulator. Activation of homomeric P2X3 receptors contributes to acute nociception and activation of heteromeric P2X2/3 receptors appears to modulate

Advances in Pharmacology, Volume 75
ISSN 1054-3589
http://dx.doi.org/10.1016/bs.apha.2015.09.001

longer-lasting nociceptive sensitivity associated with nerve injury or chronic inflammation. In neuropathic pain activation of P2X4, P2X7, and $P2Y_{12}$ receptors on microglia may serve to maintain nociceptive sensitivity through complex neural–glial cell interactions and antagonists to these receptors reduce neuropathic pain. Potential therapeutic approaches involving purinergic mechanisms will be discussed.

ABBREVIATIONS

5-HT 5-hydroxytryptamine
ADP adenosine 5′-diphosphate
AK adenosine kinase
ATP adenosine 5′-triphosphate
BDNF brain-derived neurotrophic factor
CFA complete Freund's adjuvant
CGRP calcitonin gene-related peptide
$cPLA_2$ cytosolic phospholipase A_2
DRG dorsal root ganglia
E-NPP ecto-nucleotide pyrophosphatase/phosphodiesterases
E-NTPDases ecto-nucleoside triphosphate diphosphohydrolases
IB_4 isolectin B_4
IBS irritable bowel syndrome
IL interleukin
LPS lipopolysaccharide
MAPK mitogen-activated protein kinase
NEBs neuroepithelial bodies
NGF nerve growth factor
p38 phospho38
PPADS pyridoxalphosphate-6-azophenyl-2′,4′-disulfonic acid
SMARs subepithelial receptor-like endings associated with smooth muscle
SP substance P
TM transmembrane
TNF-α tumour necrosis factor-α
TNP-ATP 2′,3′-O-(2,4,6-trinitrophenyl)-ATP
TRPV1 transient receptor potential vanilloid 1
UTP uridine 5′-triphosphate
α,β-meATP α,β-methylene ATP

1. INTRODUCTION

The purinergic signaling hypothesis was presented in 1972, namely that adenosine 5′-triphosphate (ATP) is an extracellular signaling molecule (Burnstock, 1972). ATP was shown to be a transmitter in nonadrenergic, noncholinergic nerves supplying the gut (Burnstock, Campbell, Satchell, & Smythe, 1970), and bladder (Burnstock, Dumsday, & Smythe,

1972). Later, ATP was recognized as a cotransmitter in nerves in both peripheral and central nervous systems (Burnstock, 2007a). Receptors for purines and pyrimidines were shown to be widely expressed on non-neuronal as well as nerve cells (see Burnstock & Knight, 2004).

Until recently, apart from vesicular release from nerves (e.g., Pankratov, Lalo, Verkhratsky, & North, 2006), it was assumed that the source of extracellular ATP acting on purinoceptors was damaged or dying cells. However, it is now recognized that ATP release from healthy cells is a physiological mechanism (see Bodin & Burnstock, 2001; Dubyak, 2006). ATP is released from most cell types during mechanical deformation in response to shear stress, stretch, or osmotic swelling, as well as to hypoxia and various agents. Exocytotic vesicular release of ATP from nerves and from endothelial cells (Burnstock, 1999), urothelial cells (Knight, Bodin, De Groat, & Burnstock, 2002), osteoblasts (Romanello et al., 2005), fibroblasts (Boudreault & Grygorczyk, 2004), and astrocytes (Montana, Malarkey, Verderio, Matteoli, & Parpura, 2006) is one of the ATP transport mechanisms. In addition, there is evidence for ATP transport via connexin or pannexin hemichannels, ATP-binding cassette transporters, plasmalemmal voltage-dependent anion channels, and P2X7 receptors (Dubyak, 2006; Lazarowski, 2012; Scemes, Suadicani, Dahl, & Spray, 2007). ATP release from endothelial cells is increased during acute inflammation (Bodin & Burnstock, 1998). While adenosine is largely produced by ectoenzymatic breakdown of ATP, there may be subpopulations of neurons and/or glial cells that release adenosine directly (Wall & Dale, 2007). Probes for real-time measurement of ATP and adenosine release in biological tissues have been described (Llaudet, Hatz, Droniou, & Dale, 2005; Nakamura et al., 2006).

After release, nucleotides undergo rapid enzymatic degradation (Yegutkin, 2014; Zimmermann, 2001). Ecto-nucleotidase families include the ecto-nucleoside triphosphate diphosphohydrolases (E-NTPDases, CD39), ecto-nucleotide pyrophosphatase/phosphodiesterases (E-NPP), alkaline phosphatases, and ecto-5′-nucleotidase (CD73). E-NTPDases and E-NPPs hydrolyze ATP and adenosine 5′-diphosphate (ADP) to adenosine monophosphate that is further hydrolyzed by CD73 to adenosine.

Two families of purinoceptors called P1 and P2 (for adenosine and ATP/ADP, respectively) were recognized in 1978 (Burnstock, 1978). In 1985 a proposal suggesting a pharmacological basis for distinguishing two types of P2 receptor (P2X and P2Y) was made (Burnstock & Kennedy, 1985). On the basis of studies of transduction mechanisms and the cloning of nucleotide receptors, it was proposed that purinoceptors should belong to two major families: a P2X family of ligand-gated ion channel receptors and a P2Y family of G protein-coupled receptors (Abbracchio & Burnstock, 1994). Currently, seven P2X subunits (P2X1–7) and eight P2Y receptor subtypes ($P2Y_1$, $P2Y_2$, $P2Y_4$, $P2Y_6$, $P2Y_{11}$, $P2Y_{12}$, $P2Y_{13}$, and $P2Y_{14}$) are recognized, including receptors that are sensitive to pyrimidines as well as purines (Burnstock, 2007b; Ralevic & Burnstock, 1998). Four subtypes of P1 receptors were cloned, namely, A_1, A_{2A}, A_{2B}, and A_3 (see Fredholm, IJzerman, Jacobson, Klotz, & Linden, 2001). Selective agonists and antagonists are available for the P1 receptor subtypes (Jacobson & Gao, 2006). P2X1–7 receptor subunits have been cloned and characterized, with intracellular NH_2- and COOH-termini and two transmembrane (TM)-spanning regions, one involved with channel gating and the other lining the ion pore (Chen et al., 1995; Egan, Samways, & Li, 2006; Lewis et al., 1995; North, 2002). P2X receptors involve three subunits that form a stretched trimer (Nicke et al., 1998). P2X receptor subunits can combine to form either homomultimers or heteromultimers (Burnstock, 2007b; North, 2002; Volonté, Amadio, D'Ambrosi, Colpi, & Burnstock, 2006). Heteromultimers have been established for P2X2/3, P2X4/6, P2X1/5, and P2X2/6 receptors. P2X7 receptors possess small cation channels, but on prolonged exposure to high concentrations of agonist, large channels (pores) are activated that allow the passage of larger molecular weight molecules (Garcia-Marcos, Pochet, Marino, & Dehaye, 2006). P2X7 receptors are localized on immune cells and glia. They mediate proinflammatory cytokine release, cell proliferation, and apoptosis. The metabotropic P2Y receptors have a subunit topology of an extracellular NH_2-terminus and intracellular COOH-terminus and seven TM-spanning regions (Abbracchio et al., 2006). $P2Y_1$, $P2Y_{12}$, and $P2Y_{13}$ receptors are activated principally by nucleoside diphosphates, while $P2Y_2$, $P2Y_4$, and $P2Y_6$ receptors are activated by both purine and pyrimidine nucleotides. P2Y receptor subtypes can form heterodimeric complexes (Ecke et al., 2008). Adenosine A_1 receptors can form a heteromeric complex with $P2Y_1$ receptors (Fischer & Krügel, 2007), while dopamine D_1 and adenosine A_1 receptors have been shown to form functionally interactive heteromeric complexes. Selective agonists and antagonists for most of the P2Y receptor subtypes are already available (Abbracchio et al., 2006).

There were early reports that pain was produced by injection of ATP into human skin blisters (Bleehen & Keele, 1977; Collier, James, & Schneider, 1966). Claims were made for ATP involvement in migraine (Burnstock, 1981) and for involvement in pain pathways in the spinal cord (Jahr & Jessell, 1983; Salter & Henry, 1985). P2X3 ionotropic ion channel purinergic receptors were cloned in 1995 (Chen et al., 1995) and shown to be localized predominantly on small nociceptive sensory neurons in dorsal root ganglia (DRG) together with P2X2/3 heteromultimer receptors (Bradbury, Burnstock, & McMahon, 1998; Burnstock, 2007a, 2009a). Burnstock (1996) put forward a unifying purinergic hypothesis for the initiation of pain, proposing that ATP released as a cotransmitter with noradrenaline, and neuropeptide Y from sympathetic nerve terminal varicosities might be involved in sympathetic pain (causalgia and reflex sympathetic dystrophy). Further, it was suggested that ATP released from vascular endothelial cells of microvessels during reactive hyperemia is associated with pain in migraine, angina, and ischemia; and that high levels of ATP are released from tumor cells, damaged during abrasive activity to reach P2X3 receptors on nociceptive sensory nerves. The involvement of purinergic signaling in pain has been reinforced by an increasing number of papers. Nociceptive fibers expressing P2X3 receptors were shown to arise largely from the population of small neurons in the DRG that labeled with the isolectin B_4 (IB_4) (Bradbury et al., 1998; Vulchanova et al., 2001). Decreased sensitivity to noxious stimuli associated with the loss of IB_4-binding neurons expressing P2X3 receptors indicated that these sensory neurons are essential for the signaling of acute pain (Vulchanova et al., 1996). The central projections of these primary afferent neurons are in inner lamina II of the dorsal horn where there are peripheral projections to skin, tooth pulp, tongue, and subepithelial regions of visceral organs (see Fig. 1; Burnstock & Wood, 1996). P2X3 and P2X2/3 receptors on sensory neurons are the predominant P2 receptor subtypes involved in the initiation of nociception. However, P2Y receptors are also present (Nakayama, Yamashita, Konishi, Kazama, & Kokubun, 2004; Ruan & Burnstock, 2003), which are involved in modulation of pain transmission (Gerevich et al., 2004; Malin & Molliver, 2010). P2Y receptors potentiate pain induced by chemical or physical stimuli via capsaicin-sensitive, transient receptor potential vanilloid 1 (TRPV1) channels (Lakshmi & Joshi, 2005). It was proposed that the functional interaction between $P2Y_2$ receptors and TRPV1 channels of nociceptors could underlie ATP-induced inflammatory pain. In mice-lacking TRPV1 receptors, ATP-induced hyperalgesia was abolished. The involvement of adenosine has also been proposed (Burnstock & Sawynok, 2010; Sawynok & Liu, 2003). Reviews concerned with different aspects of purinergic signaling and pain are available (Bele & Fabbretti, 2015; Burnstock, 2001b, 2006, 2009c, 2012; Burnstock & Sawynok, 2010; Donnelly-Roberts, McGaraughty, Shieh, Honore, & Jarvis, 2008; Hanani, 2012; Jarvis, 2010; Krames, 2014; Magni & Ceruti, 2014; Tsuda, Beggs, Salter, & Inoue, 2013; Tsuda, Tozaki-Saitoh, & Inoue, 2010).

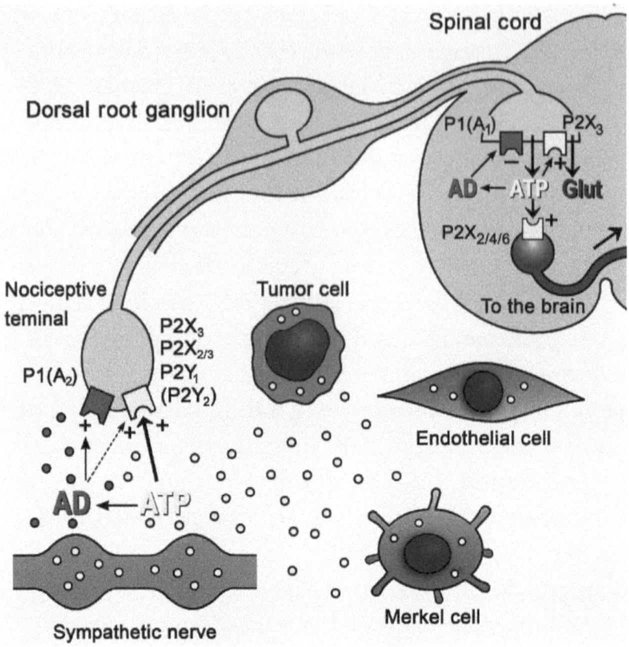

Figure 1 Hypothetical schematic of the roles of purine nucleotides and nucleosides in pain pathways. At sensory nerve terminals in the periphery, $P2X_3$ and $P2X_{2/3}$ receptors have been identified as the principal P2X purinoceptors present, although recent studies have also shown expression of $P2Y_1$ and possibly $P2Y_2$ receptors on a subpopulation of $P2X_3$ receptor-immunopositive fibers. Other known P2X purinoceptor subtypes (1–7) are also expressed at low levels in dorsal root ganglia. Although less potent than ATP, adenosine (AD) also appears to act on sensory terminals, probably directly via $P1(A_2)$ purinoceptors; however, it also acts synergistically (broken line) to potentiate $P2X_{2/3}$ receptor activation, which also may be true for 5-hydroxytryptamine, capsaicin, and protons. At synapses in sensory pathways in the CNS, ATP appears to act postsynaptically via $P2X_2$, $P2X_4$, and/or $P2X_6$ purinoceptor subtypes, perhaps as heteromultimers, and after breakdown to adenosine, it acts as a prejunctional inhibitor of transmission via $P1(A_2)$ purinoceptors. $P2X_3$ receptors on the central projections of primary afferent neurons in lamina II of the dorsal horn mediate facilitation of glutamate and probably also ATP release. Sources of ATP acting on $P2X_3$ and $P2X_{2/3}$ receptors on sensory terminals include sympathetic nerves, endothelial, Merkel, and tumor cells. *Modified from Burnstock and Wood (1996) and reproduced with permission of Elsevier.*

2. PURINERGIC MECHANOSENSORY TRANSDUCTION AND PAIN

It was proposed that purinergic mechanosensory transduction occurred in visceral tubes and sacs, including ureter, bladder, and gut (Burnstock, 1999). ATP released from epithelial cells during distension was suggested to act on P2X3 homomeric and P2X2/3 heteromeric receptors on subepithelial sensory nerves initiating impulses in sensory pathways to pain centers in the central nervous system (Fig. 2A). There is evidence supporting this hypothesis in various organs.

2.1 Urinary Bladder

There was early evidence for ATP release from rabbit urinary bladder epithelial cells by hydrostatic pressure changes (Ferguson, Kennedy, & Burton, 1997). The authors speculated that this may be the basis of a sensory mechanism. Exposure to α,β-methylene ATP (α,β-meATP), which desensitizes the ATP receptors, significantly reduced the activity of mechanosensitive pelvic nerve afferents in an *in vitro* model of rat urinary bladder (Namasivayam, Eardley, & Morrison, 1999). Mice lacking the P2X3 receptor exhibited reduced inflammatory pain and marked urinary bladder hyporeflexia with reduced voiding frequency and increased voiding volume (Cockayne et al., 2000). This suggested that P2X3 receptors are involved in purinergic mechanosensory transduction underlying both pain and physiological voiding reflexes. Later, using P2X2 knockout mice and P2X2/P2X3 double knockout mice, P2X2 receptors were also shown to play a role in mediating the sensory effect of ATP (Cockayne et al., 2005). A study of purinergic mechanosensory transduction in the mouse urinary bladder showed that ATP was released from urothelial cells during distension, and further that activity initiated in pelvic sensory nerves was mimicked by ATP and α,β-meATP (Vlaskovska et al., 2001). Sensory nerve activity was attenuated by P2X3 antagonists and in P2X3 knockout mice and P2X3 receptors were shown to be expressed by suburothelial sensory nerve fibers. Single unit analysis of sensory fibers in the mouse urinary bladder showed that there were both low- and high-threshold fibers sensitive to ATP contributing to physiological and nociceptive mechanosensory transduction, respectively (Rong, Spyer, & Burnstock, 2002). The roles of ATP released from urothelial cells and suburothelial myofibroblasts on various bladder functions have been discussed in several articles (Lazzeri, 2006; Sui, Wu, & Fry, 2006).

Intravesical application of ATP stimulated the micturition reflex in awake, freely moving rats, probably by stimulating suburothelial C-fibers (Pandita & Andersson, 2002). ATP has also been shown to induce a dose-dependent hypereflexia in conscious and anesthetized mice, which was dose dependently inhibited by the P2X3 receptors antagonist 2′,3′-*O*-(2,4,6-trinitrophenyl)-ATP (TNP-ATP) (Hu, Gever, Nunn, Ford, & Zhu, 2004). P2X1 and P2X3 receptors play a role in the micturition reflex

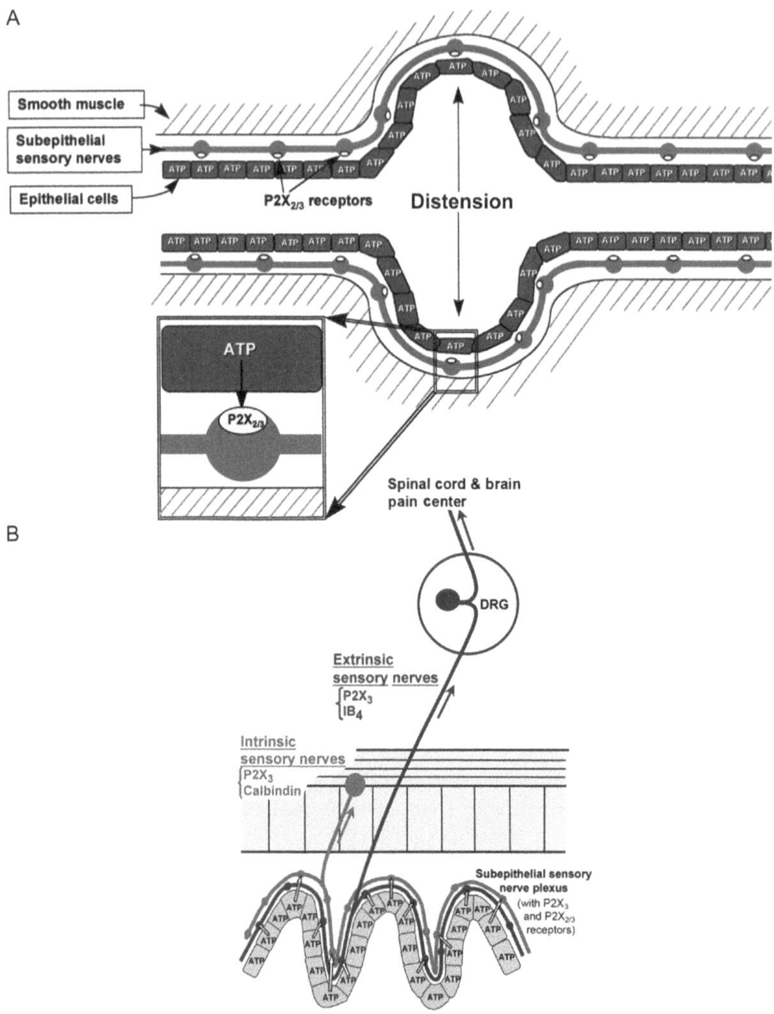

Figure 2 Purinergic mechanosensory transduction. (A) Schematic representation of hypothesis for purinergic mechanosensory transduction in tubes (e.g., ureter, vagina, salivary and bile ducts, gut) and sacs (e.g., urinary and gall bladders, and lung). It is proposed that distension leads to release of ATP from epithelium lining the tube or sac, which then acts on $P2X_3$ and/or $P2X_{2/3}$ receptors on subepithelial sensory nerves to convey sensory/nociceptive information to the CNS. (B) Schematic of a novel hypothesis about purinergic mechanosensory transduction in the gut. It is proposed that ATP released from mucosal epithelial cells during moderate distension acts preferentially on $P2X_3$ and/or $P2X_{2/3}$ receptors on low-threshold subepithelial intrinsic sensory nerve fibers (labeled with calbindin) to modulate peristaltic reflexes. ATP released during extreme (colic) distension also acts on $P2X_3$ and/or $P2X_{2/3}$ receptors on high-threshold extrinsic sensory nerve fibers (labeled with isolectin B4 (IB_4)) that send messages via the dorsal root ganglia (DRG) to pain centers in the central nervous system. *Panel (A) Modified from Burnstock (1999), reproduced with permission from Blackwell Publishing and panel (B) from Burnstock (2001c), reproduced with permission from Wiley-Liss, Inc.*

in female urethane-anesthetized rats (King, Knowles, Burnstock, & Ramage, 2004). P2X3 receptor blockade raised the pressure and volume thresholds for the reflex, while P2X1 receptor antagonism diminished motor activity related to voiding. Cyclophosphamide-induced rat bladder inflammation (a model for interstitial cystitis) sensitized and enhanced P2X3 and P2X2/3 receptor function (Dang, Lamb, Cohen, Bielefeldt, & Gebhart, 2008). Botulinum toxin A had antinociceptive effects in treating interstitial cystitis. It inhibited distension-mediated release of ATP by the urothelium in conditions of bladder inflammation (Smith, Vemulakonda, Kiss, Boone, & Somogyi, 2005) as well as ATP release from parasympathetic nerves as a cotransmitter with acetylcholine (Mackenzie, Burnstock, & Dolly, 1982). Trigonal injection of botulinum toxin A was found to be effective in reducing pain in patients with refractory bladder pain syndrome/interstitial cystitis (Pinto et al., 2010). Endogenous control of bladder activity via presynaptic P2X3 and P2X2/3 receptors in the spinal cord has been reported (Kaan, Yip, Grist, et al., 2010). $P2Y_2$ receptors were shown to sensitize mouse bladder sensory neurons facilitating purinergic nociceptive currents (Chen, Molliver, & Gebhart, 2010). In a later paper, however, it was proposed that expression of $P2Y_2$ receptors on nociceptive sensory neurons provided a mechanism to prevent excessive ATP signaling through P2X3 receptors (Mo, Peleshok, Cao, Ribeiro-da-Silva, & Séguéla, 2013).

2.2 Ureter

The passage through the ureter of a kidney stone causes severe pain. Immunostaining of P2X3 receptors was shown on sensory nerves in the subepithelial region (Lee, Bardini, & Burnstock, 2000). Distension of the ureter of both guinea pig and humans resulted in substantial ATP release from the urothelium in a pressure-dependent manner (Calvert, Thompson, & Burnstock, 2008; Knight et al., 2002). No urothelial cell damage was shown to occur during distension using scanning electron microscopy. Further, after removal of the urothelium, there was no ATP release during distension. Release of ATP from urothelial cells was, at least partly, vesicular. Distension of the ureter resulted in an initial rapid then maintained increase in afferent nerve discharge using a guinea pig preparation perfused *in vitro* (Rong & Burnstock, 2004). The rapid increase was mimicked by intraluminal application of ATP or α,β-meATP, while TNP-ATP attenuated the nerve discharge. The maintained increase in activity was partly due to adenosine.

2.3 Gut

It was proposed that purinergic mechanosensory transduction in the gut initiated both physiological reflex modulation of peristalsis via intrinsic sensory fibers and nociception via extrinsic sensory fibers (Burnstock, 2001a,b; Fig. 2A). Support for this hypothesis was obtained from a rat pelvic sensory nerve-colorectal preparation, where distension of the colorectum led to pressure-dependent increase in release of ATP from mucosal epithelial cells and evoked pelvic nerve excitation (Wynn, Rong, Xiang, & Burnstock, 2003). This excitation was mimicked by application of ATP and α,β-meATP and was attenuated by the P2X3 and P2X2/3 antagonist TNP-ATP. Potentiation of the sensory discharge was produced by ARL-67156, an ATPase inhibitor. Both low- and high-threshold fiber activities were antagonized by α,β-meATP desensitization in single fiber analysis experiments. Interactions of ATP with other mediators including 5-hydroxytryptamine (5-HT), bradykinin, prostaglandins, and substance P (SP) that activate pelvic afferent fibers in the rat colorectum have been reported (Wynn & Burnstock, 2006). Receptors to these substances (including ATP) are potential targets for drug treatment to attenuate the inappropriate visceral sensation and subsequent reflex activities that underlie abnormal bowel function and visceral pain (see Holzer, 2004; Kirkup, Brunsden, & Grundy, 2001). Forty percent of lumbar splanchnic afferents responded to α,β-meATP compared with only 7% of pelvic nerve afferents (Brierley et al., 2005).

In a model of colitis, ATP release and P2X3 and P2X2/3 receptor-mediated nociceptive sensory nerve responses were enhanced (Wynn, Bei, Ruan, & Burnstock, 2004). The excitability of visceral afferent nerves was enhanced following injury or ischemia and during inflammation in irritable bowel syndrome (IBS) (Shinoda, Feng, & Gebhart, 2009). Chronic functional visceral hyperalgesia was induced in a rat model for IBS induced by colonic injection of 0.5% acetic acid (Xu, Shenoy, Winston, Mittal, & Pasricha, 2008). It was associated with potentiation of ATP-evoked responses and enhanced expression of P2X3 receptors in colon sensory neurons. Colorectal hypersensitivity in IBS involved purinergic signaling in colorectal DRG neurons (Shinoda, La, Bielefeldt, & Gebhart, 2010). Colonic afferents are sensitized by products from immune cells to mechanical stimuli in IBS (Hughes, Brierley, & Blackshaw, 2009). Activation of spinal A_1 receptors has been shown to modulate visceral hyperalgesia (Zahn, Straub, Wenk, & Pogatzki-Zahn, 2007). Both peripheral and central roles for P2X3 receptors are involved in colon mechanosensitivity and colon hypersensitivity (Shinoda et al., 2009). Intestinal afferent hypersensitivity in a murine model of post-infectious bowel disease was shown to involve P2X2/3 receptor activation (Rong, Keating, Sun, Dong, & Grundy, 2009). α,β-MeATP-stimulated mechanosensitive mucosal receptors in mouse stomach and oesophagus leading to activity in vagal afferent nerves (Page, Martin, & Blackshaw, 2002). Sensitizing effects of P2X3 receptor agonists on mechanosensory function in esophagitis was reported (Page, O'Donnell, & Blackshaw, 2000). Purinergic mechanosensory transduction has also been considered in reflex control of intestinal secretion (Cooke, Wunderlich, & Christofi, 2003). ATP released from mucosal epithelial cells was claimed to act on $P2Y_1$ receptors on enterochromaffin cells to release 5-HT, leading to regulation of secretion either directly or via intrinsic reflex activity.

2.4 Skin

Sensory nerve fibers expressing P2X3 receptors innervate the skin (Burnstock, Knight, & Greig, 2012; Jimenez-Andrade et al., 2010). Nociceptive sensory nerve terminals in the skin are activated by ATP and α,β-meATP (Hamilton, McMahon, & Lewin, 2001). The study describes increases in inflammatory conditions due to increase in number and responsiveness of P2X3 and P2X2/3 receptors. Calcium waves mediated by extracellular ATP in human epidermal keratinocytes produce $[Ca^{2+}]_i$ elevation in DRG neurons, indicating a dynamic cross talk mediated by extracellular ATP between skin and sensory neurons (Koizumi et al., 2004). Action potential firing and inward currents in nociceptive fibers caused by skin cell damage was abolished by blockade of P2X receptors or enzymatic degradation of ATP (Cook & McCleskey, 2002). Sensitization of large mechanosensitive afferent endings was produced by locally released ATP via P2 receptors, leading to increased nociceptive responses to pressure or touch (Zhang, Chen, & Zhao, 2001). It was suggested that this mechanism, together with changes in the dorsal horn, contributes to touch-evoked pain (Zhang et al., 2001). ATP is involved in fast nociceptive signals, while persistent pain after tissue damage involves bradykinin, prostaglandin and serotonin. Nevertheless, persistent pain during inflammation may also involve sensitization and/or increase of P2X receptors. ATP was more effective in exciting nociceptors in inflamed compared to normal skin (Hamilton et al., 2001). It was suggested that this was due to upregulation of P2X2 and

P2X3 receptors on DRG neurons (Xu & Huang, 2002). The mechanical sensitivity of IB_4-positive nociceptive afferents (which express P2X3 and P2X2/3 receptors) was changed by the enhanced expression of glial cell-derived neurotrophic factor in the skin (Albers, Woodbury, Ritter, Davis, & Koerber, 2006). $P2Y_2$ receptors on the terminals of capsaicin-sensitive cutaneous mouse sensory neurons mediate nociceptive transmission and P2Y signaling may contribute to mechanotransduction in low-threshold Aβ fibers (Stucky, Medler, & Molliver, 2004). Hyperalgesia produced by complete Freund's adjuvant (CFA) and carrageenan-induced inflammation in rats was reduced by treatment with oxidized ATP, an inhibitor of P2X7 receptors (Fulgenzi et al., 2005). A pathogenic role for keratinocyte-derived ATP in irritant dermatitis has been reported (Mizumoto, Mummert, Shalhevet, & Takashima, 2003). Cutaneous sensory neurons expressing Mrgprd G protein-coupled receptors sense extracellular ATP and are putative nociceptors (Dong, Han, Zylka, Simon, & Anderson, 2001; Dussor, Zylka, Anderson, & McCleskey, 2008). It was suggested that these nociceptors in the outer epidermis respond indirectly to external stimuli by detecting ATP release in the skin. Prolonged mechanical allodynia in the lower lip skin produced by partial injury of the rat mental nerve, a branch of the trigeminal nerve, and P2X3 immunoreactive C-fibers showed a transient decrease in density of innervation (Taylor & Ribeiro-da-Silva, 2011). P2X3 receptors mediated ectopic mechanical allodynia with inflamed lower lip in mice (Yasuda et al., 2012).

P2X2, P2X3, and $P2Y_1$ receptors are abundantly expressed on sensory nerve terminals in the tongue (Bo et al., 1999; Kataoka, Toyono, Seta, Ogura, & Toyoshima, 2004). ATP and α,β-meATP excite trigeminal lingual nerve terminals in an *in vitro* preparation of intra-arterially perfused rat, mimicking nociceptive responses to noxious mechanical stimulation and high temperature (Rong, Burnstock, & Spyer, 2000). A purinergic mechanosensory transduction mechanism for the initiation of pain was proposed.

A hypothesis was presented that purinergic mechanosensory transduction is the physiological basis for initiation of the response to acupuncture (Burnstock, 2009b, 2014). Release of ATP from keratinocytes is produced by mechanical disturbance by acupuncture needles in the skin, heat, electrical current, or laser treatment. ATP would then activate P2X3 and/or P2X2/3 receptors on sensory fibers supplying the skin to activate sensory pathways leading to modulation of pain pathways as well as influencing autonomic motor neuron activity in the brainstem.

Pain from burns is a common problem. Puerarin, the active ingredient extracted from the traditional Chinese medicine Ge-gen (*Radix Puerariae*, RP) has been used to relieve angina chest pain. It was claimed to reduce the hyperalgesia mediated by P2X3 receptors after burn injury in the rat (Li et al., 2011). Tetramethylpyrazine, the active ingredient in another Chinese medicine used for treating inflammatory pain caused by injury, also reduced burn pain via DRG P2X3 receptors (Gao et al., 2010). Pine oil blocked ATP-activated pain pathways and was used against second degree burns (Clark et al., 2014).

2.5 Tooth Pain

P2X3 receptors were shown to be involved in the development and maintenance of tooth movement-induced pain (Yang et al., 2009). Nociception was claimed to be mediated by P2X3 and P2X2/3 receptors on sensory afferents in tooth pulp (Alavi, Dubyak, & Burnstock, 2001; Cook, Vulchanova, Hargreaves, Elde, & McCleskey, 1997; Renton, Yiangou, Baecker, Ford, & Anand, 2003), probably activated by ATP released by mechanical distension or inflammation of odontoblasts (Shibukawa et al., 2015). Application of mustard oil to the tooth pulp in anesthetized rats produced long-lasting central sensitization. The mustard oil sensitization was reversibly attenuated by TNP-ATP (Hu, Chiang, Hu, Dostrovsky, & Sessle, 2002).

2.6 Heart

An ATP-triggered vagal reflex has been described in the heart leading to suppression of sinus node automaticity and atrioventricular nodal conduction (Pelleg & Hurt, 1990). This is likely to be mediated by P2X2/3 receptors located on vagal sensory nerve terminals in the left ventricle, suggesting that ATP is released from ischemic myocytes (Xu, Kussmaul, Kurnik, Al-Ahdav, & Pelleg, 2005). P2X3 receptors on sensory fibers have been implicated in the heart originating in the nodose ganglion in nociception associated with myocardial ischemic injury (Wang et al., 2008).

2.7 Lung

In the lung pulmonary neuroepithelial bodies (NEBs) are oxygen sensors, especially in early development before the carotid system has matured (Brouns, Van Genechten, Burnstock, Timmermans, & Adriaensen, 2003). Subepithelial receptor-like endings associated with smooth muscle

(SMARs) expressing purinoceptors serve as sensory organs in the lung. P2X3 and P2X2/3 receptors are expressed on a subpopulation of vagal sensory fibers that supply NEBs and SMARs with their origin in nodose ganglia (Brouns, De Proost, Pintelon, Timmermans, & Adriaensen, 2006). High concentrations of ATP are present in the secretory vesicles of NEBs, indicated by quinacrine staining. It has been suggested that ATP is released from these cells in response to both mechanical stimulation during high-pressure ventilation and during hypoxia (Rich, Douillet, Mahler, Husain, & Boucher, 2003). Both TRPV1 and P2X receptors mediate sensory transduction of pulmonary reactive oxygen species by capsaicin-sensitive vagal lung afferent fibers (Ruan, Lin, Lin, & Kou, 2005). Vagal C-fibers innervating the pulmonary system are derived from cell bodies situated in both the jugular (superior) vagal ganglion neurons, which project fibers to the extrapulmonary airways (larynx, trachea, bronchus) and the lung parenchymal tissue, and nodose (inferior) neurons, which innervate primarily structures within the lungs. Only the nodose C-fibers responded to α,β-meATP. Vagal afferent purinergic signaling may be partly responsible for the hyperactivity associated with asthma and chronic obstructive pulmonary disease (Adriaensen & Timmermans, 2004). P2X7 receptor function is regulated by Th1 and Th2 cytokines, suggesting a role for P2X7 receptors in pulmonary diseases, including lung hypersensitivity associated with chronic inflammatory responses (Lemaire & Leduc, 2004).

2.8 Musculoskeletal Systems and Joints

ATP has been claimed to excite or sensitize myofascial nociceptors (Bland-Ward & Humphrey, 1997). Infusion of a combination of ATP, serotonin, histamine, and prostaglandin E_2 produced prolonged muscle pain and tenderness in human muscle (Mørk, Ashina, Bendtsen, Olesen, & Jensen, 2003). P2 receptors on the endings of thin fiber muscle afferents mediate both metabolic and mechanoreceptor components of the exercise pressor reflex (Hanna & Kaufman, 2003). ATP is an effective stimulant of group IV receptors in mechanically sensitive muscle afferents (Li & Sinoway, 2002). The muscle pressor response evoked by mechanically sensitive muscle stretch was enhanced by ATP and attenuated by pyridoxalphosphate-6-azophenyl-2′,4′-disulfonic acid (PPADS) (Li & Sinoway, 2002). Intramuscular injections of ATP excited a subpopulation of unmyelinated (group IV) muscle afferent fibers (Hoheisel, Reinöhl, Unger, & Mense, 2004), implicating P2X2 or P2X2/3 receptors that are sensitive to acidic pH. ATP acting on P2X3 receptors on sensory nerve fibers in masseter muscle was claimed to play an important role in pressure pain and mechanical hyperalgesia caused by excessive muscular contraction (Shinoda, Ozaki, & Sugiura, 2008). Sustained facilitation of cranial nociception was induced by ATP via P2X receptors on neck muscle nociceptors in mice (Makowska, Panfil, & Ellrich, 2006). This may play a role in the pathophysiology of tension-type headache (Ristić & Ellrich, 2012). Nociceptive information from the orofacial region via P2X3 receptors on afferent fibers reaches trigeminal brainstem sensory nuclei (Kim et al., 2008 see also Chiang, Dostrovsky, Iwata, & Sessle, 2011; Lim & Mitchell, 2012; Shinoda & Iwata, 2013).

ATP is a stimulant of articular nociceptors in the knee joint via P2X3 receptors (Dowd, McQueen, Chessell, & Humphrey, 1998; Seino et al., 2006) and also to some extent in the lumbar intervertebral disc (Aoki et al., 2003). $P2Y_2$ receptor mRNA is expressed in human knee joints. ATP is released by mechanical stimulation from both cultured normal and osteoarthritic chondrocytes and $P2Y_2$ receptor mRNA was expressed by these cells (Millward-Sadler, Wright, Flatman, & Salter, 2004). Ankle joint movement affects postoperative pain via peripheral and central A_1 receptors (Martins, Mazzardo-Martins, Cidral-Filho, Stramosk, & Santos, 2013). Sensory nerve fibers arising from the trigeminal ganglion supplying the temporomandibular joint have abundant receptors that respond to ATP and retrograde tracing revealed that 52% of neurons supplying this joint exhibited P2X3 receptors (Ichikawa et al., 2004). Temporomandibular joint P2X3 and P2X2/3 receptors are involved in carrageenan-induced inflammatory hyperalgesia in rats (Teixeira, Oliveira, Nociti, et al., 2010). The pain produced when monoarthritis was induced by injection of CFA into the unilateral temporomandibular joint of the rat was associated with an increase in P2X3 receptor-positive small neurons in the trigeminal ganglion (Shinoda, Ozaki, Asai, Nagamine, & Sugiura, 2005). P2X receptor activation in rat temporomandibular joint induced nociception, and antagonism by PPADS decreased carrageenan-induced inflammatory hyperalgesia (Oliveira et al., 2005). Oxidized ATP inhibits inflammatory pain in arthritic rats by inhibition of the P2X7 receptor (Dell'Antonio, Quattrini, Cin, Fulgenzi, & Ferrero, 2002).

3. NEUROPATHIC AND INFLAMMATORY PAIN

In a seminal study published in Nature in 2003, expression of P2X4 receptors on spinal cord microglia was shown to be increased in neuropathic pain, which was reduced after use of P2X4 antisense oligonucleotides (Tsuda et al., 2003). An explosion of work focused on purinergic signaling in neuropathic pain has followed (Burnstock, 2006; Inoue, 2007; McGaraughty & Jarvis, 2006; Nakatsuka & Gu, 2006). P2X7 and $P2Y_{12}$ receptors on microglia have also been shown to be involved in neuropathic pain (see Horváth et al., 2014; Jarvis, 2010; Smith, 2010; Tsuda et al., 2010). The underlying mechanisms involving P2X4, P2X7, and $P2Y_{12}$ receptors are being investigated (see Trang & Salter, 2012; Tsuda, Inoue, & Salter, 2005). ATP serves as an acute danger signal and is a mediator of inflammation and immunity (Di Virgilio, Boeynaems, & Robson, 2009). Rapamycin, an inhibitor of the mTOR pathway in nerves, reduced pain in a neuropathic pain model; the mTOR pathway is involved in ADP-evoked astrocyte activation and ATP release in the spinal dorsal horn (Cui et al., 2014).

Adenosine has also been claimed to be a potential analgesic target for inflammatory and neuropathic pain (Burnstock & Sawynok, 2010; Dickenson, Suzuki, & Reeve, 2000; Sawynok & Liu, 2003), particularly via A_1 and A_{2A} receptors (Korboukh et al., 2012; Loram et al., 2009; Sowa, Voss, & Zylka, 2010; Vincenzi et al., 2014; Zylka, 2011). However, it was reported that chronic pain in rats was controlled by A_3 adenosine agonists (Chen et al., 2012; Little et al., 2015; Paoletta et al., 2013).

3.1 P2X3 and P2X2/3 Receptors

P2X3 and P2X2/3 receptors are involved in neuropathic and inflammatory pain (Lu et al., 2010, and see Giniatullin & Nistri, 2013; Noguchi & Okubo, 2011; Wirkner, Sperlágh, & Illes, 2007), probably those located on primary afferent nerve terminals in inner lamina 2 of the spinal cord (Vulchanova et al., 1998) and in the trigeminal brainstem sensory nuclei (Kim et al., 2008). It has been suggested that ATP coreleased with γ-aminobutyric acid in spinal interneurons may be involved in modulation of nociceptive pathways (Jo & Schlichter, 1999). In the inner lamina 2 of the dorsal horn of the spinal cord P2X3 receptors on terminals of primary afferent nerves mediate facilitation of glutamate release (Gu & MacDermott, 1997). Thermal hyperalgesia may be mediated by spinal P2X3 receptors via activation of *N*-methyl-*D*-aspartate receptors (Tsuda, Ueno, & Inoue, 1999). It has been claimed that supraspinal P2X3 and P2X2/3 receptors play an inhibitory role in pain transmission (Fukui, Nakagawa, Minami, Satoh, & Kaneko, 2006). Intrathecal administration of ATP produces long-lasting allodynia via P2X2/3 receptors (Nakagawa et al., 2007). Spinal P2X2 and P2X3 receptors were reported to be involved in neuropathic pain in a mouse model of chronic constriction injury (Ueno et al., 2003). It has been suggested that P2X3/P2X2/3 receptor-dependent cytosolic phospholipase A_2 ($cPLA_2$) activity in primary sensory neurons is a key event in neuropathic pain and that $cPLA_2$ might be a potential target for treating neuropathic pain (Tsuda, Hasegawa, & Inoue, 2007). Sensitization of P2X3 receptors rather than a change in ATP release appears to be responsible for neuropathic pain and allodynia (Chen, Li, Wang, Gu, & Huang, 2005). The P2X3 and P2X2/3 receptor antagonism that reduces inflammatory hyperalgesia and chemogenic nociception was claimed to be mediated by the spinal opioid system (McGaraughty et al., 2005; Oliveira, Pelegrini-da-Silva, Tambeli, & Parada, 2009).

Antisense oligonucleotides have been used to downregulate the P2X3 receptor, and inhibition of the development of mechanical hyperalgesia as well as significant reversal of established hyperalgesia were observed in models of neuropathic (partial sciatic nerve ligation) and inflammatory (CFA) pain (Barclay et al., 2002; Honore et al., 2002; Stone & Vulchanova, 2003). P2X3 antisense oligonucleotides or antagonists were less effective for treating discogenic (lumbar intervertebral disc) than cutaneous tissue pain (Aoki et al., 2003). In the chronically compressed DRG, there is upregulation of P2X3 receptors (Xiang et al., 2008). The expression of P2X3 receptors in the rat DRG is reduced by cyclooxygenase inhibitors and hyperalgesia is attenuated following chronic constriction injury (Wang et al., 2010). Vascular endothelial growth factor is involved in neuropathic pain transmission mediated by P2X2/3 receptors on primary sensory neurons (Lin et al., 2010). The sensitivity to ATP of satellite cells in sensory ganglia is increased 500-fold after axotomy or inflammation, which is likely to contribute to chronic pain (Hanani, Kushnir, & Cherkas, 2007). P2X3 and P2X2/3 receptor antagonists reduced spontaneous firing and evoked responses of spinal nociceptive neurons in inflamed rats (Xu, Chu, Brederson, Jarvis, & McGaraughty, 2012).

ATP, via P2X3 receptors, caused sensitization of trigeminal ganglion nociceptive neurons (Masterson & Durham, 2010) and P2X3 receptors expressed by nociceptive trigeminal neurons were sensitized by SP (Park et al., 2010). ATP-mediated mechanical allodynia was facilitated by low pH via the activation of P2X3 receptors, while thermal hyperalgesia induced by ATP was mediated primarily by $P2Y_1$ receptors under low pH conditions (Seo et al., 2011).

Endothelin-1 induces hyperalgesia in rats that is enhanced by repeated mechanical stimulation at the site of administration. This effect was produced by its action on vascular endothelial cells, sensitizing them to mechanical stimulation and associated release of ATP, which then acts on P2X3 receptors on nociceptors (Joseph, Green, Bogen, Alvarez, & Levine, 2013; Joseph, Green, & Levine, 2014). P2X3 receptor-mediated peripheral pain signal transduction was attenuated by 17β-estradiol via estrogen receptor-α and GPR30 receptors (Lu et al., 2013; Ma et al., 2011). Pregabalin is an antiepileptic drug used for the treatment of neuropathic pain, which appears to be due to its inhibition of P2X3 receptor expression in the spinal dorsal horn (Yu, Fu, Zhang, Liu, & Cui, 2013). Neuropathic pain sensitization was mediated by P2X3 receptors in resiniferatoxin-induced neuropathy (Hsieh, Chiang, Lue, & Hsieh, 2012; Lin, Fu, Hsiao, & Hsieh, 2013).

3.2 P2X4 Receptors

There have been a number of papers concerned with the role and underlying mechanisms involved in P2X4 receptor activation of spinal microglia in neuropathic pain following the initial discovery by Tsuda et al. (2003) (see Beggs, Trang, & Salter, 2012; Inoue, 2007; Trang, Beggs, & Salter, 2006, 2011; Tsuda et al., 2005; Tsuda, Masuda, Tozaki-Saitoh, & Inoue, 2013). Brain-derived neurotrophic factor (BDNF) is released from microglia by the stimulation of P2X4 receptors (Coull et al., 2005; Trang & Salter, 2012; Fig. 3). Upregulation of microglial P2X4 receptors and neuropathic pain has been claimed to involve increase in spinal fibronectin/integrin following peripheral nerve injury (Tsuda, Toyomitsu, et al., 2008). Ligands for toll-like receptors and nucleotide-binding oligomerization domain 2 receptors stimulate microglial P2X4 receptor upregulation, indicating that microglia sense the presence of inflammatory stimulation using multiple recognition systems (Guo, Guo, Wendel, & Schluesener, 2006). An important role in the pathogenesis of neuropathic pain is played by Lyn tyrosine kinase and it is required to mediate nerve injury-induced upregulation of P2X4 receptors (Tsuda, Tozaki-Saitoh, et al., 2008).

Enhancement of pain behavior after nerve injury requires both P2X4 receptors and phospho38 (p38) mitogen-activated protein kinase (MAPK) (Tsuda, Mizokoshi, Shigemoto-Mogami, Koizumi, & Inoue, 2004). ATP activates p38 or ERK1/2 MAPKs resulting in the release of tumor necrosis factor-α (TNF-α) and interleukin (IL)-6. The level of p38 was increased in microglia in rats displaying allodynia and intraspinal administration of the p38 inhibitor, SB203580, suppressed allodynia. This suggests that neuropathic pain hypersensitivity depends on the activation of the p38 signaling

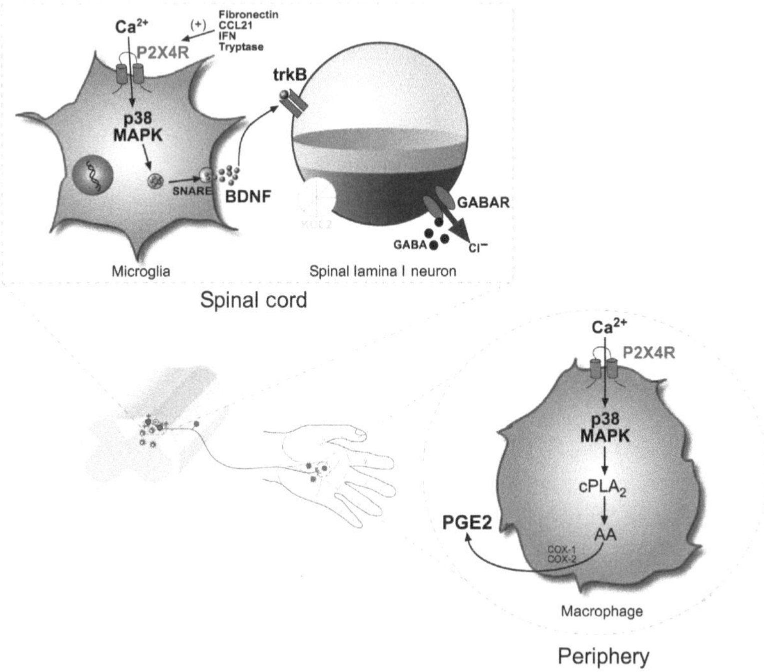

Figure 3 P2X4 receptor(R)-p38 MAPK is a core signaling pathway through which spinal microglia and peripheral macrophages contribute to neuropathic pain and inflammatory pain. (A) Following injury to a peripheral nerve, expression of P2X4R is upregulated in microglia that reside in the spinal dorsal horn. Several factors have recently been implicated in the upregulation of microglial P2X4R: the fibronectin-Lyn kinase signaling cascade, cytokine IFN-γ, tryptase released from mast cells, and the chemokine CCL21. Influx of Ca^{2+} through ATP-stimulated P2X4R activates p38-MAPK and drives the synthesis and SNARE-dependent release of BDNF. Acting on its cognate receptor, trkB, BDNF released from microglia signals to dorsal horn lamina I neurons to downregulate the K^+–Cl^- cotransporter KCC2, resulting in aberrant nociceptive output that underlies pain hypersensitivity characterized by hyperalgesia, allodynia, and spontaneous pain. (B) Like microglia, peripheral macrophages constitutively express P2X4R. Inflammatory challenges that activate P2X4R on macrophages trigger Ca^{2+} influx and p38 MAPK phosphorylation. In macrophages, the P2X4R-p38 MAPK pathway is a signaling hub that activates cytosolic phospholipase A_2 ($cPLA_2$), which liberates arachidonic acid (AA) resulting in a cyclooxygenase (COX)-dependent synthesis and release of prostaglandin E2 (PGE2), a key substrate that sensitizes primary sensory neurons and leads to hyperexcitability of peripheral nociceptive pathways that is a hallmark of inflammatory pain. *Reproduced from Trang and Salter (2012), with permission from Springer.*

pathway in microglia in the dorsal horn following peripheral nerve injury. Platelet-activating factor, released from activated microglia, is a potent inducer of tactile allodynia and thermal hyperalgesia after intrathecal injection into the spinal cord and it was suggested that this response is mediated by

ATP (Morita et al., 2004). Systemic and intracerebro-ventricular infection of proinflammatory bacterial lipopolysaccharide (LPS) results in thermal hyperalgesia and tactile allodynia and LPS has been shown to enhance responses to low concentrations of ATP mediated by P2X4 receptors (Raouf, Chabot-Doré, Ase, Blais, & Séguéla, 2007).

Mechanical hyperalgesia induced by peripheral nerve injury in P2X4 receptor-deficient mice is lacking and they show impaired BDNF release from microglia and reduced neuropathic pain (Ulmann et al., 2008). Mechanical allodynia and upregulation of P2X4 receptors in spinal microglia is a feature of experimental autoimmune neuritis (Zhang, Zhang, Fauser, & Schluesener, 2008). Morphine tolerance is attenuated by inhibition of microglial P2X4 receptors (Horvath, Romero-Sandoval, & De Leo, 2010). Cells in the nucleus pulposus secrete inflammatory cytokines, including IL-1β and TNF-α, which play a major role in the development of neuropathic pain and the expression of P2X4 receptors in the DRG was increased (Otoshi, Kikuchi, Konno, & Sekiguchi, 2010). Prostaglandin E2 release from macrophages is mediated by P2X4 receptors to initiate inflammatory pain (Ulmann, Hirbec, & Rassendren, 2010). Interferon regulatory factor-5, which is induced in spinal microglia after peripheral nerve injury, is responsible for direct transcriptional control of P2X4 receptors (Masuda et al., 2014). Dexmedetomidine, a selective α_2-adrenoceptor agonist, which has been used for sedation and analgesia, reduced pain in the spared nerve injury neuropathic pain rat model, which is related to reduced expression of P2X4 receptors and BDNF in microglia of the spinal dorsal horn (Zhou, Wu, Chen, Liu, & Miao, 2014).

3.3 P2X7 Receptors

P2X7 receptors were first expressed in a mouse microglial cell line, NTW8 (Chessell, Michel, & Humphrey, 1997), and later on rat brain microglia (Yu et al., 2008). Relief of inflammation-induced mechanical hyperalgesia in rats with the P2X7 receptor antagonist, oxidized ATP, was reported (Dell'Antonio et al., 2002). In P2X7 knockout mice, chronic inflammatory and neuropathic pain was abolished, as was release of IL-1β (Chessell et al., 2005). The authors suggested that the P2X7 receptor, via regulation of mature IL-1β production, plays an upstream transductional role in the development of neuropathic and inflammatory pain (see also Clark et al., 2010).

P2X7 receptor blockade reduced nociception in animal models of persistent neuropathic and inflammatory pain (Donnelly-Roberts et al., 2008; Hughes, Hatcher, & Chessell, 2007; Nelson et al., 2008). These findings together with growing evidence supporting the role of P2X7 receptor modulation in proinflammatory IL-1 processing (Ferrari et al., 2006) suggest a specific role for P2X7 receptors in neural–glial cell interactions associated with ongoing pain (Donnelly-Roberts & Jarvis, 2007).

P2X4 and P2X7 receptor knockout mice have a common pain phenotype, but this phenotype appears to be conferred via different mechanisms (Chessell et al., 2006). P2X7 receptor activation through the p38 MAPK system leads to TNF-α production in microglia and treatment with inhibitors of either TNF-α or p38 results in reduction of hyperalgesia (see Teixeira, Oliveira, Parada, & Tambeli, 2010). Immune cells expressing P2X7 receptors play a pivotal role in changes in pain thresholds (Chessell et al., 2005). After injury in a neuropathic pain model, there was increase in expression of P2X7 receptor mRNA and protein in spinal microglia (Kobayashi, Takahashi, Miyagawa, Yamanaka, & Noguchi, 2011). In an acute inflammatory pain model, P2X7 receptors on microglia *in vivo* were claimed to play a major role in the development of sensitization of nociceptive neurons in rat medullary dorsal horn (Itoh et al., 2011). Activation of P2X7 receptors releases glutamate in the spinal cord, which contributes to mechanical allodynia following partial nerve ligation of the sciatic nerve (Andó & Sperlágh, 2013). Oxaliplatin, an anticancer drug, which has been shown to induce painful neuropathy, causes P2X7 receptor activation (Massicot et al., 2013). The P2X7 receptor antagonist, A438079, prevented the effects on allodynia induced by paclitaxel, another anticancer drug (Ochi-ishi et al., 2014). Peripheral P2X7 receptor activation induced mechanical hyperalgesia via inflammatory mediators, especially bradykinin (Teixeira, de Oliveira-Fusaro, Parada, & Tambeli, 2014). Some of the P2X7 receptor single nucleotide polymorphisms correlate with pain sensitivity, including that in a diabetic pain patient population (Ursu et al., 2014).

3.4 P2Y Receptors

The role of metabotropic P2Y receptors in pain has been less investigated compared to P2X receptors (see Gerevich & Illes, 2004). However, $P2Y_1$, $P2Y_2$, $P2Y_4$, and $P2Y_6$ receptor mRNA is expressed in DRG neurons, suggesting that these receptors may be involved in peripheral somatosensory transmission (Burnstock, 2007a; Moriyama et al., 2003). Activation of uridine 5′-triphosphate (UTP)-sensitive $P2Y_2$ and/or $P2Y_4$ receptors and uridine diphosphate-sensitive $P2Y_6$ receptors produced inhibition of spinal pain transmission (Okada, Nakagawa, Minami, & Satoh, 2002). $P2Y_1$ and $P2Y_4$ receptors were identified on small diameter sensory neurons, a subpopulation of which also expressed P2X3 receptors (Ruan & Burnstock, 2003) and TRPV1 receptors (Gerevich et al., 2004). $P2Y_1$ receptor activation of DRG neurons modulated currents generated through *N*-type ($Ca_v2.2$) calcium channels and P2X3 receptors (Gerevich, Müller, & Illes, 2005). $P2Y_1$ receptor-related inhibition of *N*-type calcium channels or P2X3 receptors could result in decreased release of nociceptive transmitters into the spinal cord (Burnstock, 2007a).

After peripheral axotomy, $P2Y_1$ receptor mRNA was upregulated in the lumbar DRG, indicating that $P2Y_1$ receptors may contribute to heightened somatosensory sensitivity (Xiao et al., 2002). Peripheral $P2Y_1$ receptor blockade prevented induction of thermal hyperalgesia via modulation of TRPV1 expression in carrageenan-induced inflammatory pain in rats (Kwon et al., 2014). In isolated skin-nerve preparations, 54% of cutaneous C-fibers and 12% of A-mechanoreceptors responded to UTP via $P2Y_2$ receptors (Stucky et al., 2004). However, an additional 22–26% of large diameter Aβ fibers responded to UTP, which suggests that $P2Y_2$ receptors may be directly involved in the transmission of low-threshold mechanical inputs to the spinal cord. Activation of the hetero-oligomeric $P2Y_2/A_1$ receptor complex (Suzuki, Namba, Tsuga, & Nakata, 2006) may also modulate the antinociceptive effects of A_1 receptor agonists (McGaraughty & Jarvis, 2006). In bulbo-spinal nociceptive modulation, it has been suggested that while on-cells preferentially express P2X receptors, off-cells express P2Y receptors in the rostral ventromedial medulla (Selden, Carlson, Cetas, Close, & Heinricher, 2007). P2Y receptor activation inhibits P2X3 receptor channels via G protein-dependent facilitation of their desensitization (Gerevich et al., 2007).

$P2Y_{12}$ receptors are expressed on microglia (Haynes et al., 2006) and are involved in neuropathic pain after peripheral nerve injury. Intrathecal administration of the $P2Y_{12}$ receptor antagonist, AR-C69931MX, prevented the development of tactile allodynia (Tozaki-Saitoh et al., 2008). Activation of $P2Y_{12}$ receptors by ATP is via the p38 MAPK pathway (Kobayashi et al., 2008). It was suggested that $P2Y_6$ and $P2Y_{11}$ receptors may be involved in neuropathic pain (Barragán-Iglesias et al., 2014).

However, evidence has been presented that $P2Y_6$ receptor antagonists had no effect on neuropathic pain behavior in mice (Syhr et al., 2014).

4. CANCER PAIN

Purinergic mechanisms are of interest in relation to cancer pain (Burnstock, 1996; Gilchrist et al., 2005; Mantyh, Clohisy, Koltzenburg, & Hunt, 2002). The unusually high levels of ATP contained in tumor cells (Maehara, Kusumoto, Anai, Kusumoto, & Sugimachi, 1987) may be released by mechanical stress to activate P2X3 receptors on nearby nociceptive sensory nerve fibers (Burnstock, 1996). In a bone cancer pain model, there is increased expression of P2X3 receptors on calcitonin gene-related peptide (CGRP) immunoreactive epidermal sensory nerve fibers (Gilchrist et al., 2005). This is of interest by analogy with that described for increased P2X3 receptor expression on CGRP neurons in a model of inflammatory colitis (Wynn et al., 2004). There is also increased expression of P2X3 receptors in other cancers that involve mechanically sensitive tumors (Mantyh et al., 2002). In bone tumors antagonists that block the mechanically gated channels and/or ATP receptors in the richly innervated periosteum may reduce movement-associated pain. In a rat model of squamous cell carcinoma of the lower gingiva, increased expression of P2X3 receptors was reported to be associated with thermal and mechanical hyperalgesia (Nagamine et al., 2006).

P2X receptor activity is controlled by opioids in rat sensory neurons, and P2X receptors on sensory neurons cocultured with cancer cells showed a decrease in opioid sensitivity (Chizhmakov et al., 2009). After orthotopic inoculation of B16-BL6 melanoma cells into the hind paw of mice, spontaneous licking of the tumor-bearing paw, an indicator of pain, was reported; this was blocked by P2X3 receptor antagonists (Fujita, Andoh, Sasaki, Saiki, & Kuraishi, 2010). Cisplatin is a drug used for the treatment of malignancies, but unfortunately with a side effect of pain. Following repeated injections of cisplatin in rats, mechanical allodynia, and hyperalgesia were observed (Authier, Fialip, Eschalier, & Coudoré, 2000). Cisplatin induced upregulation of P2X3 receptors in DRG and in muscle afferents in rats (Hori, Ozaki, Suzuki, & Sugiura, 2010). Minodronic acid used for the treatment of bone metastases exerted an analgesic effect in pain models and was shown to antagonize purinergic P2X2/3 receptor function (Kakimoto et al., 2008). Systemic antagonism of P2X3 and P2X2/3 receptors attenuated bone cancer pain in rats (Kaan, Yip, Patel, et al., 2010). The neuronal calcium sensor protein, visinin-like protein 1, caused upregulation of P2X3 receptors in DRG neurons, contributing to bone cancer pain in rats (Liu et al., 2013). Pain was caused by ATP secreted by head and neck squamous carcinoma cells acting via P2X2/3 heteromultimer receptors (Ye et al., 2014). Pain hypersensitivity associated with bone cancer pain was reduced by activation of K_{ATP} channels at the spinal cord level (Xia et al., 2014). Reviews about purinergic signaling and cancer pain are available (Bele & Fabbretti, 2015; Burnstock & Di Virgilio, 2013; Franceschini & Adinolfi, 2014).

5. MIGRAINE

The involvement of ATP in migraine was first considered in relation to the vascular theory of this disorder, where it was suggested that ATP released from endothelial cells during reactive hyperemia activated P2X3 receptors on nociceptive sensory fibers in the adventitia following cerebral vascular vasospasm (not associated with pain) (Burnstock, 1989). P2X3 receptor involvement in neuronal dysfunction in brain areas that mediate nociception such as the trigeminal nucleus and thalamus has also been considered (Ambalavanar & Dessem, 2009; Ambalavanar, Moritani, & Dessem, 2005; Fabbretti et al., 2006). Upregulation of nociceptive P2X3 receptors on trigeminal neurons by the migraine mediators CGRP and nerve growth factor (NGF) has been reported (Fabbretti et al., 2006; Giniatullin, Nistri, & Fabbretti, 2008). Anti-NGF treatment suppressed responses evoked by P2X3 receptor activation in an *in vivo* model of mouse trigeminal pain (D'Arco et al., 2007). A review concluded that ATP has a role in sensitization of primary afferents at both peripheral and central terminals in mechanisms underlying migraine headache (Jennings & Cho, 2007). A possible role of adenosine in migraine has been discussed (Shapiro, 2007). Plasma adenosine has been shown to rise during migraine attacks and adenosine triggered migraine attacks while dipyridamole, an adenosine uptake inhibitor, increased migraine attack frequency.

Genetic deletion and antagonists of the P2X7 receptor reduced migraine in a mouse animal model (Gölöncsér & Sperlágh, 2014). Mouse trigeminal sensory neurons from a transgenic familial hemiplegic migraine type-1 model, exhibited a lower firing threshold and generated more action potentials in response to α,β-meATP, acting via P2X3 receptors (Hullugundi, Ansuini, Ferrari, van den Maagdenberg, & Nistri, 2014). Purinergic receptors, expressed in rat middle meningeal arteries, may play a role in migraine

(Haanes & Edvinsson, 2014). The role of ion channels in migraine, including P2X3 receptors, has been reviewed (Yan & Dussor, 2014).

6. THERAPEUTIC DEVELOPMENTS

There is much interest in developing selective P2X3, P2X2/3, P2X4, P2X7, and $P2Y_{12}$ receptor antagonists that are orally bioavailable, can cross the blood–brain barrier, and do not degrade *in vivo* for the treatment of acute and neuropathic pain (see Carter et al., 2009; Ford, 2012; Gever, Cockayne, Dillon, Burnstock, & Ford, 2006; Gever et al., 2010; Jahangir et al., 2009). Reviews about the involvement and therapeutic potential of purinergic drugs for gastrointestinal diseases and pain are available (Moynes, Lucas, Beyak, & Lomax, 2014; Ochoa-Cortes, Liñán-Rico, Jacobson, & Christofi, 2014). TNP-ATP, a trinitrophenyl-substituted nucleotide, is a very potent antagonist at both P2X3 and P2X2/3 receptors, but breaks down quickly *in vivo* (Burnstock, 2007a). A-317491 (synthesized by Abbott Laboratories) (Jarvis et al., 2002; Sharp et al., 2006) and compound RO3 (synthesized by Roche Palo Alto) (Gever et al., 2006) and its derivative AF-353 (Gever et al., 2010) are effective P2X3 and P2X2/3 antagonists. Systemic administration of A-317491 reduced nociception in inflammatory and neuropathic pain models (Jarvis et al., 2002). Traditional Chinese medicines, such as tetramethylpyrazine, sodium ferulate, and puerarin, have been reported to antagonize P2X3 and P2X2/3 receptors to reduce pain (Gao et al., 2008; Liang, Xu, Li, & Gao, 2010; Persson, Xu, Wiesenfeld-Hallin, Devor, & Fried, 2010). Also, a Chinese herbal medicine used as an analgesic for centuries, lappaconitine, acting on P2X3 receptors in rat DRG reduced neuropathic pain (Ou et al., 2011). Emodin (3-methyl-1,6,8-trihydroxyanthraquinone), an active anthraquinone constituent of rhubarb extract, reduced neuropathic pain mediated by P2X3 receptors in primary sensory nerves (Gao et al., 2011). Other P2X3 antagonists for the treatment of neuropathic pain have been reviewed (Cantin et al., 2012). Combined antisense and RNA interference-mediated treatment for specific inhibition of the recombinant rat P2X3 receptor has been recommended as a promising pain therapy (Hemmings-Mieszczak, Dorn, Natt, Hall, & Wishart, 2003). P2X3 double-stranded short interfering RNA relieves chronic neuropathic pain and is a new avenue for therapeutic pain strategies (Dorn et al., 2004). P2X3 receptors are highly expressed on trigeminal primary afferent neurons, suggesting that they may be effective targets for craniofacial pain therapies (Ambalavanar & Dessem, 2009). Silencing C-terminal Src inhibitory kinase in trigeminal neurons potentiated P2X3 receptor responses, identifying a potential target for trigeminal pain suppression (D'Arco et al., 2009). P2X3 receptors have been claimed to be useful targets for the treatment of pain in chronic prostatitis (Zhang et al., 2011). Clinical trials for some P2X3 receptor antagonists are in progress (see Ford, 2012; Gever et al., 2006, 2010) and reduced pain sensation was noted in a suramin phase 1 cancer clinical trial (Ho, Huo, Lu, Newman, & Levin, 1992).

ATP is released during cortical spreading into the cerebral spinal fluid (Schock et al., 2007). It may be involved in activation and sensitization of primary afferent fibers in the trigeminal ganglia via P2X3 receptors, suggesting that this may be a target for migraine treatment (see Burnstock, 2009a). P2X3 receptors are known to be expressed exclusively by a subset of trigeminal and spinal sensory neurons (Chen et al., 1995) and again were proposed as promising candidates for antimigraine drug development (Fabbretti, 2010; Waeber & Moskowitz, 2003; Wirkner et al., 2007). P2X3 receptor activity of mouse sensory nerves mediating trigeminal pain is enhanced by the familial hemiplegic migraine calcium channel mutation R192Q (Nair et al., 2010). $P2Y_1$ receptor interaction with P2X3 receptors on trigeminal neurons after sensitization of these neurons with algogenic stimuli (e.g., NGF, BDNF, or bradykinin) has been suggested and may represent a new potential target for antimigraine drugs (Fumagalli, Ceruti, Verderio, & Abbracchio, 2006). A_1 receptor stimulation has also been considered for migraine treatment (Humphrey, 2007). It has also been claimed that A_{2A} receptor gene variation may contribute to the pathogenesis of migraine (Hohoff et al., 2007).

The P2X7 receptor is a major target for inflammatory and neuropathic pain (Alves, Bezerra, Faria, Ferreira, & da Silva Frutuoso, 2013; Bhattacharya, Neff, & Wickenden, 2011; Donnelly-Roberts et al., 2008; Ferrari et al., 2006; Romagnoli et al., 2008; Tsuda, Tozaki-Saitoh, & Inoue, 2012). A number of P2X7 receptor antagonists have been used including: oxidized ATP, Brilliant Blue G, the tyrosine derivatives KN-62 and KN-04, cyclic imides, adamantane and benzamide derivatives (Gunosewoyo, Coster, & Kassiou, 2007), compound 4g (Romagnoli et al., 2007), chelerythrine and other benzophenenanthidine alkaloids (Shemon, Sluyter, Conigrave, & Wiley, 2004), U73122 and U73343 (Takenouchi, Ogihara, Sato, & Kitani, 2005). More recently, compounds such as cyanoguanidines and aminotetrazoles have been introduced (Shieh, Jarvis, Lee, & Perner, 2006). Systemic administration of the P2X7 receptor-selective antagonists A-438079 and A-740003 had dose-dependent antinociceptive effects in models of neuropathic (Honore et al., 2006; McGaraughty et al., 2007; Nelson et al., 2006) and inflammatory (Honore et al., 2006) pain. A-740003 was more potent than A-438079 in reducing mechanical allodynia 2 weeks after spinal L_5/L_6 nerve ligation. The antinociceptive effects of P2X7 antagonists in inflammatory pain models are not secondary to an anti-inflammatory effect, since A-740003 was more effective in reducing nociception than paw edema. The antinociceptive action of A-438079 is due to blocking mechanical and thermal inputs to spinal neurons (McGaraughty et al., 2007). Spontaneous activity of all classes of spinal neurons was reduced by A-438079 in neuropathic, but not sham rats.

Selective P2X4 antagonists were only available relatively recently. A series of benzofuro-1,4-diazepin-2-ones were reported to be effective P2X4 antagonists in a Bayer Health Care, AG patent (see Shieh et al., 2006). The microglia-to-neuron P2X4 receptor–BDNF–K^+–Cl^- cotransporter pathway could be a therapeutic target for preventing hyperalgesia without affecting morphine analgesia (Ferrini et al., 2013). Antidepressants have been claimed to be effective in relieving neuropathic pain. Some antidepressants, in particular paroxetine, was an effective antagonist to P2X4 receptors in transfected cells and preliminary clinical studies showed that it was successfully used against chronic pain (Nagata et al., 2009). Carbamazepine derivatives have recently been shown to have potent P2X4 receptor blocking activities offering a promising development for the treatment of neuropathic pain (Tian et al., 2014). Peripheral administration of A_1 receptor agonists leads to antinociception against mechanical hyperalgesia (Aley, Green, & Levine, 1995; Taiwo & Levine, 1990). A_2 receptor antagonists have been claimed to produce antinociception in pain models (Yoon et al., 2006). Reviews describing the development of adenosine receptor ligands as antinociceptive and anti-inflammatory drugs are available (Akkari, Burbiel, Hockemeyer, & Müller, 2006; Burnstock & Sawynok, 2010). Other therapeutic approaches to pain are being considered, including the use of agents that control the expression of receptors and others that inhibit ATP breakdown by selective inhibition of the known ecto-nucleotidases. In addition, agents are being developed that will be able to enhance or inhibit ATP release, another useful way forward as a therapeutic strategy. An adenosine kinase (AK) inhibitor, A-134974, alleviated tactile allodynia via spinal sites in peripheral nerve-injured rats, increasing the growing evidence that AK inhibitors may be useful analgesic agents (Zhu et al., 2001).

Table 1 Purinoceptor Subtypes Involved in Acute and Chronic Neuropathic and Inflammatory Pain

Receptor Subtype	Distribution	Function
P2X3/P2X2/3	Terminals of nociceptive sensory nerves	Mediation of acute and chronic visceral, musculoskeletal, and dermal pain initiated by purinergic mechanosensory transduction and cancer
	Sensory nerves in CNS	Mediation of neuropathic and inflammatory pain, including migraine
P2X4	Microglia in CNS	Mediation of neuropathic pain
P2X7	Microglia	Mediation of neuropathic pain
	Tumor cells	Mediation of cancer cell death
$P2Y_{12}$	Microglia	Mediation of neuropathic pain
P1		
A_1 agonists	Presynaptic terminals of peripheral and central neurons	Inhibitory modulation of pain pathways
A_2 antagonists		Antinociception

7. CONCLUSION

The subtypes of purinoceptors involved in acute and chronic neuropathic and inflammatory pain are summarized in Table 1. Therapeutic strategies involving purinergic drugs are being explored, involving P2X3, P2X2/3, P2X4, P2X7, and $P2Y_{12}$ receptor antagonists and A_1 receptor agonists. While there is clearly purinergic multi-receptor involvement in pain pathology, the precise roles and interactions with other antinociceptive agents are still to be resolved.

CONFLICT OF INTEREST

The author confirms that these article contents have no conflict of interest.

ACKNOWLEDGMENT

The author thanks Dr. Gillian E. Knight for her excellent editorial assistance.

REFERENCES

Abbracchio, M. P., & Burnstock, G. (1994). Purinoceptors: Are there families of P_{2X} and P_{2Y} purinoceptors? *Pharmacology and Therapeutics*, *64*, 445–475.

Abbracchio, M. P., Burnstock, G., Boeynaems, J.-M., Barnard, E. A., Boyer, J. L., Kennedy, C., et al. (2006). International Union of Pharmacology. Update and subclassification of the P2Y G protein-coupled nucleotide receptors: From molecular mechanisms and pathophysiology to therapy. *Pharmacological Reviews*, *58*, 281–341.

Adriaensen, D., & Timmermans, J. P. (2004). Purinergic signalling in the lung: Important in asthma and COPD? *Current Opinion in Pharmacology*, *4*, 207–214.

Akkari, R., Burbiel, J. C., Hockemeyer, J., & Müller, C. E. (2006). Recent progress in the development of adenosine receptor ligands as antiinflammatory drugs. *Current Topics in Medicinal Chemistry*, *6*, 1375–1399.

Alavi, A. M., Dubyak, G. R., & Burnstock, G. (2001). Immunohistochemical evidence for ATP receptors in human dental pulp. *Journal of Dental Research*, *80*, 476–483.

Albers, K. M., Woodbury, C. J., Ritter, A. M., Davis, B. M., & Koerber, H. R. (2006). Glial cell-line-derived neurotrophic factor expression in skin alters the mechanical sensitivity of cutaneous nociceptors. *Journal of Neuroscience*, *26*, 2981–2990.

Aley, K. O., Green, P. G., & Levine, J. D. (1995). Opioid and adenosine peripheral antinociception are subject to tolerance and withdrawal. *Journal of Neuroscience*, *15*, 8031–8038.

Alves, L. A., Bezerra, R. J., Faria, R. X., Ferreira, L. G., & da Silva Frutuoso, V. (2013). Physiological roles and potential therapeutic applications of the P2X7 receptor in inflammation and pain. *Molecules*, *18*, 10953–10972.

Ambalavanar, R., & Dessem, D. (2009). Emerging peripheral receptor targets for deep-tissue craniofacial pain therapies. *Journal of Dental Research*, *88*, 201–211.

Ambalavanar, R., Moritani, M., & Dessem, D. (2005). Trigeminal $P2X_3$ receptor expression differs from dorsal root ganglion and is modulated by deep tissue inflammation. *Pain*, *117*, 280–291.

Andó, R. D., & Sperlágh, B. (2013). The role of glutamate release mediated by extrasynaptic P2X7 receptors in animal models of neuropathic pain. *Brain Research Bulletin*, *93*, 80–85.

Aoki, Y., Ohtori, S., Takahashi, K., Ino, H., Ozawa, T., Douya, H., et al. (2003). $P2X_3$-immunoreactive primary sensory neurons innervating lumbar intervertebral disc in rats. *Brain Research*, *989*, 214–220.

Authier, N., Fialip, J., Eschalier, A., & Coudoré, F. (2000). Assessment of allodynia and hyperalgesia after cisplatin administration to rats. *Neuroscience Letters*, *291*, 73–76.

Barclay, J., Patel, S., Dorn, G., Wotherspoon, G., Moffatt, S., Eunson, L., et al. (2002). Functional downregulation of $P2X_3$ receptor subunit in rat sensory neurons reveals a significant role in chronic neuropathic and inflammatory pain. *Journal of Neuroscience*, *22*, 8139–8147.

Barragán-Iglesias, P., Pineda-Farias, J. B., Cervantes-Durán, C., Bravo-Hernández, M., Rocha-González, H. I., Murbartián, J., et al. (2014). Role of spinal $P2Y_6$ and $P2Y_{11}$ receptors in neuropathic pain in rats: Possible involvement of glial cells. *Molecular Pain*, *10*, 29.

Beggs, S., Trang, T., & Salter, M. W. (2012). $P2X4R^+$ microglia drive neuropathic pain. *Nature Neuroscience*, *15*, 1068–1073.

Bele, T., & Fabbretti, E. (2015). P2X receptors, sensory neurons and pain. *Current Medicinal Chemistry*, *22*, 845–850.

Bhattacharya, A., Neff, R. A., & Wickenden, A. D. (2011). The physiology, pharmacology and future of P2X7 as an analgesic drug target: Hype or promise? *Current Pharmaceutical Biotechnology*, *12*, 1698–1706.

Bland-Ward, P. A., & Humphrey, P. P. A. (1997). Acute nociception mediated by hindpaw P2X receptor activation in the rat. *British Journal of Pharmacology*, *122*, 365–371.

Bleehen, T., & Keele, C. A. (1977). Observations on the algogenic actions of adenosine compounds on human blister base preparation. *Pain, 3*, 367–377.
Bo, X., Alavi, A., Xiang, Z., Oglesby, I., Ford, A., & Burnstock, G. (1999). Localization of ATP-gated $P2X_2$ and $P2X_3$ receptor immunoreactive nerves in rat taste buds. *Neuroreport, 10*, 1107–1111.
Bodin, P., & Burnstock, G. (1998). Increased release of ATP from endothelial cells during acute inflammation. *Inflammation Research, 47*, 351–354.
Bodin, P., & Burnstock, G. (2001). Purinergic signalling: ATP release. *Neurochemical Research, 26*, 959–969.
Boudreault, F., & Grygorczyk, R. (2004). Cell swelling-induced ATP release is tightly dependent on intracellular calcium elevations. *Journal of Physiology, 561*, 499–513.
Bradbury, E. J., Burnstock, G., & McMahon, S. B. (1998). The expression of $P2X_3$ purinoceptors in sensory neurons: Effects of axotomy and glial-derived neurotrophic factor. *Molecular and Cellular Neurosciences, 12*, 256–268.
Brierley, S. M., Carter, R., Jones, W., III, Xu, L., Robinson, D. R., Hicks, G. A., et al. (2005). Differential chemosensory function and receptor expression of splanchnic and pelvic colonic afferents in mice. *Journal of Physiology, 567*, 267–281.
Brouns, I., De Proost, I., Pintelon, I., Timmermans, J. P., & Adriaensen, D. (2006). Sensory receptors in the airways: Neurochemical coding of smooth muscle-associated airway receptors and pulmonary neuroepithelial body innervation. *Autonomic Neuroscience, 126–127*, 307–319.
Brouns, I., Van Genechten, J., Burnstock, G., Timmermans, J.-P., & Adriaensen, D. (2003). Ontogenesis of $P2X_3$ receptor-expressing nerve fibres in the rat lung, with special reference to neuroepithelial bodies. *Biomedical Research, 14*, 80–86.
Burnstock, G. (1972). Purinergic nerves. *Pharmacological Reviews, 24*, 509–581.
Burnstock, G. (1978). A basis for distinguishing two types of purinergic receptor. In R. W. Straub & L. Bolis (Eds.), *Cell membrane receptors for drugs and hormones: A multidisciplinary approach* (pp. 107–118). New York: Raven Press.
Burnstock, G. (1981). Pathophysiology of migraine: A new hypothesis. *Lancet, 317*, 1397–1399.
Burnstock, G. (1989). The role of adenosine triphosphate in migraine. *Biomedicine and Pharmacotherapy, 43*, 727–736.
Burnstock, G. (1996). A unifying purinergic hypothesis for the initiation of pain. *Lancet, 347*, 1604–1605.
Burnstock, G. (1999). Release of vasoactive substances from endothelial cells by shear stress and purinergic mechanosensory transduction. *Journal of Anatomy, 194*, 335–342.
Burnstock, G. (2001a). Purinergic signalling in gut. In M. P. Abbracchio & M. Williams (Eds.), *Handbook of experimental pharmacology: Vol. 151/II. Purinergic and pyrimidinergic signalling II—Cardiovascular, respiratory, immune, metabolic and gastrointestinal tract function* (pp. 141–238). Berlin: Springer-Verlag.
Burnstock, G. (2001b). Purine-mediated signalling in pain and visceral perception. *Trends in Pharmacological Sciences, 22*, 182–188.
Burnstock, G. (2001c). Expanding field of purinergic signaling. *Drug Development Research, 52*, 1–10.
Burnstock, G. (2006). Pathophysiology and therapeutic potential of purinergic signalling. *Pharmacological Reviews, 58*, 58–86.
Burnstock, G. (2007a). Physiology and pathophysiology of purinergic neurotransmission. *Physiological Reviews, 87*, 659–797.
Burnstock, G. (2007b). Purine and pyrimidine receptors. *Cellular and Molecular Life Sciences, 64*, 1471–1483.
Burnstock, G. (2009a). Purines and sensory nerves. *Handbook of Experimental Pharmacology, 194*, 333–392.

Burnstock, G. (2009b). Acupuncture: A novel hypothesis for the involvement of purinergic signalling. *Medical Hypotheses, 73*, 470–472.
Burnstock, G. (2009c). Purinergic mechanosensory transduction and visceral pain. *Molecular Pain, 5*, 69.
Burnstock, G. (2012). Targeting the visceral purinergic system for pain control. *Current Opinion in Pharmacology, 12*, 80–86.
Burnstock, G. (2014). Purinergic signalling in acupuncture. *Science, 346*, S23–S25.
Burnstock, G., Campbell, G., Satchell, D., & Smythe, A. (1970). Evidence that adenosine triphosphate or a related nucleotide is the transmitter substance released by non-adrenergic inhibitory nerves in the gut. *British Journal of Pharmacology, 40*, 668–688.
Burnstock, G., & Di Virgilio, F. (2013). Purinergic signalling in cancer. *Purinergic Signalling, 9*, 491–540.
Burnstock, G., Dumsday, B., & Smythe, A. (1972). Atropine resistant excitation of the urinary bladder: The possibility of transmission via nerves releasing a purine nucleotide. *British Journal of Pharmacology, 44*, 451–461.
Burnstock, G., & Kennedy, C. (1985). Is there a basis for distinguishing two types of P_2-purinoceptor?. *General Pharmacology, 16*, 433–440.
Burnstock, G., & Knight, G. E. (2004). Cellular distribution and functions of P2 receptor subtypes in different systems. *International Review of Cytology, 240*, 31–304.
Burnstock, G., Knight, G. E., & Greig, A. V. H. (2012). Purinergic signalling in healthy and diseased skin. *Journal of Investigative Dermatology, 132*, 526–546.
Burnstock, G., & Sawynok, J. (2010). ATP and adenosine receptors and pain. In P. Beaulieu, D. Lussier, F. Porreca, & A. H. Dickenson (Eds.), *Pharmacology of pain* (pp. 303–326). Seattle: IASP Press.
Burnstock, G., & Wood, J. N. (1996). Purinergic receptors: Their role in nociception and primary afferent neurotransmission. *Current Opinion in Neurobiology, 6*, 526–532.
Calvert, R. C., Thompson, C. S., & Burnstock, G. (2008). ATP release from the human ureter on distension and $P2X_3$ receptor expression on suburothelial sensory nerves. *Purinergic Signalling, 4*, 377–381.
Cantin, L. D., Bayrakdarian, M., Buon, C., Grazzini, E., Hu, Y. J., Labrecque, J., et al. (2012). Discovery of P2X3 selective antagonists for the treatment of chronic pain. *Bioorganic & Medicinal Chemistry Letters, 22*, 2565–2571.
Carter, D. S., Alam, M., Cai, H., Dillon, M. P., Ford, A. P., Gever, J. R., et al. (2009). Identification and SAR of novel diaminopyrimidines. Part 1: The discovery of RO-4, a dual $P2X_3/P2X_{2/3}$ antagonist for the treatment of pain. *Bioorganic & Medicinal Chemistry Letters, 19*, 1628–1631.
Chen, C. C., Akopian, A. N., Sivilotti, L., Colquhoun, D., Burnstock, G., & Wood, J. N. (1995). A P2X purinoceptor expressed by a subset of sensory neurons. *Nature, 377*, 428–431.
Chen, Z., Janes, K., Chen, C., Doyle, T., Bryant, L., Tosh, D. K., et al. (2012). Controlling murine and rat chronic pain through A_3 adenosine receptor activation. *FASEB Journal, 26*, 1855–1865.
Chen, Y., Li, G. W., Wang, C., Gu, Y., & Huang, L. Y. (2005). Mechanisms underlying enhanced P2X receptor-mediated responses in the neuropathic pain state. *Pain, 119*, 38–48.
Chen, X., Molliver, D. C., & Gebhart, G. F. (2010). The $P2Y_2$ receptor sensitizes mouse bladder sensory neurons and facilitates purinergic currents. *Journal of Neuroscience, 30*, 2365–2372.
Chessell, I. P., Hatcher, J. P., Bountra, C., Michel, A. D., Hughes, J. P., Green, P., et al. (2005). Disruption of the $P2X_7$ purinoceptor gene abolishes chronic inflammatory and neuropathic pain. *Pain, 114*, 386–396.

Chessell, I. P., Hatcher, J. P., Hughes, J. P., Ulmann, L., Green, P., Mander, P. K., et al. (2006). The role of $P2X_7$ and $P2X_4$ in pain processing; common or divergent pathways? *Purinergic Signalling, 2*, 46–47.

Chessell, I. P., Michel, A. D., & Humphrey, P. P. (1997). Properties of the pore-forming $P2X_7$ purinoceptor in mouse NTW8 microglial cells. *British Journal of Pharmacology, 121*, 1429–1437.

Chiang, C. Y., Dostrovsky, J. O., Iwata, K., & Sessle, B. J. (2011). Role of glia in orofacial pain. *The Neuroscientist, 17*, 303–320.

Chizhmakov, I., Mamenko, N., Volkova, T., Khasabova, I., Simone, D. A., & Krishtal, O. (2009). P2X receptors in sensory neurons co-cultured with cancer cells exhibit a decrease in opioid sensitivity. *European Journal of Neuroscience, 29*, 76–86.

Clark, S. P., Bollag, W. B., Westlund, K. N., Ma, F., Falls, G., Xie, D., et al. (2014). Pine oil effects on chemical and thermal injury in mice and cultured mouse dorsal root ganglion neurons. *Phytotherapy Research, 28*, 252–260.

Clark, A. K., Staniland, A. A., Marchand, F., Kaan, T. K., McMahon, S. B., & Malcangio, M. (2010). P2X7-dependent release of interleukin-1β and nociception in the spinal cord following lipopolysaccharide. *Journal of Neuroscience, 30*, 573–582.

Cockayne, D. A., Dunn, P. M., Zhong, Y., Hamilton, S. G., Cain, G. R., Knight, G., et al. (2005). $P2X_2$ knockout mice and $P2X_2$/$P2X_3$ double knockout mice reveal a role for the $P2X_2$ receptor subunit in mediating multiple sensory effects of ATP. *Journal of Physiology, 567*, 621–639.

Cockayne, D. A., Hamilton, S. G., Zhu, Q.-M., Dunn, P. M., Zhong, Y., Novakovic, S., et al. (2000). Urinary bladder hyporeflexia and reduced pain-related behaviour in $P2X_3$-deficient mice. *Nature, 407*, 1011–1015.

Collier, H. O., James, G. W. L., & Schneider, C. (1966). Antagonism by aspirin and fenamates of bronchoconstriction and nociception induced by adenosine-5′-triphosphate. *Nature, 212*, 411–412.

Cook, S. P., & McCleskey, E. W. (2002). Cell damage excites nociceptors through release of cytosolic ATP. *Pain, 95*, 41–47.

Cook, S. P., Vulchanova, L., Hargreaves, K. M., Elde, R., & McCleskey, E. W. (1997). Distinct ATP receptors on pain-sensing and stretch-sensing neurons. *Nature, 387*, 505–508.

Cooke, H. J., Wunderlich, J., & Christofi, F. L. (2003). "The force be with you": ATP in gut mechanosensory transduction. *News in Physiological Science, 18*, 43–49.

Coull, J. A., Beggs, S., Boudreau, D., Boivin, D., Tsuda, M., Inoue, K., et al. (2005). BDNF from microglia causes the shift in neuronal anion gradient underlying neuropathic pain. *Nature, 438*, 1017–1021.

Cui, J., He, W., Yi, B., Zhao, H., Lu, K., Ruan, H., et al. (2014). mTOR pathway is involved in ADP-evoked astrocyte activation and ATP release in the spinal dorsal horn in a rat neuropathic pain model. *Neuroscience, 275*, 395–403.

Dang, K., Lamb, K., Cohen, M., Bielefeldt, K., & Gebhart, G. F. (2008). Cyclophosphamide-induced bladder inflammation sensitizes and enhances P2X receptor function in rat bladder sensory neurons. *Journal of Neurophysiology, 99*, 49–59.

D'Arco, M., Giniatullin, R., Leone, V., Carloni, P., Birsa, N., Nair, A., et al. (2009). The C-terminal Src inhibitory kinase (Csk)-mediated tyrosine phosphorylation is a novel molecular mechanism to limit $P2X_3$ receptor function in mouse sensory neurons. *Journal of Biological Chemistry, 284*, 21393–21401.

D'Arco, M., Giniatullin, R., Simonetti, M., Fabbro, A., Nair, A., Nistri, A., et al. (2007). Neutralization of nerve growth factor induces plasticity of ATP-sensitive $P2X_3$ receptors of nociceptive trigeminal ganglion neurons. *Journal of Neuroscience, 27*, 8190–8201.

Dell'Antonio, G., Quattrini, A., Cin, E. D., Fulgenzi, A., & Ferrero, M. E. (2002). Relief of inflammatory pain in rats by local use of the selective P2X7 ATP receptor inhibitor, oxidized ATP. *Arthritis and Rheumatism, 46*, 3378–3385.

Di Virgilio, F., Boeynaems, J. M., & Robson, S. C. (2009). Extracellular nucleotides as negative modulators of immunity. *Current Opinion in Pharmacology, 9*, 507–513.

Dickenson, A. H., Suzuki, R., & Reeve, A. J. (2000). Adenosine as a potential analgesic target in inflammatory and neuropathic pains. *CNS Drugs, 13*, 77–85.

Dong, X., Han, S., Zylka, M. J., Simon, M. I., & Anderson, D. J. (2001). A diverse family of GPCRs expressed in specific subsets of nociceptive sensory neurons. *Cell, 106*, 619–632.

Donnelly-Roberts, D. L., & Jarvis, M. F. (2007). Discovery of $P2X_7$ receptor-selective antagonists offers new insights into $P2X_7$ receptor function and indicates a role in chronic pain states. *British Journal of Pharmacology, 151*, 571–579.

Donnelly-Roberts, D., McGaraughty, S., Shieh, C. C., Honore, P., & Jarvis, M. F. (2008). Painful purinergic receptors. *Journal of Pharmacology and Experimental Therapeutics, 324*, 409–415.

Dorn, G., Patel, S., Wotherspoon, G., Hemmings-Mieszczak, M., Barclay, J., Natt, F. J., et al. (2004). siRNA relieves chronic neuropathic pain. *Nucleic Acids Research, 32*, e49.

Dowd, E., McQueen, D. S., Chessell, I. P., & Humphrey, P. P. A. (1998). P2X receptor-mediated excitation of nociceptive afferents in the normal and arthritic rat knee joint. *British Journal of Pharmacology, 125*, 341–346.

Dubyak, G. R. (2006). ATP release mechanisms. In G. Burnstock & T. R. Arnett (Eds.), *Nucleotides and regulation of bone cell function* (pp. 99–158). Boca Raton, Florida: Taylor & Francis Group.

Dussor, G., Zylka, M. J., Anderson, D. J., & McCleskey, E. W. (2008). Cutaneous sensory neurons expressing the Mrgprd receptor sense extracellular ATP and are putative nociceptors. *Journal of Neurophysiology, 99*, 1581–1589.

Ecke, D., Hanck, T., Tulapurkar, M. E., Schafer, R., Kassack, M., Stricker, R., et al. (2008). Hetero-oligomerization of the $P2Y_{11}$ receptor with the $P2Y_1$ receptor controls the internalization and ligand selectivity of the $P2Y_{11}$ receptor. *Biochemical Journal, 409*, 107–116.

Egan, T. M., Samways, D. S., & Li, Z. (2006). Biophysics of P2X receptors. *Pflügers Archives—European Journal of Physiology, 452*, 501–512.

Fabbretti, E. (2010). ATP-mediated signalling in trigeminal neurons of an animal model of migraine. *Purinergic Signalling, 6*, S7.

Fabbretti, E., D'Arco, M., Fabbro, A., Simonetti, M., Nistri, A., & Giniatullin, R. (2006). Delayed upregulation of ATP $P2X_3$ receptors of trigeminal sensory neurons by calcitonin gene-related peptide. *Journal of Neuroscience, 26*, 6163–6171.

Ferguson, D. R., Kennedy, I., & Burton, T. J. (1997). ATP is released from rabbit urinary bladder epithelial cells by hydrostatic pressure changes—A possible sensory mechanism? *Journal of Physiology, 505*, 503–511.

Ferrari, D., Pizzirani, C., Adinolfi, E., Lemoli, R. M., Curti, A., Idzko, M., et al. (2006). The $P2X_7$ receptor: A key player in IL-1 processing and release. *Journal of Immunology, 176*, 3877–3883.

Ferrini, F., Trang, T., Mattioli, T. A., Laffray, S., Del'Guidice, T., Lorenzo, L. E., et al. (2013). Morphine hyperalgesia gated through microglia-mediated disruption of neuronal Cl^- homeostasis. *Nature Neuroscience, 16*, 183–192.

Fischer, W., & Krügel, U. (2007). P2Y receptors: Focus on structural, pharmacological and functional aspects in the brain. *Current Medicinal Chemistry, 14*, 2429–2455.

Ford, A. P. (2012). In pursuit of P2X3 antagonists: Novel therapeutics for chronic pain and afferent sensitization. *Purinergic Signalling, 8*, 3–26.

Franceschini, A., & Adinolfi, E. (2014). P2X receptors: New players in cancer pain. *World Journal of Biological Chemistry, 5*, 429–436.

Fredholm, B. B., IJzerman, A. P., Jacobson, K. A., Klotz, K. N., & Linden, J. (2001). International Union of Pharmacology. XXV. Nomenclature and classification of adenosine receptors. *Pharmacological Reviews, 53*, 527–552.

Fujita, M., Andoh, T., Sasaki, A., Saiki, I., & Kuraishi, Y. (2010). Involvement of peripheral adenosine 5′-triphosphate and P2X purinoceptor in pain-related behavior produced by orthotopic melanoma inoculation in mice. *European Journal of Neuroscience*, *31*, 1629–1636.

Fukui, M., Nakagawa, T., Minami, M., Satoh, M., & Kaneko, S. (2006). Inhibitory role of supraspinal $P2X_3/P2X_{2/3}$ subtypes on nociception in rats. *Molecular Pain*, *2*, 19.

Fulgenzi, A., Dell'Antonio, G., Foglieni, C., Dal Cin, E., Ticozzi, P., Franzone, J. S., et al. (2005). Inhibition of chemokine expression in rat inflamed paws by systemic use of the antihyperalgesic oxidized ATP. *BMC Immunology*, *6*, 18.

Fumagalli, M., Ceruti, S., Verderio, C., & Abbracchio, M. P. (2006). ATP as a neurotransmitter of pain in migraine: A functional role for P2Y receptors in primary cultures from mouse trigeminal sensory ganglia. *Purinergic Signalling*, *2*, 120–121.

Gao, Y., Liu, H., Deng, L., Zhu, G., Xu, C., Li, G., et al. (2011). Effect of emodin on neuropathic pain transmission mediated by P2X $_{2/3}$ receptor of primary sensory neurons. *Brain Research Bulletin*, *84*, 406–413.

Gao, Y., Xu, C., Liang, S., Zhang, A., Mu, S., Wang, Y., et al. (2008). Effect of tetramethylpyrazine on primary afferent transmission mediated by $P2X_3$ receptor in neuropathic pain states. *Brain Research Bulletin*, *77*, 27–32.

Gao, Y., Xu, C., Yu, K., Li, G., Wan, F., Liu, S., et al. (2010). Effect of tetramethylpyrazine on DRG neuron $P2X_3$ receptor involved in transmitting pain after burn. *Burns*, *36*, 127–134.

Garcia-Marcos, M., Pochet, S., Marino, A., & Dehaye, J. P. (2006). $P2X_7$ and phospholipid signalling: The search of the "missing link" in epithelial cells. *Cellular Signalling*, *18*, 2098–2104.

Gerevich, Z., Borvendeg, S. J., Schröder, W., Franke, H., Wirkner, K., Nörenberg, W., et al. (2004). Inhibition of N-type voltage-activated calcium channels in rat dorsal root ganglion neurons by P2Y receptors is a possible mechanism of ADP-induced analgesia. *Journal of Neuroscience*, *24*, 797–807.

Gerevich, Z., & Illes, P. (2004). P2Y receptors and pain transmission. *Purinergic Signalling*, *1*, 3–10.

Gerevich, Z., Müller, C., & Illes, P. (2005). Metabotropic $P2Y_1$ receptors inhibit $P2X_3$ receptor-channels in rat dorsal root ganglion neurons. *European Journal of Pharmacology*, *521*, 34–38.

Gerevich, Z., Zadori, Z., Müller, C., Wirkner, K., Schröder, W., Rubini, P., et al. (2007). Metabotropic P2Y receptors inhibit $P2X_3$ receptor-channels via G protein-dependent facilitation of their desensitization. *British Journal of Pharmacology*, *151*, 226–236.

Gever, J., Cockayne, D. A., Dillon, M. P., Burnstock, G., & Ford, A. P. D. W. (2006). Pharmacology of P2X channels. *Pflügers Archives—European Journal of Physiology*, *452*, 537.

Gever, J. R., Rothschild, S., Henningsen, R., Martin, R., Hackos, D., Panicker, S., et al. (2010). AF-353, a novel, potent orally bioavailable P2X3/P2X2/3 receptor antagonist. *British Journal of Pharmacology*, *160*, 1387–1398.

Gilchrist, L. S., Cain, D. M., Harding-Rose, C., Kov, A. N., Wendelschafer-Crabb, G., Kennedy, W. R., et al. (2005). Re-organization of $P2X_3$ receptor localization on epidermal nerve fibers in a murine model of cancer pain. *Brain Research*, *1044*, 197–205.

Giniatullin, R., & Nistri, A. (2013). Desensitization properties of P2X3 receptors shaping pain signaling. *Frontiers in Cellular Neuroscience*, *7*, 245.

Giniatullin, R., Nistri, A., & Fabbretti, E. (2008). Molecular mechanisms of sensitization of pain-transducing $P2X_3$ receptors by the migraine mediators CGRP and NGF. *Molecular Neurobiology*, *37*, 83–90.

Gölöncsér, F., & Sperlágh, B. (2014). Effect of genetic deletion and pharmacological antagonism of P2X7 receptors in a mouse animal model of migraine. *The Journal of Headache and Pain*, *15*, 24.

Gu, J. G., & MacDermott, A. B. (1997). Activation of ATP P2X receptors elicits glutamate release from sensory neuron synapses. *Nature, 389*, 749–753.
Gunosewoyo, H., Coster, M. J., & Kassiou, M. (2007). Molecular probes for $P2X_7$ receptor studies. *Current Medicinal Chemistry, 14*, 1505–1523.
Guo, L. H., Guo, K. T., Wendel, H. P., & Schluesener, H. J. (2006). Combinations of TLR and NOD2 ligands stimulate rat microglial P2X4R expression. *Biochemical and Biophysical Research Communications, 349*, 1156–1162.
Haanes, K. A., & Edvinsson, L. (2014). Expression and characterization of purinergic receptors in rat middle meningeal artery-potential role in migraine. *PLoS One, 9*, e108782.
Hamilton, S. G., McMahon, S. B., & Lewin, G. R. (2001). Selective activation of nociceptors by P2X receptor agonists in normal and inflamed rat skin. *Journal of Physiology, 534*, 437–445.
Hanani, M. (2012). Intercellular communication in sensory ganglia by purinergic receptors and gap junctions: Implications for chronic pain. *Brain Research, 1487*, 183–191.
Hanani, M., Kushnir, R., & Cherkas, P. S. (2007). Nerve damage or inflammation augment purinergic signalling in satellite glial cells in mouse sensory ganglia. In *Proceedings of the VII European meeting, glial cells in health and disease, London* (pp. 83–86).
Hanna, R. L., & Kaufman, M. P. (2003). Role played by purinergic receptors on muscle afferents in evoking the exercise pressor reflex. *Journal of Applied Physiology, 94*, 1437–1445.
Haynes, S. E., Hollopeter, G., Yang, G., Kurpius, D., Dailey, M. E., Gan, W. B., et al. (2006). The $P2Y_{12}$ receptor regulates microglial activation by extracellular nucleotides. *Nature Neuroscience, 9*, 1512–1519.
Hemmings-Mieszczak, M., Dorn, G., Natt, F. J., Hall, J., & Wishart, W. L. (2003). Independent combinatorial effect of antisense oligonucleotides and RNAi-mediated specific inhibition of the recombinant rat P2X3 receptor. *Nucleic Acids Research, 31*, 2117–2126.
Ho, B. T., Huo, Y. Y., Lu, J. G., Newman, R. A., & Levin, V. A. (1992). Analgesic activity of anticancer agent suramin. *Anti-Cancer Drugs, 3*, 91–94.
Hoheisel, U., Reinöhl, J., Unger, T., & Mense, S. (2004). Acidic pH and capsaicin activate mechanosensitive group IV muscle receptors in the rat. *Pain, 110*, 149–157.
Hohoff, C., Marziniak, M., Lesch, K. P., Deckert, J., Sommer, C., & Mossner, R. (2007). An adenosine A_{2A} receptor gene haplotype is associated with migraine with aura. *Cephalalgia, 27*, 177–181.
Holzer, P. (2004). Gastrointestinal pain in functional bowel disorders: Sensory neurons as novel drug targets. *Expert Opinion on Therapeutic Targets, 8*, 107–123.
Honore, P., Donnelly-Roberts, D., Namovic, M. T., Hsieh, G., Zhu, C. Z., Mikusa, J. P., et al. (2006). A-740003 [N-(1-{[(cyanoimino)(5-quinolinylamino) methyl]amino}-2,2-dimethylpropyl)-2-(3,4-dimethoxyphenyl)acetamide], a novel and selective $P2X_7$ receptor antagonist, dose-dependently reduces neuropathic pain in the rat. *The Journal of Pharmacology and Experimental Therapeutics, 319*, 1376–1385.
Honore, P., Kage, K., Mikusa, J., Watt, A. T., Johnston, J. F., Wyatt, J. R., et al. (2002). Analgesic profile of intrathecal $P2X_3$ antisense oligonucleotide treatment in chronic inflammatory and neuropathic pain states in rats. *Pain, 99*, 11–19.
Hori, K., Ozaki, N., Suzuki, S., & Sugiura, Y. (2010). Upregulations of $P2X_3$ and ASIC3 involve in hyperalgesia induced by cisplatin administration in rats. *Pain, 149*, 393–405.
Horváth, G., Gölöncsér, F., Csölle, C., Király, K., Andó, R. D., Baranyi, M., et al. (2014). Central $P2Y_{12}$ receptor blockade alleviates inflammatory and neuropathic pain and cytokine production in rodents. *Neurobiology of Disease, 70*, 162–178.
Horvath, R. J., Romero-Sandoval, E. A., & De Leo, J. A. (2010). Inhibition of microglial $P2X_4$ receptors attenuates morphine tolerance, Iba1, GFAP and μ opioid receptor protein expression while enhancing perivascular microglial ED2. *Pain, 150*, 401–413.

Hsieh, Y. L., Chiang, H., Lue, J. H., & Hsieh, S. T. (2012). P2X3-mediated peripheral sensitization of neuropathic pain in resiniferatoxin-induced neuropathy. *Experimental Neurology, 235*, 316–325.

Hu, B., Chiang, C. Y., Hu, J. W., Dostrovsky, J. O., & Sessle, B. J. (2002). P2X receptors in trigeminal subnucleus caudalis modulate central sensitization in trigeminal subnucleus oralis. *Journal of Neurophysiology, 88*, 1614–1624.

Hu, S. T., Gever, J., Nunn, P. A., Ford, A. P., & Zhu, Q.-M. (2004). Cystometric studies with ATP, PPADS and TNP-ATP in conscious and anaesthetised C57BL/6 mice. *Journal of Urology, 171*, 461–462.

Hughes, P. A., Brierley, S. M., & Blackshaw, L. A. (2009). Post-inflammatory modification of colonic afferent mechanosensitivity. *Clinical and Experimental Pharmacology and Physiology, 36*, 1034–1040.

Hughes, J. P., Hatcher, J. P., & Chessell, I. P. (2007). The role of $P2X_7$ in pain and inflammation. *Purinergic Signalling, 3*, 163–169.

Hullugundi, S. K., Ansuini, A., Ferrari, M. D., van den Maagdenberg, A. M., & Nistri, A. (2014). A hyperexcitability phenotype in mouse trigeminal sensory neurons expressing the R192Q *CACNA1A* missense mutation of familial hemiplegic migraine type-1. *Neuroscience, 266*, 244–254.

Humphrey, P. P. A. (2007). The discovery of a new drug class for the acute treatment of migraine. *Headache, 47*(Suppl. 1), S10–S19.

Ichikawa, H., Fukunaga, T., Jin, H. W., Fujita, M., Takano-Yamamoto, T., & Sugimoto, T. (2004). VR1-, VRL-1- and $P2X_3$ receptor-immunoreactive innervation of the rat temporomandibular joint. *Brain Research, 1008*, 131–136.

Inoue, K. (2007). P2 receptors and chronic pain. *Purinergic Signalling, 3*, 135–144.

Itoh, K., Chiang, C. Y., Li, Z., Lee, J. C., Dostrovsky, J. O., & Sessle, B. J. (2011). Central sensitization of nociceptive neurons in rat medullary dorsal horn involves purinergic P2X7 receptors. *Neuroscience, 192*, 721–731.

Jacobson, K. A., & Gao, Z. G. (2006). Adenosine receptors as therapeutic targets. *Nature Reviews Drug Discovery, 5*, 247–264.

Jahangir, A., Alam, M., Carter, D. S., Dillon, M. P., Bois, D. J., Ford, A. P., et al. (2009). Identification and SAR of novel diaminopyrimidines. Part 2: The discovery of RO-51, a potent and selective, dual $P2X_3/P2X_{2/3}$ antagonist for the treatment of pain. *Bioorganic & Medicinal Chemistry Letters, 19*, 1632–1635.

Jahr, C. E., & Jessell, T. M. (1983). ATP excites a subpopulation of rat dorsal horn neurones. *Nature, 304*, 730–733.

Jarvis, M. F. (2010). The neural-glial purinergic receptor ensemble in chronic pain states. *Trends in Neurosciences, 33*, 48–57.

Jarvis, M. F., Burgard, E. C., McGaraughty, S., Honore, P., Lynch, K., Brennan, T. J., et al. (2002). A-317491, a novel potent and selective non-nucleotide antagonist of $P2X_3$ and $P2X_{2/3}$ receptors, reduces chronic inflammatory and neuropathic pain in the rat. *Proceedings of the National Academy of Sciences of the United States of America, 99*, 17179–17184.

Jennings, E. A., & Cho, H.-J. (2007). Peripheral sensitization in migraine-role for P2X purinergic receptors in the dura-vascular sensory pathway. *Drug Development Research, 68*, 321–328.

Jimenez-Andrade, J. M., Mantyh, W. G., Bloom, A. P., Xu, H., Ferng, A. S., Dussor, G., et al. (2010). A phenotypically restricted set of primary afferent nerve fibers innervate the bone versus skin: Therapeutic opportunity for treating skeletal pain. *Bone, 46*, 306–313.

Jo, Y. H., & Schlichter, R. (1999). Synaptic corelease of ATP and GABA in cultured spinal neurons. *Nature Neuroscience, 2*, 241–245.

Joseph, E. K., Green, P. G., Bogen, O., Alvarez, P., & Levine, J. D. (2013). Vascular endothelial cells mediate mechanical stimulation-induced enhancement of endothelin hyperalgesia via activation of $P2X_{2/3}$ receptors on nociceptors. *Journal of Neuroscience, 33*, 2849–2859.

Joseph, E. K., Green, P. G., & Levine, J. D. (2014). ATP release mechanisms of endothelial cell-mediated stimulus-dependent hyperalgesia. *The Journal of Pain, 15*, 771–777.

Kaan, T. K., Yip, P. K., Grist, J., Cefalu, J. S., Nunn, P. A., Ford, A. P., et al. (2010a). Endogenous purinergic control of bladder activity via presynaptic $P2X_3$ and $P2X_{2/3}$ receptors in the spinal cord. *Journal of Neuroscience, 30*, 4503–4507.

Kaan, T. K., Yip, P. K., Patel, S., Davies, M., Marchand, F., Cockayne, D. A., et al. (2010b). Systemic blockade of P2X3 and P2X2/3 receptors attenuates bone cancer pain behaviour in rats. *Brain, 133*, 2549–2564.

Kakimoto, S., Nagakura, Y., Tamura, S., Watabiki, T., Shibasaki, K., Tanaka, S., et al. (2008). Minodronic acid, a third-generation bisphosphonate, antagonizes purinergic $P2X_{2/3}$ receptor function and exerts an analgesic effect in pain models. *European Journal of Pharmacology, 589*, 98–101.

Kataoka, S., Toyono, T., Seta, Y., Ogura, T., & Toyoshima, K. (2004). Expression of $P2Y_1$ receptors in rat taste buds. *Histochemistry and Cell Biology, 121*, 419–426.

Kim, Y. S., Paik, S. K., Cho, Y. S., Shin, H. S., Bae, J. Y., Moritani, M., et al. (2008). Expression of $P2X_3$ receptor in the trigeminal sensory nuclei of the rat. *Journal of Comparative Neurology, 506*, 627–639.

King, B. F., Knowles, I., Burnstock, G., & Ramage, A. (2004). Investigation of the effects of P2 purinoceptor ligands on the micturition reflex in female urethane-anaesthetised rats. *British Journal of Pharmacology, 142*, 519–530.

Kirkup, A. J., Brunsden, A. M., & Grundy, D. (2001). Receptors and transmission in the brain-gut axis: Potential for novel therapies. I. Receptors on visceral afferents. *American Journal of Physiology. Gastrointestinal and Liver Physiology, 280*, G787–G794.

Knight, G. E., Bodin, P., De Groat, W. C., & Burnstock, G. (2002). ATP is released from guinea pig ureter epithelium on distension. *American Journal of Physiology Renal Physiology, 282*, F281–F288.

Kobayashi, K., Takahashi, E., Miyagawa, Y., Yamanaka, H., & Noguchi, K. (2011). Induction of the P2X7 receptor in spinal microglia in a neuropathic pain model. *Neuroscience Letters, 504*, 57–61.

Kobayashi, K., Yamanaka, H., Fukuoka, T., Dai, Y., Obata, K., & Noguchi, K. (2008). $P2Y_{12}$ receptor upregulation in activated microglia is a gateway of p38 signaling and neuropathic pain. *Journal of Neuroscience, 28*, 2892–2902.

Koizumi, S., Fujishita, K., Inoue, K., Shigemoto-Mogami, Y., Tsuda, M., & Inoue, K. (2004). Ca^{2+} waves in keratinocytes are transmitted to sensory neurons: The involvement of extracellular ATP and $P2Y_2$ receptor activation. *Biochemical Journal, 380*, 329–338.

Korboukh, I., Hull-Ryde, E. A., Rittiner, J. E., Randhawa, A. S., Coleman, J., Fitzpatrick, B. J., et al. (2012). Orally active adenosine A_1 receptor agonists with antinociceptive effects in mice. *Journal of Medicinal Chemistry, 55*, 6467–6477.

Krames, E. S. (2014). The role of the dorsal root ganglion in the development of neuropathic pain. *Pain Medicine, 15*, 1669–1685.

Kwon, S. G., Roh, D. H., Yoon, S. Y., Moon, J. Y., Choi, S. R., Choi, H. S., et al. (2014). Blockade of peripheral P2Y1 receptors prevents the induction of thermal hyperalgesia via modulation of TRPV1 expression in carrageenan-induced inflammatory pain rats: Involvement of p38 MAPK phosphorylation in DRGs. *Neuropharmacology, 79*, 368–379.

Lakshmi, S., & Joshi, P. G. (2005). Co-activation of $P2Y_2$ receptor and TRPV channel by ATP: Implications for ATP induced pain. *Cell and Molecular Neurobiology, 25*, 819–832.

Lazarowski, E. R. (2012). Vesicular and conductive mechanisms of nucleotide release. *Purinergic Signalling, 8*, 359–373.

Lazzeri, M. (2006). The physiological function of the urothelium—More than a simple barrier. *Urology International*, *76*, 289–295.

Lee, H. Y., Bardini, M., & Burnstock, G. (2000). Distribution of P2X receptors in the urinary bladder and the ureter of the rat. *Journal of Urology*, *163*, 2002–2007.

Lemaire, I., & Leduc, N. (2004). Purinergic $P2X_7$ receptor function in lung alveolar macrophages: Pharmacologic characterisation and bidirectional regulation by Th1 and Th2 cytokines. *Drug Development Research*, *59*, 118–127.

Lewis, C., Neidhart, S., Holy, C., North, R. A., Buell, G., & Surprenant, A. (1995). Coexpression of $P2X_2$ and $P2X_3$ receptor subunits can account for ATP-gated currents in sensory neurons. *Nature*, *377*, 432–435.

Li, J., & Sinoway, L. I. (2002). ATP stimulates chemically sensitive and sensitizes mechanically sensitive afferents. *American Journal of Physiology Heart and Circulatory Physiology*, *283*, H2636–H2643.

Li, X., Zhang, J., Gao, Y., Yang, Y., Xu, C., Li, G., et al. (2011). Puerarin alleviates burn-related procedural pain mediated by P2X $_3$ receptors. *Purinergic Signalling*, *7*, 489–497.

Liang, S., Xu, C., Li, G., & Gao, Y. (2010). P2X receptors and modulation of pain transmission: Focus on effects of drugs and compounds used in traditional Chinese medicine. *Neurochemistry International*, *57*, 705–712.

Lim, J. C., & Mitchell, C. H. (2012). Inflammation, pain, and pressure-purinergic signaling in oral tissues. *Journal of Dental Research*, *91*, 1103–1109.

Lin, C. L., Fu, Y. S., Hsiao, T. H., & Hsieh, Y. L. (2013). Enhancement of purinergic signalling by excessive endogenous ATP in resiniferatoxin (RTX) neuropathy. *Purinergic Signalling*, *9*, 249–257.

Lin, J., Li, G., Den, X., Xu, C., Liu, S., Gao, Y., et al. (2010). VEGF and its receptor-2 involved in neuropathic pain transmission mediated by $P2X_{2/3}$ receptor of primary sensory neurons. *Brain Research Bulletin*, *83*, 284–291.

Little, J. W., Ford, A., Symons-Liguori, A. M., Chen, Z., Janes, K., Doyle, T., et al. (2015). Endogenous adenosine A_3 receptor activation selectively alleviates persistent pain states. *Brain*, *138*, 28–35.

Liu, M., Yang, H., Fang, D., Yang, J. J., Cai, J., Wan, Y., et al. (2013). Upregulation of P2X3 receptors by neuronal calcium sensor protein VILIP-1 in dorsal root ganglions contributes to the bone cancer pain in rats. *Pain*, *154*, 1551–1568.

Llaudet, E., Hatz, S., Droniou, M., & Dale, N. (2005). Microelectrode biosensor for real-time measurement of ATP in biological tissue. *Analytical Chemistry*, 77, 3267–3273.

Loram, L. C., Harrison, J. A., Sloane, E. M., Hutchinson, M. R., Sholar, P., Taylor, F. R., et al. (2009). Enduring reversal of neuropathic pain by a single intrathecal injection of adenosine 2A receptor agonists: A novel therapy for neuropathic pain. *Journal of Neuroscience*, *29*, 14015–14025.

Lu, Y., Jiang, Q., Yu, L. H., Su, D. F., Burnstock, G., & Ma, B. (2013). 17β-Estradiol rapidly attenuates P2X3 receptor-mediated peripheral pain signal transduction via ER and GPR30. *Endocrinology*, *154*, 2421–2433.

Lu, Z. J., Miao, X. R., Wu, J. X., Wang, X. Y., Miao, Q., & Yu, W. F. (2010). Acute PAR2 activation reduces α, β-MeATP sensitive currents in rat dorsal root ganglion neurons. *Neuroreport*, *21*, 227–232.

Ma, B., Yu, L., Fan, J., Cong, B., He, P., Ni, X., et al. (2011). Estrogen modulation of peripheral pain signal transduction: Involvement of $P2X_3$ receptors. *Purinergic Signalling*, 7, 73–83.

Mackenzie, I., Burnstock, G., & Dolly, J. O. (1982). The effects of purified botulinum neurotoxin type A on cholinergic, adrenergic and non-adrenergic, atropine-resistant autonomic neuromuscular transmission. *Neuroscience*, 7, 997–1006.

Maehara, Y., Kusumoto, H., Anai, H., Kusumoto, T., & Sugimachi, K. (1987). Human tumor tissues have higher ATP contents than normal tissues. *Clinica Chimica Acta, 169*, 341–343.

Magni, G., & Ceruti, S. (2014). The purinergic system and glial cells: Emerging costars in nociception. *BioMed Research International, 2014*, 495789.

Makowska, A., Panfil, C., & Ellrich, J. (2006). ATP induces sustained facilitation of craniofacial nociception through P2X receptors on neck muscle nociceptors in mice. *Cephalalgia, 26*, 697–706.

Malin, S. A., & Molliver, D. C. (2010). Gi- and Gq-coupled ADP (P2Y) receptors act in opposition to modulate nociceptive signaling and inflammatory pain behavior. *Molecular Pain, 6*, 21.

Mantyh, P. W., Clohisy, D. R., Koltzenburg, M., & Hunt, S. P. (2002). Molecular mechanisms of cancer pain. *Nature Reviews Cancer, 2*, 201–209.

Martins, D. F., Mazzardo-Martins, L., Cidral-Filho, F. J., Stramosk, J., & Santos, A. R. (2013). Ankle joint mobilization affects postoperative pain through peripheral and central adenosine A_1 receptors. *Physical Therapy, 93*, 401–412.

Massicot, F., Hache, G., David, L., Chen, D., Leuxe, C., Garnier-Legrand, L., et al. (2013). P2X7 cell death receptor activation and mitochondrial impairment in oxaliplatin-induced apoptosis and neuronal injury: Cellular mechanisms and *in vivo* approach. *PLoS One, 8*, e66830.

Masterson, C. G., & Durham, P. L. (2010). DHE repression of ATP-mediated sensitization of trigeminal ganglion neurons. *Headache, 50*, 1424–1439.

Masuda, T., Iwamoto, S., Yoshinaga, R., Tozaki-Saitoh, H., Nishiyama, A., Mak, T. W., et al. (2014). Transcription factor IRF5 drives $P2X4R^+$-reactive microglia gating neuropathic pain. *Nature Communications, 5*, 3771.

McGaraughty, S., Chu, K. L., Namovic, M. T., Donnelly-Roberts, D. L., Harris, R. R., Zhang, X. F., et al. (2007). $P2X_7$-related modulation of pathological nociception in rats. *Neuroscience, 146*, 1817–1828.

McGaraughty, S., Honore, P., Wismer, C. T., Mikusa, J., Zhu, C. Z., McDonald, H. A., et al. (2005). Endogenous opioid mechanisms partially mediate $P2X_3/P2X_{2/3}$-related antinociception in rat models of inflammatory and chemogenic pain but not neuropathic pain. *British Journal of Pharmacology, 146*, 180–188.

McGaraughty, S., & Jarvis, M. F. (2006). Purinergic control of neuropathic pain. *Drug Development Research, 67*, 376–388.

Millward-Sadler, S. J., Wright, M. O., Flatman, P. W., & Salter, D. M. (2004). ATP in the mechanotransduction pathway of normal human chondrocytes. *Biorheology, 41*, 567–575.

Mizumoto, N., Mummert, M. E., Shalhevet, D., & Takashima, A. (2003). Keratinocyte ATP release assay for testing skin-irritating potentials of structurally diverse chemicals. *Journal of Investigative Dermatology, 121*, 1066–1072.

Mo, G., Peleshok, J. C., Cao, C. Q., Ribeiro-da-Silva, A., & Séguéla, P. (2013). Control of P2X3 channel function by metabotropic P2Y2 UTP receptors in primary sensory neurons. *Molecular Pharmacology, 83*, 640–647.

Montana, V., Malarkey, E. B., Verderio, C., Matteoli, M., & Parpura, V. (2006). Vesicular transmitter release from astrocytes. *Glia, 54*, 700–715.

Morita, K., Morioka, N., Abdin, J., Kitayama, S., Nakata, Y., & Dohi, T. (2004). Development of tactile allodynia and thermal hyperalgesia by intrathecally administered platelet-activating factor in mice. *Pain, 111*, 351–359.

Moriyama, T., Iida, T., Kobayashi, K., Higashi, T., Fukuoka, T., Tsumura, H., et al. (2003). Possible involvement of $P2Y_2$ metabotropic receptors in ATP-induced transient receptor potential vanilloid receptor 1-mediated thermal hypersensitivity. *Journal of Neuroscience, 23*, 6058–6062.

Mørk, H., Ashina, M., Bendtsen, L., Olesen, J., & Jensen, R. (2003). Experimental muscle pain and tenderness following infusion of endogenous substances in humans. *European Journal of Pain, 7*, 145–153.

Moynes, D. M., Lucas, G. H., Beyak, M. J., & Lomax, A. E. (2014). Effects of inflammation on the innervation of the colon. *Toxicologic Pathology, 42*, 111–117.

Nagamine, K., Ozaki, N., Shinoda, M., Asai, H., Nishiguchi, H., Mitsudo, K., et al. (2006). Mechanical allodynia and thermal hyperalgesia induced by experimental squamous cell carcinoma of the lower gingiva in rats. *The Journal of Pain, 7*, 659–670.

Nagata, K., Imai, T., Yamashita, T., Tsuda, M., Tozaki-Saitoh, H., & Inoue, K. (2009). Antidepressants inhibit $P2X_4$ receptor function: A possible involvement in neuropathic pain relief. *Molecular Pain, 5*, 20.

Nair, A., Simonetti, M., Birsa, N., Ferrari, M. D., van den Maagdenberg, A. M., Giniatullin, R., et al. (2010). Familial hemiplegic migraine $Ca_v2.1$ channel mutation R192Q enhances ATP-gated $P2X_3$ receptor activity of mouse sensory ganglion neurons mediating trigeminal pain. *Molecular Pain, 6*, 48.

Nakagawa, T., Wakamatsu, K., Zhang, N., Maeda, S., Minami, M., Satoh, M., et al. (2007). Intrathecal administration of ATP produces long-lasting allodynia in rats: Differential mechanisms in the phase of the induction and maintenance. *Neuroscience, 147*, 445–455.

Nakamura, M., Mie, M., Funabashi, H., Yamamoto, K., Ando, J., & Kobatake, E. (2006). Cell-surface-localized ATP detection with immobilized firefly luciferase. *Analytical Biochemistry, 352*, 61–67.

Nakatsuka, T., & Gu, J. G. (2006). P2X purinoceptors and sensory transmission. *Pflügers Archives—European Journal of Physiology, 452*, 598–607.

Nakayama, S., Yamashita, T., Konishi, M., Kazama, H., & Kokubun, S. (2004). P2Y-mediated Ca^{2+} response is spatiotemporally graded and synchronized in sensory neurons: A two-photon photolysis study. *FASEB Journal, 18*, 1562–1564.

Namasivayam, S., Eardley, I., & Morrison, J. F. B. (1999). Purinergic sensory neurotransmission in the urinary bladder: An *in vitro* study in the rat. *BJU International, 84*, 854–860.

Nelson, D. W., Gregg, R. J., Kort, M. E., Perez-Medrano, A., Voight, E. A., Wang, Y., et al. (2006). Structure-activity relationship studies on a series of novel, substituted 1-benzyl-5-phenyltetrazole $P2X_7$ antagonists. *Journal of Medicinal Chemistry, 49*, 3659–3666.

Nelson, D. W., Sarris, K., Kalvin, D. M., Namovic, M. T., Grayson, G., Donnelly-Roberts, D. L., et al. (2008). Structure-activity relationship studies on N'-aryl carbohydrazide $P2X_7$ antagonists. *Journal of Medicinal Chemistry, 51*, 3030–3034.

Nicke, A., Baumert, H. G., Rettinger, J., Eichele, A., Lambrecht, G., Mutschler, E., et al. (1998). $P2X_1$ and $P2X_3$ receptors form stable trimers: A novel structural motif of ligand-gated ion channels. *EMBO Journal, 17*, 3016–3028.

Noguchi, K., & Okubo, M. (2011). Leukotrienes in nociceptive pathway and neuropathic/inflammatory pain. *Biological & Pharmaceutical Bulletin, 34*, 1163–1169.

North, R. A. (2002). Molecular physiology of P2X receptors. *Physiological Reviews, 82*, 1013–1067.

Ochi-ishi, R., Nagata, K., Inoue, T., Tozaki-Saitoh, H., Tsuda, M., & Inoue, K. (2014). Involvement of the chemokine CCL3 and the purinoceptor P2X7 in the spinal cord in paclitaxel-induced mechanical allodynia. *Molecular Pain, 10*, 53.

Ochoa-Cortes, F., Liñán-Rico, A., Jacobson, K. A., & Christofi, F. L. (2014). Potential for developing purinergic drugs for gastrointestinal diseases. *Inflammatory Bowel Disease, 20*, 1259–1287.

Okada, M., Nakagawa, T., Minami, M., & Satoh, M. (2002). Analgesic effects of intrathecal administration of P2Y nucleotide receptor agonists UTP and UDP in normal and neuropathic pain model rats. *Journal of Pharmacology and Experimental Therapeutics, 303*, 66–73.

Oliveira, M. C., Parada, C. A., Veiga, M. C., Rodrigues, L. R., Barros, S. P., & Tambeli, C. H. (2005). Evidence for the involvement of endogenous ATP and P2X receptors in TMJ pain. *European Journal of Pain*, *9*, 87–93.
Oliveira, M. C., Pelegrini-da-Silva, A., Tambeli, C. H., & Parada, C. A. (2009). Peripheral mechanisms underlying the essential role of P2X3,2/3 receptors in the development of inflammatory hyperalgesia. *Pain*, *141*, 127–134.
Otoshi, K., Kikuchi, S., Konno, S., & Sekiguchi, M. (2010). The reactions of glial cells and endoneurial macrophages in the dorsal root ganglion and their contribution to pain-related behavior after application of nucleus pulposus onto the nerve root in rats. *Spine*, *35*, 264–271.
Ou, S., Zhao, Y. D., Xiao, Z., Wen, H. Z., Cui, J., & Ruan, H. Z. (2011). Effect of lappaconitine on neuropathic pain mediated by $P2X_3$ receptor in rat dorsal root ganglion. *Neurochemistry International*, *58*, 564–573.
Page, A. J., Martin, C. M., & Blackshaw, L. A. (2002). Vagal mechanoreceptors and chemoreceptors in mouse stomach and esophagus. *Journal of Neurophysiology*, *87*, 2095–2103.
Page, A. J., O'Donnell, T. A., & Blackshaw, L. A. (2000). P2X purinoceptor-induced sensitization of ferret vagal mechanoreceptors in oesophageal inflammation. *Journal of Physiology (London)*, *523*, 403–411.
Pandita, R. K., & Andersson, K. E. (2002). Intravesical adenosine triphosphate stimulates the micturition reflex in awake, freely moving rats. *Journal of Urology*, *168*, 1230–1234.
Pankratov, Y., Lalo, U., Verkhratsky, A., & North, R. A. (2006). Vesicular release of ATP at central synapses. *Pflügers Archives—European Journal of Physiology*, *452*, 589–597.
Paoletta, S., Tosh, D. K., Finley, A., Gizewski, E. T., Moss, S. M., Gao, Z. G., et al. (2013). Rational design of sulfonated A_3 adenosine receptor-selective nucleosides as pharmacological tools to study chronic neuropathic pain. *Journal of Medicinal Chemistry*, *56*, 5949–5963.
Park, C. K., Bae, J. H., Kim, H. Y., Jo, H. J., Kim, Y. H., Jung, S. J., et al. (2010). Substance P sensitizes P2X3 in nociceptive trigeminal neurons. *Journal of Dental Research*, *89*, 1154–1159.
Pelleg, A., & Hurt, C. M. (1990). Evidence for ATP-triggered vagal reflex in the canine heart in vivo. *Annals of the New York Academy of Sciences*, *603*, 441–442.
Persson, A. K., Xu, X. J., Wiesenfeld-Hallin, Z., Devor, M., & Fried, K. (2010). Expression of DRG candidate pain molecules after nerve injury—A comparative study among five inbred mouse strains with contrasting pain phenotypes. *Journal of the Peripheral Nervous System*, *15*, 26–39.
Pinto, R., Lopes, T., Frias, B., Silva, A., Silva, J. A., Silva, C. M., et al. (2010). Trigonal injection of botulinum toxin A in patients with refractory bladder pain syndrome/interstitial cystitis. *European Urology*, *58*, 360–365.
Ralevic, V., & Burnstock, G. (1998). Receptors for purines and pyrimidines. *Pharmacological Reviews*, *50*, 413–492.
Raouf, R., Chabot-Doré, A. J., Ase, A. R., Blais, D., & Séguéla, P. (2007). Differential regulation of microglial $P2X_4$ and $P2X_7$ ATP receptors following LPS-induced activation. *Neuropharmacology*, *53*, 496–504.
Renton, T., Yiangou, Y., Baecker, P. A., Ford, A. P., & Anand, P. (2003). Capsaicin receptor VR1 and ATP purinoceptor $P2X_3$ in painful and nonpainful human tooth pulp. *Journal of Orofacial Pain*, *17*, 245–250.
Rich, P. B., Douillet, C. D., Mahler, S. A., Husain, S. A., & Boucher, R. C. (2003). Adenosine triphosphate is released during injurious mechanical ventilation and contributes to lung edema. *Journal of Trauma*, *55*, 290–297.
Ristić, D., & Ellrich, J. (2012). P2X7 receptor blockade reverses purinergic facilitation of neck muscle nociception in mice. *Cephalalgia*, *32*, 544–553.

Romagnoli, R., Baraldi, P. G., Carrion, M. D., Cara, C. L., Preti, D., Cruz-Lopez, O., et al. (2007). From tyrosine to glycine: Synthesis and biological activity of potent antagonists of the purinergic $P2X_7$ receptor. *Journal of Medicinal Chemistry, 50*, 3706–3715.

Romagnoli, R., Baraldi, P. G., Cruz-Lopez, O., Lopez-Cara, C., Preti, D., Borea, P. A., et al. (2008). The $P2X_7$ receptor as a therapeutic target. *Expert Opinion on Therapeutic Targets, 12*, 647–661.

Romanello, M., Codognotto, A., Bicego, M., Pines, A., Tell, G., & D'Andrea, P. (2005). Autocrine/paracrine stimulation of purinergic receptors in osteoblasts: Contribution of vesicular ATP release. *Biochemical and Biophysical Research Communications, 331*, 1429–1438.

Rong, W., & Burnstock, G. (2004). Activation of ureter nociceptors by exogenous and endogenous ATP in guinea pig. *Neuropharmacology, 47*, 1093–1101.

Rong, W., Burnstock, G., & Spyer, K. M. (2000). P2X purinoceptor-mediated excitation of trigeminal lingual nerve terminals in an *in vitro* intra-arterially perfused rat tongue preparation. *Journal of Physiology, 524*, 891–902.

Rong, W., Keating, C., Sun, B., Dong, L., & Grundy, D. (2009). Purinergic contribution to small intestinal afferent hypersensitivity in a murine model of postinfectious bowel disease. *Neurogastroenterology and Motility, 21*(665–71), e32.

Rong, W., Spyer, M., & Burnstock, G. (2002). Activation and sensitisation of low and high threshold afferent fibres mediated by P2X receptors in the mouse urinary bladder. *Journal of Physiology, 541*, 591–600.

Ruan, H.-Z., & Burnstock, G. (2003). Localisation of $P2Y_1$ and $P2Y_4$ receptors in dorsal root, nodose and trigeminal ganglia of the rat. *Histochemistry and Cell Biology, 120*, 415–426.

Ruan, T., Lin, Y. S., Lin, K. S., & Kou, Y. R. (2005). Sensory transduction of pulmonary reactive oxygen species by capsaicin-sensitive vagal lung afferent fibres in rats. *Journal of Physiology, 565*, 563–578.

Salter, M. W., & Henry, J. L. (1985). Effects of adenosine 5′-monophosphate and adenosine 5′-triphosphate on functionally identified units in the cat spinal dorsal horn. Evidence for a differential effect of adenosine 5′-triphosphate on nociceptive vs non-nociceptive units. *Neuroscience, 15*, 815–825.

Sawynok, J., & Liu, X. J. (2003). Adenosine in the spinal cord and periphery: Release and regulation of pain. *Progress in Neurobiology, 69*, 313–340.

Scemes, E., Suadicani, S. O., Dahl, G., & Spray, D. C. (2007). Connexin and pannexin mediated cell-cell communication. *Neuron Glia Biology, 3*, 199–201.

Schock, S. C., Munyao, N., Yakubchyk, Y., Sabourin, L. A., Hakim, A. M., Ventureyra, E. C., et al. (2007). Cortical spreading depression releases ATP into the extracellular space and purinergic receptor activation contributes to the induction of ischemic tolerance. *Brain Research, 1168*, 129–138.

Seino, D., Tokunaga, A., Tachibana, T., Yoshiya, S., Dai, Y., Obata, K., et al. (2006). The role of ERK signaling and the P2X receptor on mechanical pain evoked by movement of inflamed knee joint. *Pain, 123*, 193–203.

Selden, N. R., Carlson, J. D., Cetas, J., Close, L. N., & Heinricher, M. M. (2007). Purinergic actions on neurons that modulate nociception in the rostral ventromedial medulla. *Neuroscience, 146*, 1808–1816.

Seo, H. S., Roh, D. H., Kwon, S. G., Yoon, S. Y., Kang, S. Y., Moon, J. Y., et al. (2011). Acidic pH facilitates peripheral α, βmeATP-mediated nociception in rats: Differential roles of P2X, P2Y, ASIC and TRPV1 receptors in ATP-induced mechanical allodynia and thermal hyperalgesia. *Neuropharmacology, 60*, 580–586.

Shapiro, R. E. (2007). Caffeine and headaches. *Neurological Sciences, 28*(Suppl. 2), S179–S183.

Sharp, C. J., Reeve, A. J., Collins, S. D., Martindale, J. C., Summerfield, S. G., Sargent, B. S., et al. (2006). Investigation into the role of $P2X_3/P2X_{2/3}$ receptors in neuropathic pain

following chronic constriction injury in the rat: An electrophysiological study. *British Journal of Pharmacology, 148*, 845–852.
Shemon, A. N., Sluyter, R., Conigrave, A. D., & Wiley, J. S. (2004). Chelerythrine and other benzophenanthridine alkaloids block the human $P2X_7$ receptor. *British Journal of Pharmacology, 142*, 1015–1019.
Shibukawa, Y., Sato, M., Kimura, M., Sobhan, U., Shimada, M., Nishiyama, A., et al. (2015). Odontoblasts as sensory receptors: Transient receptor potential channels, pannexin-1, and ionotropic ATP receptors mediate intercellular odontoblast-neuron signal transduction. *Pflügers Archives—European Journal of Physiology, 467*, 843–863.
Shieh, C. C., Jarvis, M. F., Lee, H., & Perner, R. J. (2006). P2X receptor ligands and pain. *Expert Opinion on Therapeutic Patents, 16*, 1113–1127.
Shinoda, M., Feng, B., & Gebhart, G. F. (2009). Peripheral and central $P2X_3$ receptor contributions to colon mechanosensitivity and hypersensitivity in the mouse. *Gastroenterology, 137*, 2096–2104.
Shinoda, M., & Iwata, K. (2013). Neural communication in the trigeminal ganglion contributes to ectopic orofacial pain. *Journal of Oral Biosciences, 55*, 165–168.
Shinoda, M., La, J. H., Bielefeldt, K., & Gebhart, G. F. (2010). Altered purinergic signaling in colorectal dorsal root ganglion neurons contributes to colorectal hypersensitivity. *Journal of Neurophysiology, 104*, 3113–3123.
Shinoda, M., Ozaki, N., Asai, H., Nagamine, K., & Sugiura, Y. (2005). Changes in $P2X_3$ receptor expression in the trigeminal ganglion following monoarthritis of the temporomandibular joint in rats. *Pain, 116*, 42–51.
Shinoda, M., Ozaki, N., & Sugiura, Y. (2008). Involvement of ATP and its receptors on nociception in rat model of masseter muscle pain. *Pain, 134*, 148–157.
Smith, H. S. (2010). Activated microglia in nociception. *Pain Physician, 13*, 295–304.
Smith, C. P., Vemulakonda, V. M., Kiss, S., Boone, T. B., & Somogyi, G. T. (2005). Enhanced ATP release from rat bladder urothelium during chronic bladder inflammation: Effect of botulinum toxin A. *Neurochemistry International, 47*, 291–297.
Sowa, N. A., Voss, M. K., & Zylka, M. J. (2010). Recombinant ecto-5′-nucleotidase (CD73) has long lasting antinociceptive effects that are dependent on adenosine A_1 receptor activation. *Molecular Pain, 6*, 20.
Stone, L. S., & Vulchanova, L. (2003). The pain of antisense: In vivo application of antisense oligonucleotides for functional genomics in pain and analgesia. *Advanced Drug Delivery Reviews, 55*, 1081–1112.
Stucky, C. L., Medler, K. A., & Molliver, D. C. (2004). The P2Y agonist UTP activates cutaneous afferent fibers. *Pain, 109*, 36–44.
Sui, G. P., Wu, C., & Fry, C. H. (2006). Characterization of the purinergic receptor subtype on Guinea-pig suburothelial myofibroblasts. *BJU International, 97*, 1327–1331.
Suzuki, T., Namba, K., Tsuga, H., & Nakata, H. (2006). Regulation of pharmacology by hetero-oligomerization between A_1 adenosine receptor and $P2Y_2$ receptor. *Biochemical and Biophysical Research Communications, 351*, 559–565.
Syhr, K. M., Kallenborn-Gerhardt, W., Lu, R., Olbrich, K., Schmitz, K., Männich, J., et al. (2014). Lack of effect of a P2Y6 receptor antagonist on neuropathic pain behavior in mice. *Pharmacology, Biochemistry, and Behaviour, 124*, 389–395.
Taiwo, Y. O., & Levine, J. D. (1990). Direct cutaneous hyperalgesia induced by adenosine. *Neuroscience, 38*, 757–762.
Takenouchi, T., Ogihara, K., Sato, M., & Kitani, H. (2005). Inhibitory effects of U73122 and U73343 on Ca^{2+} influx and pore formation induced by the activation of $P2X_7$ nucleotide receptors in mouse microglial cell line. *Biochimica et Biophysica Acta, 1726*, 177–186.
Taylor, A. M., & Ribeiro-da-Silva, A. (2011). GDNF levels in the lower lip skin in a rat model of trigeminal neuropathic pain: Implications for nonpeptidergic fiber reinnervation and parasympathetic sprouting. *Pain, 152*, 1502–1510.

Teixeira, J. M., de Oliveira-Fusaro, M. C., Parada, C. A., & Tambeli, C. H. (2014). Peripheral P2X7 receptor-induced mechanical hyperalgesia is mediated by bradykinin. *Neuroscience*, *277*, 163–173.
Teixeira, J. M., Oliveira, M. C., Nociti, F. H., Jr., Clemente-Napimoga, J. T., Pelegrini-da-Silva, A., Parada, C. A., et al. (2010a). Involvement of temporomandibular joint P2X3 and P2X2/3 receptors in carrageenan-induced inflammatory hyperalgesia in rats. *European Journal of Pharmacology*, *645*, 79–85.
Teixeira, J. M., Oliveira, M. C., Parada, C. A., & Tambeli, C. H. (2010b). Peripheral mechanisms underlying the essential role of P2X7 receptors in the development of inflammatory hyperalgesia. *European Journal of Pharmacology*, *644*, 55–60.
Tian, M., Abdelrahman, A., Weinhausen, S., Hinz, S., Weyer, S., Dosa, S., et al. (2014). Carbamazepine derivatives with P2X4 receptor-blocking activity. *Bioorganic & Medicinal Chemistry*, *22*, 1077–1088.
Tozaki-Saitoh, H., Tsuda, M., Miyata, H., Ueda, K., Kohsaka, S., & Inoue, K. (2008). $P2Y_{12}$ receptors in spinal microglia are required for neuropathic pain after peripheral nerve injury. *Journal of Neuroscience*, *28*, 4949–4956.
Trang, T., Beggs, S., & Salter, M. W. (2006). Purinoceptors in microglia and neuropathic pain. *Pflügers Archives—European Journal of Physiology*, *452*, 645–652.
Trang, T., Beggs, S., & Salter, M. W. (2011). Brain-derived neurotrophic factor from microglia: A molecular substrate for neuropathic pain. *Neuron Glia Biology*, *7*, 99–108.
Trang, T., & Salter, M. W. (2012). P2X4 purinoceptor signaling in chronic pain. *Purinergic Signalling*, *8*, 621–628.
Tsuda, M., Beggs, S., Salter, M. W., & Inoue, K. (2013). Microglia and intractable chronic pain. *Glia*, *61*, 55–61.
Tsuda, M., Hasegawa, S., & Inoue, K. (2007). P2X receptors-mediated cytosolic phospholipase A2 activation in primary afferent sensory neurons contributes to neuropathic pain. *Journal of Neurochemistry*, *103*, 1408–1416.
Tsuda, M., Inoue, K., & Salter, M. W. (2005). Neuropathic pain and spinal microglia: A big problem from molecules in "small" glia. *Trends in Neurosciences*, *28*, 101–107.
Tsuda, M., Masuda, T., Tozaki-Saitoh, H., & Inoue, K. (2013). P2X4 receptors and neuropathic pain. *Frontiers in Cellular Neuroscience*, *7*, 191.
Tsuda, M., Mizokoshi, A., Shigemoto-Mogami, Y., Koizumi, S., & Inoue, K. (2004). Activation of p38 mitogen-activated protein kinase in spinal hyperactive microglia contributes to pain hypersensitivity following peripheral nerve injury. *Glia*, *45*, 89–95.
Tsuda, M., Shigemoto-Mogami, Y., Koizumi, S., Mizokoshi, A., Kohsaka, S., Salter, M. W., et al. (2003). $P2X_4$ receptors induced in spinal microglia gate tactile allodynia after nerve injury. *Nature*, *424*, 778–783.
Tsuda, M., Toyomitsu, E., Komatsu, T., Masuda, T., Kunifusa, E., Nasu-Tada, K., et al. (2008). Fibronectin/integrin system is involved in $P2X_4$ receptor upregulation in the spinal cord and neuropathic pain after nerve injury. *Glia*, *56*, 579–585.
Tsuda, M., Tozaki-Saitoh, H., & Inoue, K. (2010). Pain and purinergic signaling. *Brain Research Reviews*, *63*, 222–232.
Tsuda, M., Tozaki-Saitoh, H., & Inoue, K. (2012). Purinergic system, microglia and neuropathic pain. *Current Opinion in Pharmacology*, *12*, 74–79.
Tsuda, M., Tozaki-Saitoh, H., Masuda, T., Toyomitsu, E., Tezuka, T., Yamamoto, T., et al. (2008). Lyn tyrosine kinase is required for $P2X_4$ receptor upregulation and neuropathic pain after peripheral nerve injury. *Glia*, *56*, 50–58.
Tsuda, M., Ueno, S., & Inoue, K. (1999). In vivo pathway of thermal hyperalgesia by intrathecal administration of α, β-methylene ATP in mouse spinal cord: Involvement of the glutamate-NMDA receptor system. *British Journal of Pharmacology*, *127*, 449–456.
Ueno, S., Moriyama, T., Honda, K., Kamiya, H., Sakurada, T., & Katsuragi, T. (2003). Involvement of $P2X_2$ and $P2X_3$ receptors in neuropathic pain in a mouse model of chronic constriction injury. *Drug Development Research*, *59*, 104–111.

Ulmann, L., Hatcher, J. P., Hughes, J. P., Chaumont, S., Green, P. J., Conquet, F., et al. (2008). Up-regulation of P2X$_4$ receptors in spinal microglia after peripheral nerve injury mediates BDNF release and neuropathic pain. *Journal of Neuroscience, 28*, 11263–11268.

Ulmann, L., Hirbec, H., & Rassendren, F. (2010). P2X4 receptors mediate PGE2 release by tissue-resident macrophages and initiate inflammatory pain. *EMBO Journal, 29*, 2290–2300.

Ursu, D., Ebert, P., Langron, E., Ruble, C., Munsie, L., Zou, W., et al. (2014). Gain and loss of function of P2X$_7$ receptors: Mechanisms, pharmacology and relevance to diabetic neuropathic pain. *Molecular Pain, 10*, 37.

Vincenzi, F., Targa, M., Romagnoli, R., Merighi, S., Gessi, S., Baraldi, P. G., et al. (2014). TRR469, a potent A$_1$ adenosine receptor allosteric modulator, exhibits anti-nociceptive properties in acute and neuropathic pain models in mice. *Neuropharmacology, 81*, 6–14.

Vlaskovska, M., Kasakov, L., Rong, W., Bodin, P., Bardini, M., Cockayne, D. A., et al. (2001). P2X$_3$ knockout mice reveal a major sensory role for urothelially released ATP. *Journal of Neuroscience, 21*, 5670–5677.

Volonté, C., Amadio, S., D'Ambrosi, N., Colpi, M., & Burnstock, G. (2006). P2 receptor web: Complexity and fine-tuning. *Pharmacology and Therapeutics, 112*, 264–280.

Vulchanova, L., Arvidsson, U., Riedl, M., Wang, J., Buell, G., Surprenant, A., et al. (1996). Differential distribution of two ATP-gated channels (P2X receptors) determined by immunocytochemistry. *Proceedings of the National Academy of Sciences of the United States of America, 93*, 8063–8067.

Vulchanova, L., Olson, T. H., Stone, L. S., Riedl, M. S., Elde, R., & Honda, C. N. (2001). Cytotoxic targeting of isolectin IB4-binding sensory neurons. *Neuroscience, 108*, 143–155.

Vulchanova, L., Riedl, M. S., Shuster, S. J., Stone, L. S., Hargreaves, K. M., Buell, G., et al. (1998). P2X$_3$ is expressed by DRG neurons that terminate in inner lamina II. *European Journal of Neuroscience, 10*, 3470–3478.

Waeber, C., & Moskowitz, M. A. (2003). Therapeutic implications of central and peripheral neurologic mechanisms in migraine. *Neurology, 61*, S9–20.

Wall, M. J., & Dale, N. (2007). Auto-inhibition of rat parallel fibre-Purkinje cell synapses by activity-dependent adenosine release. *Journal of Physiology, 581*, 553–565.

Wang, Y., Li, G., Liang, S., Zhang, A., Xu, C., Gao, Y., et al. (2008). Role of P2X$_3$ receptor in myocardial ischemia injury and nociceptive sensory transmission. *Autonomic Neuroscience, 139*, 30–37.

Wang, Y., Zhang, X., Guo, Q. L., Zou, W. Y., Huang, C. S., & Yan, J. Q. (2010). Cyclooxygenase inhibitors suppress the expression of P2X$_3$ receptors in the DRG and attenuate hyperalgesia following chronic constriction injury in rats. *Neuroscience Letters, 478*, 77–81.

Wirkner, K., Sperlágh, B., & Illes, P. (2007). P2X$_3$ receptor involvement in pain states. *Molecular Neurobiology, 36*, 165–183.

Wynn, G., Bei, M., Ruan, H.-Z., & Burnstock, G. (2004). Purinergic component of mechanosensory transduction is increased in a rat model of colitis. *American Journal of Physiology Gastrointestinal and Liver Physiology, 287*, G647–G657.

Wynn, G., & Burnstock, G. (2006). Adenosine 5′-triphosphate and it's relationship with other mediators that activate pelvic afferent neurons in the rat colorectum. *Purinergic Signalling, 2*, 517–526.

Wynn, G., Rong, W., Xiang, Z., & Burnstock, G. (2003). Purinergic mechanisms contribute to mechanosensory transduction in the rat colorectum. *Gastroenterology, 125*, 1398–1409.

Xia, H., Zhang, D., Yang, S., Wang, Y., Xu, L., Wu, J., et al. (2014). Role of ATP-sensitive potassium channels in modulating nociception in rat model of bone cancer pain. *Brain Research, 1554*, 29–35.

Xiang, Z., Xiong, Y., Yan, N., Li, X., Mao, Y., Ni, X., et al. (2008). Functional up-regulation of P2X$_3$ receptors in the chronically compressed dorsal root ganglia. *Pain, 140*, 23–34.

Xiao, H. S., Huang, Q. H., Zhang, F. X., Bao, L., Lu, Y. J., Guo, C., et al. (2002). Identification of gene expression profile of dorsal root ganglion in the rat peripheral axotomy model of neuropathic pain. *Proceedings of the National Academy of Sciences of the United States of America*, *99*, 8360–8365.

Xu, J., Chu, K. L., Brederson, J. D., Jarvis, M. F., & McGaraughty, S. (2012). Spontaneous firing and evoked responses of spinal nociceptive neurons are attenuated by blockade of P2X3 and P2X2/3 receptors in inflamed rats. *Journal of Neuroscience Research*, *90*, 1597–1606.

Xu, G. Y., & Huang, L. Y. (2002). Peripheral inflammation sensitizes P2X receptor-mediated responses in rat dorsal root ganglion neurons. *Journal of Neuroscience*, *22*, 93–102.

Xu, J., Kussmaul, W., Kurnik, P. B., Al-Ahdav, M., & Pelleg, A. (2005). Electrophysiological-anatomic correlates of ATP-triggered vagal reflex in the dog. V. Role of purinergic receptors. *American Journal of Physiology Regulatory, Integrative and Comparative Physiology*, *288*, R651–R655.

Xu, G. Y., Shenoy, M., Winston, J. H., Mittal, S., & Pasricha, P. J. (2008). P2X receptor-mediated visceral hyperalgesia in a rat model of chronic visceral hypersensitivity. *Gut*, *57*, 1230–1237.

Yan, J., & Dussor, G. (2014). Ion channels and migraine. *Headache*, *54*, 619–639.

Yang, Z., Cao, Y., Wang, Y., Luo, W., Hua, X., Lu, Y., et al. (2009). Behavioural responses and expression of $P2X_3$ receptor in trigeminal ganglion after experimental tooth movement in rats. *Archives of Oral Biology*, *54*, 63–70.

Yasuda, M., Shinoda, M., Kiyomoto, M., Honda, K., Suzuki, A., Tamagawa, T., et al. (2012). $P2X_3$ receptor mediates ectopic mechanical allodynia with inflamed lower lip in mice. *Neuroscience Letters*, *528*, 67–72.

Ye, Y., Ono, K., Bernabé, D. G., Viet, C. T., Pickering, V., Dolan, J. C., et al. (2014). Adenosine triphosphate drives head and neck cancer pain through P2X2/3 heterotrimers. *Acta Neuropathologica Communications*, *2*, 62.

Yegutkin, G. G. (2014). Enzymes involved in metabolism of extracellular nucleotides and nucleosides: Functional implications and measurement of activities. *Critical Reviews in Biochemistry and Molecular Biology*, *49*, 473–497.

Yoon, M. H., Bae, H. B., Choi, J. I., Kim, S. J., Chung, S. T., & Kim, C. M. (2006). Roles of adenosine receptor subtypes in the antinociceptive effect of intrathecal adenosine in a rat formalin test. *Pharmacology*, *78*, 21–26.

Yu, J., Fu, P., Zhang, Y., Liu, S., & Cui, D. (2013). Pregabalin alters nociceptive behavior and expression level of P2X3 receptor in the spinal dorsal horn in a rat model induced by chronic compression of the dorsal root ganglion. *The Anatomical Record*, *296*, 1907–1912.

Yu, Y., Ugawa, S., Ueda, T., Ishida, Y., Inoue, K., Kyaw, N. A., et al. (2008). Cellular localization of $P2X_7$ receptor mRNA in the rat brain. *Brain Research*, *1194*, 45–55.

Zahn, P. K., Straub, H., Wenk, M., & Pogatzki-Zahn, E. M. (2007). Adenosine A1 but not A2a receptor agonist reduces hyperalgesia caused by a surgical incision in rats: A pertussis toxin-sensitive G protein-dependent process. *Anesthesiology*, *107*, 797–806.

Zhang, Y. H., Chen, Y., & Zhao, Z. Q. (2001). Alteration of spontaneous firing rate of primary myelinated afferents by ATP in adjuvant-induced inflamed rats. *Brain Research Bulletin*, *54*, 141–144.

Zhang, H., Liu, L., Lu, G., Chen, Z., Fang, Q., Yang, Z., et al. (2011). Chemical irritation of the prostate sensitizes P_2X_3 receptor-mediated responses in rat dorsal root ganglion neurons. *Neurourology and Urodynamics*, *30*, 612–618.

Zhang, Z., Zhang, Z. Y., Fauser, U., & Schluesener, H. J. (2008). Mechanical allodynia and spinal up-regulation of $P2X_4$ receptor in experimental autoimmune neuritis rats. *Neuroscience*, *152*, 495–501.

Zhou, T. T., Wu, J. R., Chen, Z. Y., Liu, Z. X., & Miao, B. (2014). Effects of dexmedetomidine on P2X4Rs, p38-MAPK and BDNF in spinal microglia in rats with spared nerve injury. *Brain Research*, *1568*, 21–30.

Zhu, C. Z., Mikusa, J., Chu, K. L., Cowart, M., Kowaluk, E. A., Jarvis, M. F., et al. (2001). A-134974: A novel adenosine kinase inhibitor, relieves tactile allodynia via spinal sites of action in peripheral nerve injured rats. *Brain Research*, *905*, 104–110.

Zimmermann, H. (2001). Ectonucleotidases: Some recent developments and a note on nomenclature. *Drug Development Research*, *52*, 44–56.

Zylka, M. J. (2011). Pain-relieving prospects for adenosine receptors and ectonucleotidases. *Trends in Molecular Medicine*, *17*, 188–196.

CHAPTER FIVE

The Role of Store-operated Calcium Channels in Pain

Frances Munoz, Huijuan Hu[1]
Department of Pharmacology and Physiology, Drexel University College of Medicine, Philadelphia, Pennsylvania, USA
[1]Corresponding author: e-mail address: hhu@drexelmed.edu

Contents

Abstract

Store-operated calcium channels (SOCCs) are calcium-selective cation channels. Recently, there has been explosive growth in establishing the molecular mechanisms that mediate store-operated Ca^{2+} entry (SOCE) and the role of this process in normal cellular function and disease states. SOCCs and its components appear to play an important role in many Ca^{2+}-dependent processes in nonexcitable cells and are implicated in several possible disorders including allergies, multiple sclerosis, cancer, and inflammatory bowel disease. Recent studies have shown that SOCCs are expressed in the central nervous system (CNS) and involved in neuronal functions and pathological conditions, including chronic pain. In this chapter, we discuss SOCE and its physiological and pathological roles in the CNS. More specifically, we discuss the expression and function of SOCCs and their downstream signaling mechanisms under chronic pain conditions.

Advances in Pharmacology, Volume 75
ISSN 1054-3589
http://dx.doi.org/10.1016/bs.apha.2015.12.005

ABBREVIATIONS

2-APB 2-aminoethyldiphenyl borate
$[Ca^{2+}]_i$ intracellular free calcium concentration
CaMKII calcium/calmodulin-dependent protein kinase II
CFA complete Freud's adjuvant
CNS central nervous system
CRAC channels Ca^{2+} release-activated Ca^{2+} channels
DRG dorsal root ganglion
ER endoplasmic reticulum
ERKs extracellular signal-regulated kinases
MAPKs mitogen-activated protein kinases
NK1 neurokinin 1
SNI spared nerve injury
SOCCs store-operated calcium channels
SOCE store-operated Ca^{2+} entry
STIM stromal interaction molecule
VGCCs voltage-gated calcium channels
YM-58483 *N*-[4-[3,5-bis(trifluoromethyl)-1H-pyrazol-1-yl] phenyl]-4-methyl-1,2,3-thiadiazole-5-carboxamide

1. INTRODUCTION

Store-operated calcium entry (SOCE) is an essential process used to replenish intracellular Ca^{2+} stores. SOCE appears to play an important role in many Ca^{2+}-dependent processes and is implicated in several disorders including allergies, multiple sclerosis, cancer, and inflammatory bowel disease (Ma, McCarl, Khalil, Luthy, & Feske, 2010; McCarl et al., 2010; Xie, Pan, Yao, Zhou, & Han, 2015). Store-operated calcium channels (SOCCs) are highly Ca^{2+}-selective cation channels that are intimately involved in the calcium influx pathway. SOCE can be activated by the release or depletion of Ca^{2+} from intracellular stores (Putney, 2010), a process that occurs via activation of the inositol triphosphate (IP_3) receptor, or through inhibition of sarcoplasmic–endoplasmic reticulum Ca-ATPase (SERCA) (Putney, 2011). SOCCs are a major mechanism for triggering Ca^{2+} influx into non-excitable cells and have been heavily investigated in immune cells (Hogan, Lewis, & Rao, 2010). In the nervous system, SOCCs are expressed in many brain regions and influence neurotransmitter release and synaptic plasticity (Baba et al., 2003; Emptage, Reid, & Fine, 2001; Skibinska-Kijek, Wisniewska, Gruszczynska-Biegala, Methner, & Kuznicki, 2009). SOCCs have been identified in spinal cord dorsal horn neurons (Xia, Pan, Gao,

Meucci, & Hu, 2014), dorsal root ganglion (DRG) neurons (Gemes et al., 2011), hippocampal neurons (Narayanan, Dougherty, & Johnston, 2010), cortical neurons (Berna-Erro et al., 2009), and Purkinje and amygdala neurons (Skibinska-Kijek et al., 2009). SOCCs have been implicated in central nervous system (CNS) diseases such as pain, ischemic stroke, Parkinson's disease, and Alzheimer's disease (Berna-Erro et al., 2009; Gemes et al., 2011; Selvaraj, Watt, & Singh, 2009; Targos, Baranska, & Pomorski, 2005). In this chapter, we highlight the recent advances in our understanding of the function of SOCCs in neurons and discuss their involvement in pain.

2. THE MOLECULAR COMPONENTS OF SOCCs IN THE CNS

There has been explosive growth in establishing the molecular mechanisms that mediate SOCE and the role of this process in both normal cellular function and disease states. Although the importance of SOCE for cellular functions has been recognized for decades, it was not until 2006 that the first molecular component of the system, Orai1, was identified and cloned. Identification and cloning of additional components of the system rapidly followed, and it is now clear that the system is comprised of three structurally related pore-forming subunits (Orai1,2,3), called calcium release-activated calcium (CRAC) channels, located in the plasma membrane, and two calcium sensors (stromal interaction molecules STIM1/2) located on the surface of the endoplasmic reticulum (ER) (Lewis, 2007; Putney, 2011). STIM1 and STIM2 are single transmembrane proteins with an EF-hand motif in the N-terminus facing the ER lumen. Depletion of calcium from the ER produces a conformational change in STIM1 and STIM2 leading to migration of these signal transducers to locations in the ER membrane adjacent to the pore-forming subunits in the plasma membrane. Association of these proteins triggers the influx of calcium into the cell, which selectively activates signal transduction pathways (Lewis, 2007). STIM1 is the key component mediating SOCE in both nonexcitable cells and neurons (Desvignes et al., 2015; Hartmann et al., 2014; Numaga-Tomita & Putney, 2013; Xia et al., 2014). In spinal cord neurons, STIM1 is a main contributor for SOCE, but STIM2 also plays a significant role (Xia et al., 2014). STIM2 is predominantly present and is also essential to induce SOCE in hippocampal neurons (Berna-Erro et al., 2009).

Of the pore-forming subunits involved in SOCE, Orai1 appears to be the only functional CRAC channel in many cell types. Nonetheless, Orai2 is capable of forming SOCCs, but Orai2-dependent SOC currents are smaller than those obtained with Orai1 when it is overexpressed in cell lines (Lis et al., 2007; Mercer et al., 2006). Orai3 can also play a role in the generating small SOC currents, but only when Orai1 protein level is reduced, or by using a more potent expression vector (Lis et al., 2007; Mercer et al., 2006). Additionally, Orai3 along with Orai1 can encode store-independent Ca^{2+} currents regulated by STIM1 and gated by either arachidonate or its metabolite, leukotriene C4 (Mignen, Thompson, & Shuttleworth, 2007, 2008). Similarly, Orai1 is the only pore-forming subunit responsible for SOCE in dorsal horn neurons, while Orai2 and Orai3 are not involved in this process (Xia et al., 2014).

3. EXPRESSION AND FUNCTION OF SOCCs IN THE NERVOUS SYSTEM

STIM and Orai isoforms are expressed in almost all mammalian tissues and are highly conserved from *Drosophila melanogaster* to humans. STIM1 and STIM2 expression has been confirmed in many neuronal tissues (Gasperini, Choi-Lundberg, Thompson, Mitchell, & Foa, 2009; Klejman et al., 2009; Steinbeck et al., 2011). Within the brain, STIM1 and STIM2 are differentially expressed in the cerebral cortex, hippocampus, and cerebellum (Kraft, 2015). We also have shown that the mRNA levels of all of the SOCC components are expressed in both spinal tissue and cultured dorsal horn neurons, and their protein levels are comparable to those in the cortex and lymph nodes (Xia et al., 2014). In addition, the expression levels of SOCCs are similar among neonatal and adult mice, though the mRNA level of STIM2 is about twofold greater than that of STIM1 in dorsal horn neurons (Xia et al., 2014). Moreover, Orai1 and Orai3 transcripts are widely expressed in the brain as well as the heart, kidney, lung, spleen, and skeletal muscle, while Orai2 transcripts are present in the brain and primary cortical neurons (Gross et al., 2007; Wissenbach, Philipp, Gross, Cavalie, & Flockerzi, 2007). Orai1 expression has also been further confirmed in the brain regions including the cerebral cortex, hippocampus, cerebellum, and spinal cord (Guzman et al., 2014). The protein and mRNA expression levels of STIM1 and Orai1 have also been demonstrated in DRG (Gemes et al., 2011). While the functional expression of SOCCs is not well defined in brain neurons, SOCE has been reported in both cortical neurons and DRG neurons (Gemes et al., 2011). We have shown that depletion of ER calcium stores by inhibition of Ca^{2+}-ATPase transiently elevated intracellular Ca^{2+}; the subsequent addition of 2 mM Ca^{2+} caused sustained responses in majority of the neurons. This sustained calcium entry is comparable to Ca^{2+} entry mediated by voltage-gated calcium channels (VGCCs) (Xia et al., 2014). Importantly, we also found that knockdown of STIM1 and STIM2 reduces SOCE, while reduction of Orai1 almost completely abolishes SOCE in dorsal horn neurons. Thus, SOCCs are indeed functional in spinal cord dorsal horn neurons.

4. PHARMACOLOGICAL AND BIOPHYSICAL PROPERTIES OF SOCCs

Pharmacological targeting of SOCCs has provided the opportunity to further understand SOCE and the respective role of these channels in disease. Early studies have shown that native SOCC or recombinant Orai1 can be blocked by $GdCl_3$, lanthanum, SKF 96365, and 2-aminoethyldiphenylborate (2-APB), establishing well-defined SOC inhibitors in nonexcitable cells (Putney, 2010). 2-APB, one of the most widely employed inhibitors, has a bifunctional effect on these channels that is dependent on the concentrations of the compound. At low micromolar concentrations, 2-APB can potentiate CRAC channel activity, while at higher concentrations the compound can directly inhibit CRAC channel activation (Peinelt, Lis, Beck, Fleig, & Penner, 2008). These inhibitors are also used to determine the pharmacological properties of SOCCs in neurons. In spinal cord dorsal horn and DRG neurons, SOCE can be abolished by $GdCl_3$, and attenuated by 2-APB and YM-58483, another relative-specific SOCE inhibitor (Gemes et al., 2011; Xia et al., 2014). We have observed that 2-APB slightly potentiated SOCE initially and then inhibited SOCE. Our unpublished data also show that SOCE is attenuated by synta-66, a newly synthesized specific inhibitor for SOCE in nonneuronal cells (Ng, di Capite, Singaravelu, & Parekh, 2008). Thus, the pharmacological properties of SOCCs in dorsal horn neurons are similar to those in nonneuronal cells.

Along with the pharmacological properties of SOCCs, the biophysical properties of these channels are important for determining their function. A distinctive feature of CRAC channels is that they conduct Ca^{2+} better than Ba^{2+} (Bakowski & Parekh, 2007; Hoth, 1995). In nonexcitable cells, STIM1- and Orai1-mediated Ca^{2+} currents display nonvoltage activation, strong inward rectification, and reversal potential (E_{rev}) >+60 mV and are highly permeable to Ca^{2+}, but not to Ba^{2+}, Cs^{+}, or other monovalent cations (DeHaven, Smyth, Boyles, & Putney, 2007; Lis et al., 2007). Additionally, the single-channel conductance of SOCCs is very small (Parekh, 2010), and in some native cell types, SOC currents are undetectable. However, SOC currents can be recorded in most dorsal horn neurons with the *N*-methyl-D-glucamine-based artificial cerebrospinal fluid solution. Activation of SOCCs induces greater inward currents than outward currents with reversal potential around +55 mV (Xia et al., 2014). SOC currents in dorsal horn neurons are drastically reduced by replacing Ca^{2+} with Ba^{2+} (Xia et al., 2014) and have similar biophysical properties as those in nonneuronal cells (Lis et al., 2007; Smyth et al., 2010). SOC currents are also detectable in dorsal horn neurons from adult mouse spinal cord slices (Xia et al., 2014).

5. SOCCs IN NEURONAL FUNCTION AND DISEASE

The functional significance of neuronal SOCE is not well established. We have found that activation SOCE produces significant membrane depolarization and even evokes action potentials in some neurons, indicating an excitatory action in spinal cord dorsal horn neurons (Xia et al., 2014). Pharmacological evidence also shows that inhibition of SOCCs attenuated tetanus-induced dendritic Ca^{2+} accumulation and long-term potentiation at Schaffer collateral-CA1 synapses in hippocampal slice preparations, suggesting that SOCCs play a role in synaptic transmission and contribute to neuronal plasticity (Baba et al., 2003; Emptage et al., 2001). However, a study has shown that activation of SOCCs increases the density of functional h channels in hippocampal pyramidal neurons which causes a decrease in intrinsic excitability (Narayanan et al., 2010), indicating an inhibitory action of SOCCs. Moreover, SOCC activation can regulate VGCCs in cortical neurons, as SOCCs suppress depolarization-induced calcium entry and subsequent currents, which leads to the internalization of the channels (Park, Shcheglovitov, & Dolmetsch, 2010). Current literature suggests that SOCE is also important for growth cone navigation (Gasperini et al., 2009; Mitchell, Gasperini, Small, & Foa, 2012). The SOCC component STIM1 is a key regulator in neuronal Ca^{2+} signaling as well as mGluR1-dependent synaptic transmission in Purkinje neurons, and its deficiency ultimately leads to impairments cerebellar motor behavior (Hartmann et al., 2014). STIM2 is involved in calcium homeostasis and regulates resting Ca^{2+} levels in the

ER as well as Ca^{2+} leakage in cortical neurons (Gruszczynska-Biegala, Pomorski, Wisniewska, & Kuznicki, 2011). In contrast to STIM proteins, the function of CRAC channels, however, is less clear. Orai2 functions as a leak channel in the ER as its reduction dramatically reduces ER calcium leak rate (Bandara, Malmersjo, & Meyer, 2013).

SOCCs have been implicated in several CNS pathological conditions, such as Alzheimer's disease, Huntington's disease, and epilepsy (Popugaeva & Bezprozvanny, 2013; Steinbeck et al., 2011; Vigont et al., 2014). A previous report has shown that STIM proteins are increased in brains of chronic epileptic rats and pharmacologic inhibition of SOCE suppressed interictal spikes and rhythmized epileptic burst activity in chronic epileptic hippocampal slices (Steinbeck et al., 2011). STIM2 has been shown to play a pivotal role in memory and the pathology of Alzheimer's disease, as a recent study demonstrated that STIM2 is required for the stabilization and creation of mushroom dendritic spines, which play an important role in the storage of memories (Sun et al., 2014). Berna-Erro et al. (2009) have reported that STIM2-deficient mice were markedly protected from neurological damage in a model of focal cerebral ischemia, suggesting that STIM2 is a critical mediator in ischemic stroke. The role of ORAI proteins in CNS diseases remains unsolved.

6. THE POTENTIAL ROLE OF SOCCs IN THE MODULATION OF PAIN

Growing evidence suggests that SOCE and its components are involved in CNS disorders. However, the role of SOCCs in pain is not well recognized. A previous study suggests that the function of SOCCs is increased in DRG neurons after spared nerve injury (SNI) (Gemes et al., 2011). In addition, we recently observed that YM-58483 decreased SNI-induced thermal and mechanical hypersensitivity and prevented the development of SNI-induced pain hypersensitivity (Gao et al., 2013). Substance P is an endogenous neurotransmitter that signals through the neurokinin 1 (NK1) receptor, a Gαq/11-protein-coupled receptor, to produce nociceptor sensitization and pain. Substance P induced a transient calcium response in the absence of Ca^{2+}; following addition of 2 mM Ca^{2+} caused robust calcium influx (Xia et al., 2014). This Ca^{2+} entry is attenuated by SOCE inhibitors YM-58483 and $GdCl_3$, and abolished by knockdown of Orai1, suggesting that SOCCs are involved in the function of NK1 receptor.

SOCCs are also thought to play a critical role in immune responses and inflammatory diseases (Shaw & Feske, 2012). A recent report suggests that Orai1 is involved in calcium entry induced by bradykinin, an inflammatory mediator that produces nociception sensitization and pain (Szteyn, Gomez, Berg, & Jeske, 2015). Additionally, YM-58483 inhibits cytokine production from immune cells and attenuates antigen-induced hypersensitivity reactions. We have demonstrated that oral administration of YM-58483 dramatically attenuated complete Freund's adjuvant (CFA)-induced thermal hyperalgesia and prevented the development of thermal and mechanical hypersensitivity in a dose-dependent manner. Analgesic effects were observed when YM-58483 administered systemically, intrathecally, and intraplantarly (Gao et al., 2013). Pretreatment with YM-58483 strongly reduced both the first and second phases of formalin-induced spontaneous nocifensive behavior dose dependently (Gao et al., 2013). Similarly, treatment with YM-58483 after the onset of collagen-induced arthritis reverses the arthritis symptoms, reduces paw edema, and attenuates mechanical and thermal hypersensitivity.

Acute pain is mediated by peripheral transducer proteins, such as TRPV1, and occurs when exposed to chemicals, heat, or noxious mechanical stimuli. However, SOCCs in peripheral pain are not well established. We have found that YM-58483 produced antinociception in acute pain induced by heat or capsaicin or mechanical stimuli at the dose of 30 mg/kg (Gao et al., 2013). These effects suggest that SOCCs may be involved in the process of nociception.

7. THE DOWNSTREAM MECHANISMS OF SOCCs INVOLVED IN PAIN

Inflammatory mediators and proinflammatory cytokines, such as TNF-α, IL-1β, and PGE-2, contribute to the generation of inflammatory pain and peripheral pain sensitization (Parada, Yeh, Joseph, & Levine, 2003; Woolf, Allchorne, Safieh-Garabedian, & Poole, 1997). We have observed that TNF-α, IL-1β, and PGE-2 levels dramatically increased in CFA-injected paw, and IL-1β, IL-6, and TNF-α levels are markedly increased in the inflamed paw of collagen-induced arthritis mice (Gao et al., 2013, 2015). YM-58483 reduced the levels of these inflammatory mediators and cytokines (Gao et al., 2013, 2015). Previous literature has also shown that YM-58483 inhibits activation-induced secretion of TNF-α in mast cells (Law et al., 2011). Thus, it is conceivable that reduction of inflammatory mediators and proinflammatory cytokines contributes to the peripheral mechanisms by which YM-58483 reduces inflammation and pain hypersensitivity.

Increasing evidence suggests that central sensitization contributes to the persistent pain. It is well established that mitogen-activated protein kinases (MAPKs) and calcium/calmodulin-dependent protein kinase II (CaMKII) pathways are involved in central sensitization (Ji, Gereau, Malcangio, & Strichartz, 2009). It has also been shown that SOCE is implicated in extracellular signal-regulated kinase (ERK) and CaMKII activation in nonneuronal cells (Voelkers et al., 2010). The most extensively studied MAPK to date is the ERK1/2 in neurons. Recently, we discovered that ERK1/2 is activated in the spinal cord after onset of arthritis, which is significantly reduced by YM-58483 10 mg/kg (Gao et al., 2015). Numerous studies have reported the activation of CaMKII in several pain models and inhibition of CaMKII attenuates pain involving central sensitization (Crown et al., 2012; Fang, Wu, Lin, & Willis, 2002). Our results reveal that CaMKII is activated in the spinal cord after onset of arthritis and YM-58483 dose dependently inhibited the CaMKII activation. Thus, our findings indicate that spinal SOCCs are also involved in central sensitization.

8. CONCLUSION

The role of SOCE is implicated in many pathological conditions such as immune disorders, allergies, and inflammatory bowel disease (Parekh, 2010). SOCCs and their respective components have also been well studied in immune and other nonexcitable cells. While SOCE has been implicated in CNS disorders (Popugaeva & Bezprozvanny, 2013; Steinbeck et al., 2011; Vigont et al., 2014), the study of SOCCs in chronic pain conditions remains a new and emerging field. Inhibition of SOCE can attenuate or completely abolish pain hypersensitivity, suggesting that SOCE plays a role in chronic pain. While much remains elusive regarding the role of SOCCs in the nervous system, current evidence encourages the possibility that SOCCs may be used as potential drug targets for neurological diseases including pain. The identification of the individual SOCC components provides new and more specific tools to allow us to explore the different key players in chronic pain conditions. Currently, our laboratory continues its focus on elucidating the mechanisms underlying SOCC activation, and its downstream targets in chronic pain conditions.

CONFLICT OF INTEREST

The authors declare no conflicts of interest.

ACKNOWLEDGMENTS

This work was supported by the NIH/NINDS Grant R21 NS077330-01A1 and R01NS087033 to H.H.

REFERENCES

Baba, A., Yasui, T., Fujisawa, S., Yamada, R. X., Yamada, M. K., Nishiyama, N., et al. (2003). Activity-evoked capacitative Ca^{2+} entry: Implications in synaptic plasticity. *The Journal of Neuroscience*, *23*(21), 7737–7741. 23/21/7737 [pii].

Bakowski, D., & Parekh, A. B. (2007). Voltage-dependent Ba^{2+} permeation through store-operated CRAC channels: Implications for channel selectivity. *Cell Calcium*, *42*(3), 333–339. http://dx.doi.org/10.1016/j.ceca.2007.01.005. S0143-4160(07)00018-8 [pii].

Bandara, S., Malmersjo, S., & Meyer, T. (2013). Regulators of calcium homeostasis identified by inference of kinetic model parameters from live single cells perturbed by siRNA. *Science Signaling*, *6*(283), ra56. http://dx.doi.org/10.1126/scisignal.2003649. 6/283/ra56 [pii].

Berna-Erro, A., Braun, A., Kraft, R., Kleinschnitz, C., Schuhmann, M. K., Stegner, D., et al. (2009). STIM2 regulates capacitive Ca^{2+} entry in neurons and plays a key role in hypoxic neuronal cell death. *Science Signaling*, *2*(93), ra67. http://dx.doi.org/10.1126/scisignal.2000522. 2/93/ra67 [pii].

Crown, E. D., Gwak, Y. S., Ye, Z., Yu Tan, H., Johnson, K. M., Xu, G. Y., et al. (2012). Calcium/calmodulin-dependent kinase II contributes to persistent central neuropathic pain following spinal cord injury. *Pain*, *153*(3), 710–721. http://dx.doi.org/10.1016/j.pain.2011.12.013. S0304-3959(11)00751-2 [pii].

DeHaven, W. I., Smyth, J. T., Boyles, R. R., & Putney, J. W., Jr. (2007). Calcium inhibition and calcium potentiation of Orai1, Orai2, and Orai3 calcium release-activated calcium channels. *The Journal of Biological Chemistry*, *282*(24), 17548–17556. http://dx.doi.org/10.1074/jbc.M611374200. M611374200 [pii].

Desvignes, L., Weidinger, C., Shaw, P., Vaeth, M., Ribierre, T., Liu, M., et al. (2015). STIM1 controls T cell-mediated immune regulation and inflammation in chronic infection. *The Journal of Clinical Investigation*, *125*(6), 2347–2362. http://dx.doi.org/10.1172/JCI80273. 80273 [pii].

Emptage, N. J., Reid, C. A., & Fine, A. (2001). Calcium stores in hippocampal synaptic boutons mediate short-term plasticity, store-operated Ca^{2+} entry, and spontaneous transmitter release. *Neuron*, *29*(1), 197–208. S0896-6273(01)00190-8 [pii].

Fang, L., Wu, J., Lin, Q., & Willis, W. D. (2002). Calcium-calmodulin-dependent protein kinase II contributes to spinal cord central sensitization. *The Journal of Neuroscience*, *22*(10), 4196–4204. 20026343 22/10/4196 [pii].

Gao, X. H., Gao, R., Tian, Y. Z., McGonigle, P., Barrett, J. E., Dai, Y., et al. (2015). A store-operated calcium channel inhibitor attenuates collagen-induced arthritis. *British Journal of Pharmacology*, *172*(12), 2991–3002. http://dx.doi.org/10.1111/bph.13104.

Gao, R., Gao, X., Xia, J., Tian, Y., Barrett, J. E., Dai, Y., et al. (2013). Potent analgesic effects of a store-operated calcium channel inhibitor. *Pain*, *154*(10), 2034–2044. http://dx.doi.org/10.1016/j.pain.2013.06.017. S0304-3959(13)00323-0 [pii].

Gasperini, R., Choi-Lundberg, D., Thompson, M. J., Mitchell, C. B., & Foa, L. (2009). Homer regulates calcium signalling in growth cone turning. *Neural Development*, *4*, 29. http://dx.doi.org/10.1186/1749-8104-4-29. 1749-8104-4-29 [pii].

Gemes, G., Bangaru, M. L., Wu, H. E., Tang, Q., Weihrauch, D., Koopmeiners, A. S., et al. (2011). Store-operated Ca^{2+} entry in sensory neurons: Functional role and the effect of painful nerve injury. *The Journal of Neuroscience*, *31*(10), 3536–3549. http://dx.doi.org/10.1523/JNEUROSCI.5053-10.2011. 31/10/3536 [pii].

Gross, S. A., Wissenbach, U., Philipp, S. E., Freichel, M., Cavalie, A., & Flockerzi, V. (2007). Murine ORAI2 splice variants form functional Ca^{2+} release-activated Ca^{2+} (CRAC) channels. *The Journal of Biological Chemistry*, *282*(27), 19375–19384. http://dx.doi.org/10.1074/jbc.M701962200. M701962200 [pii].

Gruszczynska-Biegala, J., Pomorski, P., Wisniewska, M. B., & Kuznicki, J. (2011). Differential roles for STIM1 and STIM2 in store-operated calcium entry in rat neurons. *PLoS One*, *6*(4), e19285. http://dx.doi.org/10.1371/journal.pone.0019285.

Guzman, R., Valente, E. G., Pretorius, J., Pacheco, E., Qi, M., Bennett, B. D., et al. (2014). Expression of ORAII, a plasma membrane resident subunit of the CRAC channel, in rodent and non-rodent species. *The Journal of Histochemistry and Cytochemistry*, *62*(12), 864–878. http://dx.doi.org/10.1369/0022155414554926. 0022155414554926 [pii].

Hartmann, J., Karl, R. M., Alexander, R. P., Adelsberger, H., Brill, M. S., Ruhlmann, C., et al. (2014). STIM1 controls neuronal Ca(2)(+) signaling, mGluR1-dependent synaptic transmission, and cerebellar motor behavior. *Neuron*, *82*(3), 635–644. http://dx.doi.org/10.1016/j.neuron.2014.03.027. S0896-6273(14)00257-8 [pii].

Hogan, P. G., Lewis, R. S., & Rao, A. (2010). Molecular basis of calcium signaling in lymphocytes: STIM and ORAI. *Annual Review of Immunology*, *28*, 491–533. http://dx.doi.org/10.1146/annurev.immunol.021908.132550.

Hoth, M. (1995). Calcium and barium permeation through calcium release-activated calcium (CRAC) channels. *Pflügers Archiv*, *430*(3), 315–322.

Ji, R. R., Gereau, R. W., 4th., Malcangio, M., & Strichartz, G. R. (2009). MAP kinase and pain. *Brain Research Reviews*, *60*(1), 135–148. http://dx.doi.org/10.1016/j.brainresrev.2008.12.011. S0165-0173(08)00149-5 [pii].

Klejman, M. E., Gruszczynska-Biegala, J., Skibinska-Kijek, A., Wisniewska, M. B., Misztal, K., Blazejczyk, M., et al. (2009). Expression of STIM1 in brain and puncta-like co-localization of STIM1 and ORAI1 upon depletion of Ca(2+) store in neurons. *Neurochemistry International*, *54*(1), 49–55. http://dx.doi.org/10.1016/j.neuint.2008.10.005. S0197-0186(08)00166-6 [pii].

Kraft, R. (2015). STIM and ORAI proteins in the nervous system. *Channels (Austin, TX)*, *9*(5), 245–252. http://dx.doi.org/10.1080/19336950.2015.1071747.

Law, M., Morales, J. L., Mottram, L. F., Iyer, A., Peterson, B. R., & August, A. (2011). Structural requirements for the inhibition of calcium mobilization and mast cell activation by the pyrazole derivative BTP2. *The International Journal of Biochemistry & Cell Biology*, *43*(8), 1228–1239. http://dx.doi.org/10.1016/j.biocel.2011.04.016. S1357-2725(11)00121-X [pii].

Lewis, R. S. (2007). The molecular choreography of a store-operated calcium channel. *Nature*, *446*(7133), 284–287. http://dx.doi.org/10.1038/nature05637. nature05637 [pii].

Lis, A., Peinelt, C., Beck, A., Parvez, S., Monteilh-Zoller, M., Fleig, A., et al. (2007). CRACM1, CRACM2, and CRACM3 are store-operated Ca^{2+} channels with distinct functional properties. *Current Biology*, *17*(9), 794–800. http://dx.doi.org/10.1016/j.cub.2007.03.065. S0960-9822(07)01203-1 [pii].

Ma, J., McCarl, C. A., Khalil, S., Luthy, K., & Feske, S. (2010). T-cell-specific deletion of STIM1 and STIM2 protects mice from EAE by impairing the effector functions of Th1 and Th17 cells. *European Journal of Immunology*, *40*(11), 3028–3042. http://dx.doi.org/10.1002/eji.201040614.

McCarl, C. A., Khalil, S., Ma, J., Oh-hora, M., Yamashita, M., Roether, J., et al. (2010). Store-operated Ca^{2+} entry through ORAI1 is critical for T cell-mediated autoimmunity and allograft rejection. *Journal of Immunology, 185*(10), 5845–5858. http://dx.doi.org/10.4049/jimmunol.1001796. jimmunol.1001796 [pii].

Mercer, J. C., Dehaven, W. I., Smyth, J. T., Wedel, B., Boyles, R. R., Bird, G. S., et al. (2006). Large store-operated calcium selective currents due to co-expression of Orai1 or Orai2 with the intracellular calcium sensor, Stim1. *The Journal of Biological Chemistry, 281*(34), 24979–24990. http://dx.doi.org/10.1074/jbc.M604589200. M604589200 [pii].

Mignen, O., Thompson, J. L., & Shuttleworth, T. J. (2007). STIM1 regulates Ca^{2+} entry via arachidonate-regulated Ca^{2+}-selective (ARC) channels without store depletion or translocation to the plasma membrane. *The Journal of Physiology, 579*(Pt. 3), 703–715. http://dx.doi.org/10.1113/jphysiol.2006.122432. jphysiol.2006.122432 [pii].

Mignen, O., Thompson, J. L., & Shuttleworth, T. J. (2008). Both Orai1 and Orai3 are essential components of the arachidonate-regulated Ca^{2+}-selective (ARC) channels. *The Journal of Physiology, 586*(1), 185–195. http://dx.doi.org/10.1113/jphysiol.2007.146258. jphysiol.2007.146258 [pii].

Mitchell, C. B., Gasperini, R. J., Small, D. H., & Foa, L. (2012). STIM1 is necessary for store-operated calcium entry in turning growth cones. *Journal of Neurochemistry, 122*(6), 1155–1166. http://dx.doi.org/10.1111/j.1471-4159.2012.07840.x.

Narayanan, R., Dougherty, K. J., & Johnston, D. (2010). Calcium store depletion induces persistent perisomatic increases in the functional density of h channels in hippocampal pyramidal neurons. *Neuron, 68*(5), 921–935. http://dx.doi.org/10.1016/j.neuron.2010.11.033. S0896-6273(10)00975-X [pii].

Ng, S. W., di Capite, J., Singaravelu, K., & Parekh, A. B. (2008). Sustained activation of the tyrosine kinase Syk by antigen in mast cells requires local Ca^{2+} influx through Ca^{2+} release-activated Ca^{2+} channels. *The Journal of Biological Chemistry, 283*(46), 31348–31355. http://dx.doi.org/10.1074/jbc.M804942200. M804942200 [pii].

Numaga-Tomita, T., & Putney, J. W. (2013). Role of STIM1- and Orai1-mediated Ca^{2+} entry in Ca^{2+}-induced epidermal keratinocyte differentiation. *Journal of Cell Science, 126*(Pt. 2), 605–612. http://dx.doi.org/10.1242/jcs.115980. jcs.115980 [pii].

Parada, C. A., Yeh, J. J., Joseph, E. K., & Levine, J. D. (2003). Tumor necrosis factor receptor type-1 in sensory neurons contributes to induction of chronic enhancement of inflammatory hyperalgesia in rat. *The European Journal of Neuroscience, 17*(9), 1847–1852. 2626 [pii].

Parekh, A. B. (2010). Store-operated CRAC channels: Function in health and disease. *Nature Reviews. Drug Discovery, 9*(5), 399–410. http://dx.doi.org/10.1038/nrd3136. nrd3136 [pii].

Park, C. Y., Shcheglovitov, A., & Dolmetsch, R. (2010). The CRAC channel activator STIM1 binds and inhibits L-type voltage-gated calcium channels. *Science, 330*(6000), 101–105. http://dx.doi.org/10.1126/science.1191027. 330/6000/101 [pii].

Peinelt, C., Lis, A., Beck, A., Fleig, A., & Penner, R. (2008). 2-Aminoethoxydiphenyl borate directly facilitates and indirectly inhibits STIM1-dependent gating of CRAC channels. *The Journal of Physiology, 586*(13), 3061–3073. http://dx.doi.org/10.1113/jphysiol.2008.151365. jphysiol.2008.151365 [pii].

Popugaeva, E., & Bezprozvanny, I. (2013). Role of endoplasmic reticulum Ca^{2+} signaling in the pathogenesis of Alzheimer disease. *Frontiers in Molecular Neuroscience, 6*, 29. http://dx.doi.org/10.3389/fnmol.2013.00029.

Putney, J. W. (2010). Pharmacology of store-operated calcium channels. *Molecular Interventions, 10*(4), 209–218. http://dx.doi.org/10.1124/mi.10.4.4. 10/4/209 [pii].

Putney, J. W. (2011). The physiological function of store-operated calcium entry. *Neurochemical Research, 36*(7), 1157–1165. http://dx.doi.org/10.1007/s11064-010-0383-0.

Selvaraj, S., Watt, J. A., & Singh, B. B. (2009). TRPC1 inhibits apoptotic cell degeneration induced by dopaminergic neurotoxin MPTP/MPP(+). *Cell Calcium, 46*(3), 209–218. http://dx.doi.org/10.1016/j.ceca.2009.07.008. S0143-4160(09)00121-3 [pii].

Shaw, P. J., & Feske, S. (2012). Regulation of lymphocyte function by ORAI and STIM proteins in infection and autoimmunity. *The Journal of Physiology*, *590*(Pt. 17), 4157–4167. http://dx.doi.org/10.1113/jphysiol.2012.233221. jphysiol.2012.233221 [pii].

Skibinska-Kijek, A., Wisniewska, M. B., Gruszczynska-Biegala, J., Methner, A., & Kuznicki, J. (2009). Immunolocalization of STIM1 in the mouse brain. *Acta Neurobiologiae Experimentalis (Wars)*, *69*(4), 413–428. 6930 [pii].

Smyth, J. T., Hwang, S. Y., Tomita, T., DeHaven, W. I., Mercer, J. C., & Putney, J. W. (2010). Activation and regulation of store-operated calcium entry. *Journal of Cellular and Molecular Medicine*, *14*(10), 2337–2349. http://dx.doi.org/10.1111/j.1582-4934.2010.01168.x. JCMM1168 [pii].

Steinbeck, J. A., Henke, N., Opatz, J., Gruszczynska-Biegala, J., Schneider, L., Theiss, S., et al. (2011). Store-operated calcium entry modulates neuronal network activity in a model of chronic epilepsy. *Experimental Neurology*, *232*(2), 185–194. http://dx.doi.org/10.1016/j.expneurol.2011.08.022. S0014-4886(11)00302-5 [pii].

Sun, S., Zhang, H., Liu, J., Popugaeva, E., Xu, N. J., Feske, S., et al. (2014). Reduced synaptic STIM2 expression and impaired store-operated calcium entry cause destabilization of mature spines in mutant presenilin mice. *Neuron*, *82*(1), 79–93. http://dx.doi.org/10.1016/j.neuron.2014.02.019. S0896-6273(14)00117-2 [pii].

Szteyn, K., Gomez, R., Berg, K. A., & Jeske, N. A. (2015). Divergence in endothelin-1- and bradykinin-activated store-operated calcium entry in afferent sensory neurons. *ASN Neuro*, 7.

Targos, B., Baranska, J., & Pomorski, P. (2005). Store-operated calcium entry in physiology and pathology of mammalian cells. *Acta Biochimica Polonica*, *52*(2), 397–409. 20051073 [pii].

Vigont, V. A., Zimina, O. A., Glushankova, L. N., Kolobkova, J. A., Ryazantseva, M. A., Mozhayeva, G. N., et al. (2014). STIM1 protein activates store-operated calcium channels in cellular model of Huntington's disease. *Acta Naturae*, *6*(4), 40–47.

Voelkers, M., Salz, M., Herzog, N., Frank, D., Dolatabadi, N., Frey, N., et al. (2010). Orai1 and Stim1 regulate normal and hypertrophic growth in cardiomyocytes. *Journal of Molecular and Cellular Cardiology*, *48*(6), 1329–1334. http://dx.doi.org/10.1016/j.yjmcc.2010.01.020. S0022-2828(10)00033-7 [pii].

Wissenbach, U., Philipp, S. E., Gross, S. A., Cavalie, A., & Flockerzi, V. (2007). Primary structure, chromosomal localization and expression in immune cells of the murine ORAI and STIM genes. *Cell Calcium*, *42*(4–5), 439–446. http://dx.doi.org/10.1016/j.ceca.2007.05.014. S0143-4160(07)00115-7 [pii].

Woolf, C. J., Allchorne, A., Safieh-Garabedian, B., & Poole, S. (1997). Cytokines, nerve growth factor and inflammatory hyperalgesia: The contribution of tumour necrosis factor alpha. *British Journal of Pharmacology*, *121*(3), 417–424. http://dx.doi.org/10.1038/sj.bjp.0701148.

Xia, J., Pan, R., Gao, X., Meucci, O., & Hu, H. (2014). Native store-operated calcium channels are functionally expressed in mouse spinal cord dorsal horn neurons and regulate resting calcium homeostasis. *The Journal of Physiology*, *592*(Pt. 16), 3443–3461. http://dx.doi.org/10.1113/jphysiol.2014.275065. jphysiol.2014.275065 [pii].

Xie, J., Pan, H., Yao, J., Zhou, Y., & Han, W. (2015). SOCE and cancer: Recent progress and new perspectives. *International Journal of Cancer*, http://dx.doi.org/10.1002/ijc.29840.

CHAPTER SIX

Sodium Channels in Pain and Cancer: New Therapeutic Opportunities

Ana Paula Luiz, John N. Wood[1]
Molecular Nociception Group, Wolfson Institute for Biomedical Research, University College London, London, United Kingdom
[1]Correponding author: e-mail address: j.wood@ucl.ac.uk

Contents

Abstract

Voltage-gated sodium channels (VGSCs) underpin electrical activity in the nervous system through action potential propagation. First predicted by the modeling studies of Hodgkin and Huxley, they were subsequently identified at the molecular level by groups led by Catterall and Numa. VGSC dysfunction has long been linked to neuronal and cardiac disorders with some nonselective sodium channel blockers in current use in the clinic. The lack of selectivity means that side effect issues are a major impediment to the use of broad spectrum sodium channel blockers. Nine different sodium channels are known to exist, and selective blockers are now being developed. The potential utility of these drugs to target diseases ranging from migraine, multiple sclerosis, muscle, and immune system disorders, to cancer and pain is being explored. Four channels are potential targets for pain disorders. This conclusion comes from mouse knockout studies and human mutations that prove the involvement of $Na_V1.3$, $Na_V1.7$, $Na_V1.8$, and $Na_V1.9$ in the development and maintenance of acute and chronic pain. In this chapter, we present a short overview of the possible role of $Na_V1.3$, $Na_V1.7$, $Na_V1.8$, and $Na_V1.9$ in human pain and the emerging and unexpected role of sodium channels in cancer pathogenesis.

Advances in Pharmacology, Volume 75
ISSN 1054-3589
http://dx.doi.org/10.1016/bs.apha.2015.12.006

ABBREVIATIONS

CFA complete Freund's adjuvant
DRG dorsal root ganglion
IB4$^+$ isolectin B4 positive
mRNA messenger ribonucleic acid
NGF nerve growth factor
TG trigeminal ganglion
TTX tetrodotoxin
TTX-R tetrodotoxin resistant
TTX-S tetrodotoxin sensitive
VGSCs voltage-gated sodium channels

1. INTRODUCTION

Electrical signaling within excitable cells depends upon specialized ion permeable transmembrane proteins, the voltage-gated ion channels. Among these channels, the family of voltage-gated sodium channels (VGSCs) have long been linked to neuronal and cardiac disorders, with sodium channel blockers acting as anticonvulsants, local anesthetics, and antiarrhythmics in current clinical use. Lidocaine, mexiletine, carbamazepine, lamotrigine, and phenytoin are examples of such drugs that have been widely used to treat disorders where the chosen therapeutic approach is designed to decrease neuronal excitability. However, all these blockers are largely nonselective among the various sodium channel subtypes, and this lack of selectivity contributes to their many side effects, for example, causing motor dysfunction (Krafte & Bannon, 2008). Recent research in genomics has suggested the possible participation of VGSCs in other disorders such as autism, migraine, multiple sclerosis, cancer, muscle, and immune system disorders and confirmed the strong correlation with human pain disorders (de Lera Ruiz & Kraus, 2015; Eijkelkamp et al., 2012; Waxman et al., 2014).

With the exception of the related Na_x channel that is activated by changes in sodium concentrations (Goldin et al., 2000), there are nine homologous mammalian genes that encode VGSC alpha subunits (Eijkelkamp et al., 2012; Goldin et al., 2000; Liu & Wood, 2011). The alpha subunit is responsible for the functionality of the channel, while beta subunits modulate the biophysics and trafficking of the channel (Eijkelkamp et al., 2012; Liu & Wood, 2011). In mammals, VGSCs are multimeric transmembrane complexes composed of a large pore-forming α subunit ($Na_v\alpha$) associated with two smaller β subunits ($Na_v\beta$) (Catterall, 2000; Liu & Wood,

2011). There are five $Na_v\beta$ subunits, $\beta 1$, $\beta 1B$, $\beta 2$, $\beta 3$, and $\beta 4$, which are encoded by four different genes. Subunits $\beta 1$ and $\beta 1B$ are splice variants encoded by the same *SCN1B* gene, while $\beta 2$, $\beta 3$, and $\beta 4$ are encoded by *SCN2B*, *SCN3B*, and *SCN4B* genes, respectively (Roger, Gillet, Le Guennec, & Besson, 2015).

The family of VGSCs can be subdivided on the basis of their sensitivity to activation by veratridine or batrachotoxin and blockade by tetrodotoxin (TTX), falling into TTX-sensitive (TTX-S) or TTX-resistant (TTX-R) subsets. They also have distinct tissue-specific patterns of expression and function in the nervous system, as shown in Table 1.

Among the nine members of the sodium channel family, $Na_v1.3$, $Na_v1.7$, $Na_v1.8$, and $Na_v1.9$ have been the subject of numerous studies attempting to elucidate their potential roles in pain signaling (for an in-depth review, see Cummins, Sheets, & Waxman, 2007). The development of $Na_v1.8$ Cre-recombinase mice, that enable the selective deletion of genes in small-diameter sensory neurons, has proved fruitful in the analysis of gene function in peripheral pain pathways (Foulkes et al., 2006; Fricker, Dinocourt, Eugene, Wood, & Miles, 2009; Nassar et al., 2004; Stirling et al., 2005; Wickramasinghe et al., 2008; Zhao, Nassar, Gavazzi, & Wood, 2006), where global deletion leads to lethality (like $Na_v1.7$) or widespread functional deficits. Indeed, the Cre-recombinase method has become an important instrument for achieving precise genetic manipulation in mice. Many of these desired genetic manipulations rely on Cre's ability to direct spatially and temporally specified excision of a predetermined DNA (deoxyribonucleic acid) sequence that has been flanked by *loxP* recombination sites. Success in achieving such conditional mutagenesis in mice depends both on the careful design of conditional alleles and on reliable detection of *cre* gene expression. These procedures include polymerase chain reaction, immunohistochemistry, and the use of a recombination-proficient green fluorescent protein-tagged Cre protein (Le & Sauer, 2001).

2. $NA_V1.3$

Widely present in the brain, Nav1.3 channels are upregulated and detected in dorsal root ganglion (DRG) sensory neurons following axotomy and other forms of peripheral nerve injury (Black et al., 1999; Dib-Hajj et al., 1999). A role for $Na_v1.3$ channels in inflammatory pain has not been established, and its significance in neuropathic pain remains controversial. Acute inflammation induced by carrageenan injection into

Table 1 Voltage-Gated Sodium Channel α-Subunits: Types, Encoding Genes, Main Anatomical Expression Sites, Involvement in Diseases/Syndromes, Expression Levels in DRG, and Pharmacological and Electrophysiological Features

Channel	Previous Name	Gene Symbol	Main Anatomical Expression Sites	Diseases or Syndromes	Expression in DRG	Pharmacological Features			Electrophysiological Features
						Activators	Blockers	Sensitivity to TTX	
$Na_v1.1$	Type I	*SCN1A*	CNS (very high brain levels) and PNS	Epilepsy (loss of function in interneurons), migraine, autism	Abundant	Veratridine Batrachotoxin	TTX (10 nM) Saxitoxin	TTX-s	Fast inactivation (0.7 ms)
$Na_v1.2$	Type II	*SCN2A*	CNS and PNS	Generalized epilepsies, autism, ataxia	Present	Veratridine Batrachotoxin	μ-Conotoxin (SIIIA) TTX (10 nM) Saxitoxin	TTX-s	Fast inactivation (0.8 ms)
$Na_v1.3$	Type III	*SCN3A*	CNS (high brain levels) and PNS	Epilepsy, **neuropathic pain**	Upregulated in axotomy	Veratridine Batrachotoxin	TTX (2–15 nM) Saxitoxin	TTX-s	Fast inactivation (0.8 ms)
$Na_v1.4$	SkM1	*SCN4A*	Skeletal muscle	Hyper and hypokalemic periodic paralysis, paramyotonia congenita	Absent	Veratridine Batrachotoxin	μ-Conotoxin (GIIIA and PIIIA) TTX (5 nM) Saxitoxin	TTX-s	Fast inactivation (0.6 ms)

$Na_v1.5$	Cardiac	*SCN5A*	Cardiac muscle and Purkinje fibers	Long QT, atrial fibrillation, Brugada syndrome	Present	Veratridine Batrachotoxin	TTX (2 μM)	TTX-r	Fast inactivation (1 ms)
$Na_v1.6$	PN4/ NaCH6	*SCN8A*	CNS, PNS (particularly brain and spinal cord), and smooth muscle	Conduction in cardiac SA node, mental retardation, ataxia, pancerebellar atrophy	Abundant	Veratridine Batrachotoxin	TTX (6 nM) Saxitoxin	TTX-s	Fast inactivation (1 ms)
$Na_v1.7$	PN1/NaS	*SCN9A*	CNS and PNS	**Paroxysmal extreme pain, erythermalgia, congenital indifference to pain,** anosmia	Abundant	Veratridine Batrachotoxin	TTX (4 nM) Saxitoxin ProTx-II (0.3 nM)	TTX-s	Fast inactivation (0.5 ms)
$Na_v1.8$	SNS/PN3	*SCN10A*	PNS	**Pain noxious heat and cold, small fiber neuropathy**	Abundant	–	μO-Conotoxin MrVIB TTX (60 μM)	TTX-r	Slow inactivation (6 ms)

Continued

Table 1 Voltage-Gated Sodium Channel α-Subunits: Types, Encoding Genes, Main Anatomical Expression Sites, Involvement in Diseases/Syndromes, Expression Levels in DRG, and Pharmacological and Electrophysiological Features—cont'd

Channel	Previous Name	Gene Symbol	Main Anatomical Expression Sites	Diseases or Syndromes	Expression in DRG	Pharmacological Features			Electrophysiological Features
						Activators	Blockers	Sensitivity to TTX	
$Na_v1.9$	NaN/SNS2	*SCN11A*/ *SCN12A*	PNS and spinal sensory axons	**Inflammatory pain, peripheral neuropathy, episodic chronic pain, loss-of-pain sensation**	Abundant	–	TTX (40 μM)	TTX-r	Slow inactivation (16 ms)
Na_x	NaG	*SCN6A*/ *SCN7A*	Heart, brain, glia, PNS, and smooth muscle	Abnormal NaCl intake behavior	Present	–	–	TTX-r	Concentration sensitive

The bold text means the main found correlated to pain.
DRG, dorsal root ganglia; TG, trigeminal ganglion; PNS, peripheral nervous system; CNS, central nervous system; TTX-s, tetrodotoxin-sensitive; TTX-r, tetrodotoxin-resistant.
Sources: Alexander, Mathie, and Peters (2009), Eijkelkamp et al. (2012), Faber et al. (2012), Huang et al. (2014), Lees and Shipton (2009), Leipold et al. (2013), Ogata and Ohishi (2002), Wood and Baker (2001), and Zhang et al. (2013).

the hind paw upregulated the protein and messenger ribonucleic acid (mRNA) expression of $Na_v1.3$ channels in small neurons of lumbar DRG, but same is observed for $Na_v1.7$ and $Na_v1.8$ sodium channels (Black, Liu, Tanaka, Cummins, & Waxman, 2004). The expression of $Na_v1.3$ mRNA in DRG is high in embryonic (E17) but is much lower in adult rats. Induction to high levels of mRNA of $Na_v1.3$ in DRG neurons was also observed after axotomy (Waxman, Kocsis, & Black, 1994) and in an experimental model of diabetic neuropathy. In the model of diabetic neuropathy, the change of expression of sodium channels is not only restricted to $Na_v1.3$. One and eight weeks after onset of allodynia, the mRNA for $Na_v1.6$ and $Na_v1.9$ is also upregulated, while mRNA for $Na_v1.8$ is downregulated (Craner, Klein, Renganathan, Black, & Waxman, 2002). $Na_v1.3$-null mutant mice display normal nocifensive responses to intraplantar formalin injection (an acute inflammatory insult) and their susceptibility to spinal nerve ligation-induced neuropathic pain is also unchanged (Nassar et al., 2006). Likewise, hind paw allodynia associated with spared nerve injury in rats, another model of neuropathic pain, was unaffected by treatment with $Na_v1.3$ antisense oligonucleotides (Lindia, Kohler, Martin, & Abbadie, 2005). However, intrathecal administration of a distinct $Na_v1.3$ antisense construct reduced the hyperexcitability of dorsal horn neurons and attenuated pain-related behaviors associated with both spinal cord injury and chronic constriction injury of the peripheral nerve (Hains, Saab, Klein, Craner, & Waxman, 2004). $Na_v1.3$-null mutant mice also show a reduction of cold thermosensation and mechanosensation following chronic constriction injury (Minett et al., 2014). In trigeminal ganglion (TG) neurons, the sodium channel α-subunit $Na_v1.3$, which is absent in sham-operated animals, reappears in animals with behavioral signs of neuropathic pain following partial ischemic injury to the infraorbital nerve (Eriksson et al., 2005).

3. $NA_V1.7$

$Na_v1.7$ is expressed in peripheral neurons as well as nonneuronal tissue such as the pancreas. Hypothalamic neurons, olfactory sensory neurons, and sympathetic and peripheral sensory neurons also express this channel (Habib, Wood, & Cox, 2015; Liu & Wood, 2011). Many papers have described a strong correlation between $Na_v1.7$ function and pain disorders in rodents and humans. Importantly, loss-of-function mutations lead to congenital analgesia in otherwise normal mice and humans, making $Na_v1.7$ a very attractive analgesic drug target.

In mouse experimental models, acute inflammation induced by carrageenan injection into the hind paw increases the expression of $Na_v1.7$ sodium channels in small neurons of lumbar DRG (Black et al., 2004). Mice with selective knockout of $Na_v1.7$ channels in $Na_v1.8$-positive nociceptors lose acute noxious mechanosensation and inflammatory pain (induced by nerve growth factor (NGF), formalin, complete Freund's adjuvant (CFA), and carrageenan) (Nassar et al., 2004). When $Na_v1.7$ channels are deleted in all sensory and sympathetic neurons, noxious thermosensation is lost as well, and mechanical hypersensitivity is dramatically reduced following a surgical model of neuropathic pain (Minett et al., 2012). Thus, there appears to be an important role for $Na_v1.7$ channels in sympathetic neurons during the development of some types of neuropathic pain.

$Na_v1.7$ is clearly important, but Nav1.8 and $Na_v1.3$ are also implicated in many chronic pain conditions as in models involving DRG (constriction of sciatic or spinal nerves) or TG (constriction of branches of the trigeminal nerve) changes. In neuropathic pain, $Na_v1.3$ remains upregulated and $Na_v1.7$ and $Na_v1.8$ are downregulated (Cummins et al., 2007; Dib-Hajj, Cummins, Black, & Waxman, 2007). Interestingly, pain induced by the chemotherapeutic agent oxaliplatin and cancer-induced bone pain still occurs in $Na_v1.7$-null mice (Minett et al., 2014). In humans, an example of pain developing in a congenital indifference to pain $Na_v1.7$-null female has recently been described (Minett et al., 2015).

Gain-of-function $Na_v1.7$ point mutations (L858H, T2575A, and T2543A) are already well described as the source of many erythermalgia cases (a disorder characterized by bilateral burning pain of the feet/lower legs and hands, elevated skin temperature of affected areas, and reddened extremities) and hyperexcitability of DRG neurons (Rush et al., 2006; Yang et al., 2004). Mutations in different regions of the $Na_v1.7$ gene *SCN9A* result in distinct phenotypes. In this way, the mutation at nucleotide 984 (C–A) that transforms the codon for tyrosine 328 to a stop codon is responsible for loss of function of the $Na_v1.7$ channel, characterized by congenital indifference to pain in humans (Ahmad et al., 2007; Cox et al., 2006). The mutations (c.774_775delGT and c.2488C>T) and (c.4975A>T and c.3703delATAGCATATGG) induce an inability to detect any smell (anosmia) in humans and mice. Electrophysiological data from $Na_v1.7$-null mice show that olfactory sensory neurons are still electrically active and generate odor-evoked action potentials but fail to initiate synaptic signaling to the projection neurons in the olfactory bulb (Weiss et al., 2011). All the 8 missense mutations (R996C, V1298F, V1298D, V1299F, I1461T, F1462V, T1464I, and M1627K) found in 11 families and 2 sporadic cases induced a gain of function, characterized by episodic burning pain of the rectum, ocular, and mandibular regions (paroxysmal extreme pain disorder). Functional analysis *in vitro* of the mutations (I1461T, T1464I, M1627K) revealed a reduction in fast inactivation, leading to persistent sodium current (Fertleman et al., 2006). Thus, the evidence points to a key role for $Na_v1.7$ in pain pathways.

Due to structural similarities between the nine subtypes of sodium channels, it is difficult to make subtype-selective drugs. An alternative approach is the production of specific antibodies. Lee and colleagues described a $Na_v1.7$-specific monoclonal antibody that presented significant analgesic effects in mouse models of inflammatory (formalin) and neuropathic pain (chronic constriction injury) without affecting the motor function. The same antibody was also effective in acute (compound 48/80, chloroquine, gastrin-releasing peptide) and chronic (acetone and diethyether followed by water and 2.4-dinitrofluorobenzene) models of itch (Lee et al., 2014). However, these data have not been replicated.

4. $NA_V1.8$

Present only in small-diameter sensory neurons in the periphery, $Na_v1.8$ channels appear to be important for the hyperexcitability of DRG neurons caused by $Na_v1.7$ erythermalgia mutations (Rush et al., 2006). A screen searching for *SCN10A* mutations in 104 patients with painful, predominantly small fiber neuropathy, found 7 $Na_v1.8$ mutations (p.Leu554Pro, p.Pro939Leu, p.Gln940Leu, p.Asp1056Asn, p.Ala1304Thr, p.Cys1523Tyr, and p.Gly1662Ser) in patients who did not carry mutations in $Na_v1.7$ (Faber et al., 2012). In addition, several molecules implicated in inflammatory pain increase the expression of $Na_v1.8$, including protein kinases A and C (Fitzgerald, Okuse, Wood, Dolphin, & Moss, 1999), annexin II light chain (Okuse et al., 2002), and contactin in DRG $IB4^+$ (isolectin B4 positive) neurones (Rush et al., 2005).

Knockdown of $Na_v1.8$ mRNA with antisense oligodeoxynucleotides was effective at reducing pain behaviors associated with peripheral inflammation (Joshi et al., 2006; Khasar, Gold, & Levine, 1998). $Na_v1.8$-null mice display decreases in behavioral responses to noxious cold and mechanical stimulus as well as exhibit delayed inflammatory hyperalgesia. These animals lose slowly inactivating sodium currents (Akopian et al., 1999). Mice in which $Na_v1.8$-expressing sensory neurons are ablated present deficits in inflammatory pain behavior, yet they respond normally to heat (Abrahamsen et al., 2008).

Injury caused by chronic sciatic nerve constriction upregulated $Na_v1.8$ protein (but not mRNA) expression in nerve sprouts or neuromas, suggesting a potential role for these TTX-R sodium channels in altered pain perception (Novakovic et al., 1998). In contrast, ectopic spikes induced by sciatic nerve transection were blocked by a low concentration of TTX, which argue against the participation of $Na_v1.8$ channels (TTX-R) in their production (Omana-Zapata, Khabbaz, Hunter, Clarke, & Bley, 1997). In rats submitted to spinal nerve ligation, the allodynia and thermal hyperalgesia were reduced by $Na_v1.8$ knockdown using intrathecal administration of specific antisense oligodeoxynucleotides (Lai et al., 2002). This observation is intriguing, as several studies have shown that $Na_v1.8$ mRNA, protein, and currents are substantially decreased in axotomized DRG neurons (Cummins & Waxman, 1997; Decosterd, Ji, Abdi, Tate, & Woolf, 2002; Dib-Hajj, Black, Felts, & Waxman, 1996). In addition, Joshi et al. (2006) reported that $Na_v1.8$ antisense reduces pain behaviors associated with chronic nerve constriction injury, but not pain behaviors associated with chemotherapy (using the vincristine model) or with skin incisions (Joshi et al., 2006). Finally, Dong et al. (2007) showed that small interfering RNAs that knockdown $Na_v1.8$ could reverse mechanical allodynia caused by chronic constriction injury in rats. But studies employing $Na_v1.8$-null or $Na_v1.8/Na_v1.7$-null mice concluded that these channels do not participate in neuropathic pain induced by spinal nerve ligation (Dong et al., 2007; Kerr, Souslova, McMahon, & Wood, 2001; Nassar, Levato, Stirling, & Wood, 2005).

When selective blockers of $Na_v1.8$ such as A-803467 and ambroxol were tested in rats, they successfully suppressed various pain symptoms and neuropathic pain (Gaida, Klinder, Arndt, & Weiser, 2005; Jarvis et al., 2007). In diabetic patients, it is believed that methylglyoxal (present at high levels during hyperglycemia) depolarizes sensory neurons and induces post-translational modifications in $Na_v1.8$ increasing the activity of the channel, suggesting that a selective $Na_v1.8$ blocker could be used to treat diabetic neuropathic pain conditions (de Lera Ruiz & Kraus, 2015).

In neuropathic animals, mRNAs for $Na_v1.8$ and $Na_v1.9$ are claimed to be reduced with respect to proportions of expressing neurons and to intensities, whereas the β_3 subunit mRNA is markedly upregulated (Fried, Bongenhielm, Boissonade, & Robinson, 2001; Robinson et al., 2004).

The acute visceral pain induced by intracolonic saline or intraperitoneal acetylcholine and cyclophosphamide showed diminished nociceptive behavior in $Na_v1.8$-null mice. However, weak pain and no referred hyperalgesia were observed in $Na_v1.8$-null mutants after intracolonic capsaicin (a model in which behavior is sustained by ongoing activity in nociceptors sensitized by the initial application) or mustard oil (which sensitizes nociceptors but also provokes tissue damage) (Laird, Souslova, Wood, & Cervero, 2002). Visceral pain is also an important condition, and new drug treatments for this condition are needed.

5. $NA_V1.9$

$Na_v1.9$ channels are preferentially expressed in small-diameter DRG neurons, in TG neurons, and in intrinsic myenteric neurons (mainly nociceptors). They can be present also in free nerve terminals, central terminals within the outer layers in the spinal cord and in $IB4^+$ neurons. Computer simulations suggest that $Na_v1.9$ may modulate neurotransmitter release in the dorsal horn even when present at a low density (Dib-Hajj, Black, & Waxman, 2015; Herzog, Cummins, & Waxman, 2001).

Transgenic $Na_v1.9$-null mice show reduced hypersensitivity to inflammatory hyperalgesia induced by formalin, carrageenan, CFA, and prostaglandin E_2 (Leo, D'Hooge, & Meert, 2010; Lolignier et al., 2011; Priest et al., 2005), as well as a reduced sensitivity to nociception triggered by specific inflammatory mediators such as bradykinin, serotonin, and adenosine triphosphate, while responding normally to NGF (Amaya et al., 2006). In addition, inflammation induces an upregulation of $Na_v1.9$ mRNA in DRG 7 days after intraplantar CFA injection, while axotomy of sciatic nerve causes downregulation (Dib-Hajj, Tyrrell, Black, & Waxman, 1998; Tate et al., 1998), suggesting a role for $Na_v1.9$ channels in sensory neuronal hyperexcitability associated with chronic inflammatory pain, but not with nerve injury-induced pain. Indeed, $Na_v1.9$-null mice do not show altered pain behavior in neuropathic pain induced by section of the common peroneal and tibial nerves (Amaya et al., 2006) or spinal nerve transection (Minett et al., 2014). But when investigated in the orofacial model of neuropathic pain, $Na_v1.9$-null mice do not develop mechanical or thermal heat hypersensitivity (Luiz, Kopach, Santana-Varela, & Wood, 2015). $Na_v1.9$ channels can be modulated through protein kinase C phosphorylation by intracellular second messengers that make the channel increasingly active leading to sensory neuron sensitization (Baker, 2005; Baker, Chandra, Ding, Waxman, & Wood, 2003).

Recent studies demonstrated that peripheral neuropathy is associated with several mutations in the human *SCN11A* gene encoding $Na_V1.9$ channels (I381T, K419N, A582T, A681D, A842P, L1158P, F1689L, and one additional mutation at the 3′ acceptor splice site in intron 24) and most importantly, in patients that did not carry *SCN9A* ($Na_V1.7$) or *SCN10A* ($Na_V1.8$) mutations. Two of those mutations led to a reduction in the current threshold and increased firing frequency in response to suprathreshold stimuli (Huang et al., 2014). Another two mutations in *SCN11A* (Arg225Cys and Ala808Gly) reported in patients experiencing episodic chronic pain caused an increase in the $Na_V1.9$ channel-mediated current density and hyperexcitability of nociceptive DRG neurons without changes in the resting membrane potential (Zhang et al., 2013). In contrast, Leipold and colleagues described a gain-of-function mutation in *SCN11A* (p.Leu811Pro) correlated with an unusual syndrome of loss-of-pain sensation and inclination for self-mutilation associated with gastrointestinal motility disturbances and muscle weakness (Leipold et al., 2013).

6. PHARMACOLOGICAL APPROACHES

According to the Chronic Pain Policy Coalition, in England alone chronic pain affects over 14 million people of all ages. Pain is the second most common reason given for claiming incapacity benefit, leading to £3.8 billion spent per year on incapacity benefit for this condition. With these data, it is not difficult to understand why scientists and pharmaceutical companies from all around the world are trying to improve the pain management and the quality of life of the patients.

In the field of pain, neuropathic pain is the one that is least susceptible to available treatments. The current alternative treatments are serotonin–noradrenaline reuptake inhibitors, duloxetine, venlafaxine, tricyclic antidepressants, pregabalin, and gabapentin as first-line drugs; tramadol, capsaicin 8%, and lidocaine patches as second-line drugs; and strong opioids and botulinum toxin A as third-line drugs (Finnerup et al., 2015; Gilron, Baron, & Jensen, 2015). The full analgesic potential of these agents is thus limited by numerous adverse events related to the peripheral and central nervous systems such as dizziness, sedation, constipation, nausea, vomiting, and local irritation (Finnerup et al., 2015; Gilron et al., 2015). Drugs such as carbamazepine and mexiletine present some efficacy, when $Na_V1.7$ gain-of-function mutations are present, but have a limited therapeutic window (de Lera Ruiz & Kraus, 2015).

The pharmacotherapy of neuropathic pain remains an important component of pain management. Despite recent progress in the understanding of pathophysiological mechanisms, diagnosis, and the treatment of neuropathic pain, many patients (40–50%) remain refractory to, or intolerant of, the existing pharmacological treatment (Salat, Kowalczyk, Gryzlo, Jakubowska, & Kulig, 2014). VGSCs are considered one of the contributors to abnormal and aberrant transmission that characterizes neuropathic pain. In the last few years, major efforts regarding the discovery of new sodium channel blockers useful in the treatment of neuropathic pain have focused on improving not only potency but also selectivity (Rivara & Zuliani, 2015). Many clinical trials with isoform-selective drugs for Na_v channels are in progress however, and some results are promising (see details in Table 2).

7. SODIUM CHANNELS IN CANCER

Many studies associate aspects of cancer with VGSC expression, but a causative role for these channels in cancer and metastases is still uncertain. Multiple studies have shown the functional expression of VGSCs in cell types that are not considered electrically excitable, such as astrocytes, chondrocytes, dendritic cells, endothelial cells, fibroblasts, keratinocytes, islet β-cells, lymphocytes, macrophages, microglia, oligodendrocytes, Schwann cells, T-lymphocytes, osteoblasts, odontoblasts, red blood cells, and cancer cells. In these cells, the VGSCs may play biological roles that are not related to the generation of action potentials, but which regulate migration, endosomal acidification, phagocytosis, podosome formation, insulin release, and cytokine release (Besson et al., 2015; Black & Waxman, 2013; Eren, Ozturk, Sonmez, & Oyan, 2015; Patel & Brackenbury, 2015). In some tumor cells, the functional activity of Na_v channels may be involved in regulating the proliferative, migrative, and invasive properties of cells (Besson et al., 2015; Eren et al., 2015; Patel & Brackenbury, 2015; Roger et al., 2015). Roger and colleagues in a seminal review about VGSCs and cancer suggest that the abnormal expression of $Na_v\alpha$ and $Na_v\beta$ proteins associated with aggressive features could classify some cancers as (sodium) channelopathies (Roger et al., 2015).

Functional $Na_v\alpha$ subunits have been reported to be highly overexpressed in cancer biopsies and cancer cells—prostate, breast lung (small-cell lung cancer), leukocytes (leukemia), pleura (mesothelioma), cervix, colon, and ovary—while they are undetectable in most normal tissues (see Table 3).

Table 2 Voltage-Gated Sodium Channel Inhibitors in Current Study

Company	Code	Selectivity	Clinical Phase	Indications	Results	Observations
Pfizer	PF-05089771	$Na_v1.7$	I	Erythermalgia, postoperative dental pain, OA and DPN		
			II	DPN		
Convergence Pharmaceuticals	CNV-1014802	$Na_v1.7$	III	Trigeminal neuralgia	Well tolerated, no major side effects, reduced pain severity and the number of paroxysms in all primary and secondary outcomes	Orphan-drug designation by the FDA
				NP (lumbosacral radiculopathy)	Reduced pain	
	CNV-3000223	$Na_v1.7$				Undergoing preclinical studies
	CNV-3000164	$Na_v1.7$				Undergoing preclinical studies
Xenon/Teve	XEN-402 (or TV-5070)	$Na_v1.7$	IIa	Erythermalgia	Reduced pain	
				OA		
Xenon/Genentech	GDC-0276	$Na_v1.7$	I			

Sumitomo Dainippon Pharma	DSP-2230	$Na_v1.7$/ $Na_v1.8$	I			Antiallodynic effect in animal models of neuropathic pain
Nektar Therapeutics	NKTR-171	Peripheral Na_v		NP	Significantly reduced CNS penetration versus currently approved Na_v inhibitors, no major side effects	
WEX Pharmaceuticals	TTX	Na_v TTX-S	III	Moderate to severe inadequately controlled cancer-related pain		
			II	Chemotherapy-induced NP		

OA, osteoarthritis; DPN, diabetic peripheral neuropathy; NP, neuropathic pain; CNS, central nervous system.
Source: https://patents.google.com, de Lera Ruiz and Kraus (2015), Kwong and Carr, (2015), Salat et al. (2014), and Zakrzewska et al. (2013).

Table 3 Voltage-Gated Sodium Channel in Cancer Cells

Cancer	Cell Type	Drug	Current	Invasiveness (Matrigel™)	Channel
Prostate	Rat—Mat-Ly-Lu	1 μM TTX	Full inhibition	Reduce 33%	mRNA $Na_v1.1$, $Na_v1.2$, $Na_v1.3$, $Na_v1.4$, $Na_v1.6$, $Na_v1.8$, and **mainly $Na_v1.7$**
	Human—PC-3	TTX	Reduced	Reduce	
	Human—LNCaP	1 μM TTX	–	Reduce	α1Ab subunit
	Derivate Human—LNCaP C4	1 μM TTX	–	Reduce	Overexpression α1Ab subunit
	Derivate Human—LNCaP C4-2	1 μM TTX	–	Reduce	
Breast	Human—MDA-MB-231	30 μM TTX	Full inhibition	–	mRNA $Na_v1.2$, $Na_v1.4$, and $Na_v1.8$ low level High-level **$Na_v1.5$**, $Na_v1.6$, and $Na_v1.7$
		TTX, ranolazine, phenytoin	–	Reduce (∼35%)	
		siRNA for *SCN5A*	Full inhibition	Reduce (∼35%)	
		Veratridine	–	Increase	
Leukocytes	Jurkat T cell	10 μM TTX	Inhibition	Reduce more than 90%	mRNA $Na_v1.7$ and $Na_v1.9$ low level High-level **$Na_v1.5$** and $Na_v1.6$

Lung	Human—Calu-1	5 nM to 30 μM TTX	Dose-dependent inhibition	Dose-dependent inhibition	mRNA With exception of $Na_v1.4$, all others VGSCs **Mainly $Na_v1.7$**
	Human—H23	–	–	–	mRNA **Mainly $Na_v1.7$** ($Na_v1.5$ not functional)
	Human—H460	siRNA for *SCN9A*	–	Reduce	
Colon	Human—SW620	10 μM TTX	Partial inhibition	Reduce around 50%	**Mainly $Na_v1.5$**
	Human—SW480				**Mainly $Na_v1.5$**
	Human—HT29				**Mainly $Na_v1.5$**
Cervix	Primary culture from human cervical cancer biopsies	1 μM $Na_v1.6$-specific toxin Cn2 (similar effect: 1 μM TTX)	Partial inhibition (~50%)	Reduce (~20%)	mRNA $Na_v1.2$, $Na_v1.4$, **$Na_v1.6$ (40-fold)** and $Na_v1.7$ (20-fold)
Ovary	Ovarian cancer biopsies	–	–	–	mRNA $Na_v1.1$, $Na_v1.3$, $Na_v1.4$, and **$Na_v1.5$**
	Human ovarian cancer	1 μM TTX	–	No effect	mRNA $Na_v1.2$, $Na_v1.4$, **$Na_v1.5$**, and $Na_v1.7$
	Cells lines (Caov-3 and SKOV-3)	30 μM TTX	–	Reduce (~55%)	

The bold text means the main sodium channel correlated with the cancer type described in the row.
TTX, tetrodotoxin sensitive; *SCN5A*, gene that encodes $Na_v1.5$; *SCN9A*, gene that encodes $Na_v1.7$; VGSCs, voltage-gated sodium channels.
Source: Besson et al. (2015), Driffort et al. (2014), Nelson, Yang, Dowle, Thomas, and Brackenbury (2015), Patel and Brackenbury (2015), and Roger et al. (2015).

In addition, the presence of I_{Na} was associated with the enhanced migration and the invasive phenotype of cancer cells. This potentially opens the way for the use of VGSCs as new targets in cancer therapy (Besson et al., 2015; Driffort et al., 2014; Nelson et al., 2015; Patel & Brackenbury, 2015; Roger et al., 2015).

The positive correlation with invasiveness, proliferation, and cell migration has also been described for β1 (Nelson, Millican-Slater, Forrest, & Brackenbury, 2014) and β2 subunits (Jansson et al., 2014) in breast and prostate cancer cells, respectively. As described in Table 3, the functional expression of $Na_v\alpha$ protein (mainly $Na_v1.5$–1.7) in different types of cancer cells in the plasma membrane is positive correlated with the invasive potential of the cells. In contrast, low $Na_v\alpha$ protein expression or no plasma membrane insertion occurs at the earlier stages of the carcinogenic process. In patients, the overexpression of $Na_v1.5$ in breast cancer biopsies has been associated with lymph node invasion, metastatic relapse, and decreased survival (Brackenbury, 2012; Brackenbury, Djamgoz, & Isom, 2008; Fraser et al., 2005; Roger, Besson, & Le Guennec, 2003; Yang et al., 2012).

The VGSCs could potentially act via indirect pathways in cancer cells. Possible mechanisms include regulation of the efflux of H^+, source of extracellular acidification that potentiates cell migration (Brisson et al., 2011; Eren et al., 2015; Stock & Schwab, 2009) and enhanced degradation of the extracellular matrix (cancer cell dissemination) (Cardone, Casavola, & Reshkin, 2005), as well as regulation of gene expression and intracellular calcium levels (Davis et al., 2014; Eren et al., 2015) and regulatory activity on angiogenesis (Andrikopoulos et al., 2011).

Disappointingly, a cohort study that analyzed the hypothesis that people taking VGSC-inhibiting drugs before being diagnosed with cancer live longer than those not taking these drugs showed the opposite effect. Median time to death was 8.7 years early in the group that were taking VGSC-inhibiting drugs in breast, colon, or prostate cancer (Fairhurst, Watt, Martin, Bland, & Brackenbury, 2015). However, the study evaluated the use of VGSC-inhibiting drugs for other comorbidities such as epilepsy and arrhythmia rather than cancer. The clinical conditions of the patients combined with cancer may help explain this result.

Considering the aggressive present treatments for some cancers, the use of blockers of VGSCs already approved for other diseases and with potentially less side effects than the usual chemotherapy drugs could be evaluated for the prevention and/or reduction of metastatic tumors. As cancer is among the leading causes of death and brings huge suffering for the patient and the family, any drug that can increase life expectancy is desirable.

8. CONCLUSION

VGSCs have great potential as pharmacological targets for many different disorders in the neuronal and cardiac systems. In this chapter, we have focussed on pain disorders and cancer. The main issue is to reduce the side effects and improve the selectivity of small molecule blockers or produce antibodies that are subunit specific and potent. While new drugs are under development, the use of already FDA-approved broad spectrum sodium channel blockers will continue for pain disorders, even with some side effects, and proof-of-concept clinical trials for cancer treatment seem warranted.

CONFLICT OF INTEREST

The authors have no conflict of interest to declare.

ACKNOWLEDGMENT

This work was supported by an Arthritis UK Grant (A.L.).

REFERENCES

Abrahamsen, B., Zhao, J., Asante, C. O., Cendan, C. M., Marsh, S., Martinez-Barbera, J. P., ... Wood, J. N. (2008). The cell and molecular basis of mechanical, cold, and inflammatory pain. *Science*, *321*(5889), 702–705. http://dx.doi.org/10.1126/science.1156916.

Ahmad, S., Dahllund, L., Eriksson, A. B., Hellgren, D., Karlsson, U., Lund, P. E., ... Krupp, J. J. (2007). A stop codon mutation in SCN9A causes lack of pain sensation. *Human Molecular Genetics*, *16*(17), 2114–2121. http://dx.doi.org/10.1093/hmg/ddm160.

Akopian, A. N., Souslova, V., England, S., Okuse, K., Ogata, N., Ure, J., ... Wood, J. N. (1999). The tetrodotoxin-resistant sodium channel SNS has a specialized function in pain pathways. *Nature Neuroscience*, *2*(6), 541–548. http://dx.doi.org/10.1038/9195.

Alexander, S. P. H., Mathie, A., & Peters, J. A. (2009). Guide to receptors and channels (GRAC), 4th edition. *British Journal of Pharmacology*, *158*, S1–S239. Retrieved from <Go to ISI>://WOS:000271416300001.

Amaya, F., Wang, H., Costigan, M., Allchorne, A. J., Hatcher, J. P., Egerton, J., ... Woolf, C. J. (2006). The voltage-gated sodium channel Na(v)1.9 is an effector of peripheral inflammatory pain hypersensitivity. *Journal of Neuroscience*, *26*(50), 12852–12860. http://dx.doi.org/10.1523/JNEUROSCI.4015-06.2006.

Andrikopoulos, P., Fraser, S. P., Patterson, L., Ahmad, Z., Burcu, H., Ottaviani, D., ... Djamgoz, M. B. (2011). Angiogenic functions of voltage-gated Na^+ channels in human endothelial cells: Modulation of vascular endothelial growth factor (VEGF) signaling. *Journal of Biological Chemistry*, *286*(19), 16846–16860. http://dx.doi.org/10.1074/jbc.M110.187559.

Baker, M. D. (2005). Protein kinase C mediates up-regulation of tetrodotoxin-resistant, persistent Na+ current in rat and mouse sensory neurones. *Journal of Physiology, 567*(Pt 3), 851–867. http://dx.doi.org/10.1113/jphysiol.2005.089771.

Baker, M. D., Chandra, S. Y., Ding, Y., Waxman, S. G., & Wood, J. N. (2003). GTP-induced tetrodotoxin-resistant Na+ current regulates excitability in mouse and rat small diameter sensory neurones. *Journal of Physiology, 548*(Pt 2), 373–382. http://dx.doi.org/10.1113/jphysiol.2003.039131.

Besson, P., Driffort, V., Bon, E., Gradek, F., Chevalier, S., & Roger, S. (2015). How do voltage-gated sodium channels enhance migration and invasiveness in cancer cells? *Biochim Biophys Acta, 1848*(10 Pt B), 2493–2501. http://dx.doi.org/10.1016/j.bbamem.2015.04.013.

Black, J. A., Cummins, T. R., Plumpton, C., Chen, Y. H., Hormuzdiar, W., Clare, J. J., & Waxman, S. G. (1999). Upregulation of a silent sodium channel after peripheral, but not central, nerve injury in DRG neurons. *Journal of Neurophysiology, 82*(5), 2776–2785. Retrieved from http://www.ncbi.nlm.nih.gov/pubmed/10561444.

Black, J. A., Liu, S., Tanaka, M., Cummins, T. R., & Waxman, S. G. (2004). Changes in the expression of tetrodotoxin-sensitive sodium channels within dorsal root ganglia neurons in inflammatory pain. *Pain, 108*(3), 237–247. http://dx.doi.org/10.1016/j.pain.2003.12.035.

Black, J. A., & Waxman, S. G. (2013). Noncanonical roles of voltage-gated sodium channels. *Neuron, 80*(2), 280–291. http://dx.doi.org/10.1016/j.neuron.2013.09.012.

Brackenbury, W. J. (2012). Voltage-gated sodium channels and metastatic disease. *Channels (Austin, TX), 6*(5), 352–361. http://dx.doi.org/10.4161/chan.21910.

Brackenbury, W. J., Djamgoz, M. B., & Isom, L. L. (2008). An emerging role for voltage-gated Na+ channels in cellular migration: Regulation of central nervous system development and potentiation of invasive cancers. *The Neuroscientist, 14*(6), 571–583. http://dx.doi.org/10.1177/1073858408320293.

Brisson, L., Gillet, L., Calaghan, S., Besson, P., Le Guennec, J. Y., Roger, S., & Gore, J. (2011). Na(V)1.5 enhances breast cancer cell invasiveness by increasing NHE1-dependent H(+) efflux in caveolae. *Oncogene, 30*(17), 2070–2076. http://dx.doi.org/10.1038/onc.2010.574.

Cardone, R. A., Casavola, V., & Reshkin, S. J. (2005). The role of disturbed pH dynamics and the Na+/H+ exchanger in metastasis. *Nature Reviews. Cancer, 5*(10), 786–795. http://dx.doi.org/10.1038/nrc1713.

Catterall, W. A. (2000). From ionic currents to molecular mechanisms: The structure and function of voltage-gated sodium channels. *Neuron, 26*(1), 13–25. Retrieved from http://www.ncbi.nlm.nih.gov/pubmed/10798388.

Cox, J. J., Reimann, F., Nicholas, A. K., Thornton, G., Roberts, E., Springell, K., ... Woods, C. G. (2006). An SCN9A channelopathy causes congenital inability to experience pain. *Nature, 444*(7121), 894–898. http://dx.doi.org/10.1038/nature05413.

Craner, M. J., Klein, J. P., Renganathan, M., Black, J. A., & Waxman, S. G. (2002). Changes of sodium channel expression in experimental painful diabetic neuropathy. *Annals of Neurology, 52*(6), 786–792. http://dx.doi.org/10.1002/ana.10364.

Cummins, T. R., Sheets, P. L., & Waxman, S. G. (2007). The roles of sodium channels in nociception: Implications for mechanisms of pain. *Pain, 131*(3), 243–257. http://dx.doi.org/10.1016/j.pain.2007.07.026.

Cummins, T. R., & Waxman, S. G. (1997). Downregulation of tetrodotoxin-resistant sodium currents and upregulation of a rapidly repriming tetrodotoxin-sensitive sodium current in small spinal sensory neurons after nerve injury. *Journal of Neuroscience, 17*(10), 3503–3514. Retrieved from http://www.ncbi.nlm.nih.gov/pubmed/9133375.

Davis, F. M., Azimi, I., Faville, R. A., Peters, A. A., Jalink, K., Putney, J. W., Jr., ... Monteith, G. R. (2014). Induction of epithelial-mesenchymal transition (EMT) in breast cancer cells is calcium signal dependent. *Oncogene*, *33*(18), 2307–2316. http://dx.doi.org/10.1038/onc.2013.187.

Decosterd, I., Ji, R. R., Abdi, S., Tate, S., & Woolf, C. J. (2002). The pattern of expression of the voltage-gated sodium channels Na(v)1.8 and Na(v)1.9 does not change in uninjured primary sensory neurons in experimental neuropathic pain models. *Pain*, *96*(3), 269–277. Retrieved from http://www.ncbi.nlm.nih.gov/pubmed/11972999.

de Lera Ruiz, M., & Kraus, R. L. (2015). Voltage-gated sodium channels: Structure, function, pharmacology, and clinical indications. *Journal of Medicinal Chemistry*, *58*(18), 7093–7118. http://dx.doi.org/10.1021/jm501981g.

Dib-Hajj, S., Black, J. A., Felts, P., & Waxman, S. G. (1996). Down-regulation of transcripts for Na channel alpha-SNS in spinal sensory neurons following axotomy. *Proceedings of the National Academy of Sciences of the United States of America*, *93*(25), 14950–14954. Retrieved from http://www.ncbi.nlm.nih.gov/pubmed/8962162.

Dib-Hajj, S. D., Black, J. A., & Waxman, S. G. (2015). NaV1.9: A sodium channel linked to human pain. *Nature Reviews. Neuroscience*, *16*(9), 511–519. http://dx.doi.org/10.1038/nrn3977.

Dib-Hajj, S. D., Cummins, T. R., Black, J. A., & Waxman, S. G. (2007). From genes to pain: Na v 1.7 and human pain disorders. *Trends in Neurosciences*, *30*(11), 555–563. http://dx.doi.org/10.1016/j.tins.2007.08.004.

Dib-Hajj, S. D., Fjell, J., Cummins, T. R., Zheng, Z., Fried, K., LaMotte, R., … Waxman, S. G. (1999). Plasticity of sodium channel expression in DRG neurons in the chronic constriction injury model of neuropathic pain. *Pain*, *83*(3), 591–600. Retrieved from http://www.ncbi.nlm.nih.gov/pubmed/10568868.

Dib-Hajj, S. D., Tyrrell, L., Black, J. A., & Waxman, S. G. (1998). NaN, a novel voltage-gated Na channel, is expressed preferentially in peripheral sensory neurons and down-regulated after axotomy. *Proceedings of the National Academy of Sciences of the United States of America*, *95*(15), 8963–8968. Retrieved from http://www.ncbi.nlm.nih.gov/pubmed/9671787.

Dong, X. W., Goregoaker, S., Engler, H., Zhou, X., Mark, L., Crona, J., … Priestley, T. (2007). Small interfering RNA-mediated selective knockdown of Na(V)1.8 tetrodotoxin-resistant sodium channel reverses mechanical allodynia in neuropathic rats. *Neuroscience*, *146*(2), 812–821. http://dx.doi.org/10.1016/j.neuroscience.2007.01.054.

Driffort, V., Gillet, L., Bon, E., Marionneau-Lambot, S., Oullier, T., Joulin, V., … Roger, S. (2014). Ranolazine inhibits NaV1.5-mediated breast cancer cell invasiveness and lung colonization. *Molecular Cancer*, *13*, 264. http://dx.doi.org/10.1186/1476-4598-13-264.

Eijkelkamp, N., Linley, J. E., Baker, M. D., Minett, M. S., Cregg, R., Werdehausen, R., … Wood, J. N. (2012). Neurological perspectives on voltage-gated sodium channels. *Brain*, *135*(Pt 9), 2585–2612. http://dx.doi.org/10.1093/brain/aws225.

Eren, O. O., Ozturk, M. A., Sonmez, O. U., & Oyan, B. (2015). Voltage-gated sodium channel blockers can augment the efficacy of chemotherapeutics by their inhibitory effect on epithelial-mesenchymal transition. *Medical Hypotheses*, *84*(1), 11–13. http://dx.doi.org/10.1016/j.mehy.2014.11.006.

Eriksson, J., Jablonski, A., Persson, A. K., Hao, J. X., Kouya, P. F., Wiesenfeld-Hallin, Z., … Fried, K. (2005). Behavioral changes and trigeminal ganglion sodium channel regulation in an orofacial neuropathic pain model. *Pain*, *119*(1-3), 82–94. http://dx.doi.org/10.1016/j.pain.2005.09.019.

Faber, C. G., Lauria, G., Merkies, I. S., Cheng, X., Han, C., Ahn, H. S., … Waxman, S. G. (2012). Gain-of-function Nav1.8 mutations in painful neuropathy. *Proceedings of the National Academy of Sciences of the United States of America*, *109*(47), 19444–19449. http://dx.doi.org/10.1073/pnas.1216080109.

Fairhurst, C., Watt, I., Martin, F., Bland, M., & Brackenbury, W. J. (2015). Sodium channel-inhibiting drugs and survival of breast, colon and prostate cancer: A population-based study. *Scientific Reports*, *5*, 16758. http://dx.doi.org/10.1038/srep16758.

Fertleman, C. R., Baker, M. D., Parker, K. A., Moffatt, S., Elmslie, F. V., Abrahamsen, B., ... Rees, M. (2006). SCN9A mutations in paroxysmal extreme pain disorder: Allelic variants underlie distinct channel defects and phenotypes. *Neuron*, *52*(5), 767–774. http://dx.doi.org/10.1016/j.neuron.2006.10.006.

Finnerup, N. B., Attal, N., Haroutounian, S., McNicol, E., Baron, R., Dworkin, R. H., ... Wallace, M. (2015). Pharmacotherapy for neuropathic pain in adults: A systematic review and meta-analysis. *Lancet Neurology*, *14*(2), 162–173. http://dx.doi.org/10.1016/S1474-4422(14)70251-0.

Fitzgerald, E. M., Okuse, K., Wood, J. N., Dolphin, A. C., & Moss, S. J. (1999). cAMP-dependent phosphorylation of the tetrodotoxin-resistant voltage-dependent sodium channel SNS. *Journal of Physiology*, *516*(Pt 2), 433–446. Retrieved from http://www.ncbi.nlm.nih.gov/pubmed/10087343.

Foulkes, T., Nassar, M. A., Lane, T., Matthews, E. A., Baker, M. D., Gerke, V., ... Wood, J. N. (2006). Deletion of annexin 2 light chain p11 in nociceptors causes deficits in somatosensory coding and pain behavior. *Journal of Neuroscience*, *26*(41), 10499–10507. http://dx.doi.org/10.1523/JNEUROSCI.1997-06.2006.

Fraser, S. P., Diss, J. K., Chioni, A. M., Mycielska, M. E., Pan, H., Yamaci, R. F., ... Djamgoz, M. B. (2005). Voltage-gated sodium channel expression and potentiation of human breast cancer metastasis. *Clinical Cancer Research*, *11*(15), 5381–5389. http://dx.doi.org/10.1158/1078-0432.CCR-05-0327.

Fricker, D., Dinocourt, C., Eugene, E., Wood, J. N., & Miles, R. (2009). Pyramidal cells of rodent presubiculum express a tetrodotoxin-insensitive Na+ current. *Journal of Physiology*, *587*(Pt 17), 4249–4264. http://dx.doi.org/10.1113/jphysiol.2009.175349.

Fried, K., Bongenhielm, U., Boissonade, F. M., & Robinson, P. P. (2001). Nerve injury-induced pain in the trigeminal system. *The Neuroscientist*, 7(2), 155–165. Retrieved from http://www.ncbi.nlm.nih.gov/pubmed/11496926.

Gaida, W., Klinder, K., Arndt, K., & Weiser, T. (2005). Ambroxol, a Nav1.8-preferring Na(+) channel blocker, effectively suppresses pain symptoms in animal models of chronic, neuropathic and inflammatory pain. *Neuropharmacology*, *49*(8), 1220–1227. http://dx.doi.org/10.1016/j.neuropharm.2005.08.004.

Gilron, I., Baron, R., & Jensen, T. (2015). Neuropathic pain: Principles of diagnosis and treatment. *Mayo Clinic Proceedings*, *90*(4), 532–545. http://dx.doi.org/10.1016/j.mayocp.2015.01.018.

Goldin, A. L., Barchi, R. L., Caldwell, J. H., Hofmann, F., Howe, J. R., Hunter, J. C., ... Catterall, W. A. (2000). Nomenclature of voltage-gated sodium channels. *Neuron*, *28*(2), 365–368. Retrieved from http://www.ncbi.nlm.nih.gov/pubmed/11144347..

Habib, A. M., Wood, J. N., & Cox, J. J. (2015). Sodium channels and pain. *Handbook of Experimental Pharmacology*, *227*, 39–56. http://dx.doi.org/10.1007/978-3-662-46450-2_3.

Hains, B. C., Saab, C. Y., Klein, J. P., Craner, M. J., & Waxman, S. G. (2004). Altered sodium channel expression in second-order spinal sensory neurons contributes to pain after peripheral nerve injury. *Journal of Neuroscience*, *24*(20), 4832–4839. http://dx.doi.org/10.1523/JNEUROSCI.0300-04.2004.

Herzog, R. I., Cummins, T. R., & Waxman, S. G. (2001). Persistent TTX-resistant Na+ current affects resting potential and response to depolarization in simulated spinal sensory neurons. *Journal of Neurophysiology*, *86*(3), 1351–1364. Retrieved from http://www.ncbi.nlm.nih.gov/pubmed/11535682.

Huang, J., Han, C., Estacion, M., Vasylyev, D., Hoeijmakers, J. G., Gerrits, M. M., ... Group, P. S. (2014). Gain-of-function mutations in sodium channel Na(v)1.9 in painful neuropathy. *Brain*, *137*(Pt 6), 1627–1642. http://dx.doi.org/10.1093/brain/awu079.

Jansson, K. H., Castillo, D. G., Morris, J. W., Boggs, M. E., Czymmek, K. J., Adams, E. L., ... Sikes, R. A. (2014). Identification of beta-2 as a key cell adhesion molecule in PCa cell neurotropic behavior: A novel ex vivo and biophysical approach. *PLoS One, 9*(6), e98408. http://dx.doi.org/10.1371/journal.pone.0098408.
Jarvis, M. F., Honore, P., Shieh, C. C., Chapman, M., Joshi, S., Zhang, X. F., ... Krafte, D. S. (2007). A-803467, a potent and selective Nav1.8 sodium channel blocker, attenuates neuropathic and inflammatory pain in the rat. *Proceedings of the National Academy of Sciences of the United States of America, 104*(20), 8520–8525. http://dx.doi.org/10.1073/pnas.0611364104.
Joshi, S. K., Mikusa, J. P., Hernandez, G., Baker, S., Shieh, C. C., Neelands, T., ... Honore, P. (2006). Involvement of the TTX-resistant sodium channel Nav 1.8 in inflammatory and neuropathic, but not post-operative, pain states. *Pain, 123*(1–2), 75–82. http://dx.doi.org/10.1016/j.pain.2006.02.011.
Kerr, B. J., Souslova, V., McMahon, S. B., & Wood, J. N. (2001). A role for the TTX-resistant sodium channel Nav 1.8 in NGF-induced hyperalgesia, but not neuropathic pain. *Neuroreport, 12*(14), 3077–3080. Retrieved from http://www.ncbi.nlm.nih.gov/pubmed/11568640.
Khasar, S. G., Gold, M. S., & Levine, J. D. (1998). A tetrodotoxin-resistant sodium current mediates inflammatory pain in the rat. *Neuroscience Letters, 256*(1), 17–20. Retrieved from http://www.ncbi.nlm.nih.gov/pubmed/9832206.
Krafte, D. S., & Bannon, A. W. (2008). Sodium channels and nociception: Recent concepts and therapeutic opportunities. *Current Opinion in Pharmacology, 8*(1), 50–56. http://dx.doi.org/10.1016/j.coph.2007.09.007.
Kwong, K., & Carr, M. J. (2015). Voltage-gated sodium channels. *Current Opinion in Pharmacology, 22*, 131–139. http://dx.doi.org/10.1016/j.coph.2015.04.007.
Lai, J., Gold, M. S., Kim, C. S., Bian, D., Ossipov, M. H., Hunter, J. C., & Porreca, F. (2002). Inhibition of neuropathic pain by decreased expression of the tetrodotoxin-resistant sodium channel, NaV1.8. *Pain, 95*(1–2), 143–152. Retrieved from http://www.ncbi.nlm.nih.gov/pubmed/11790477.
Laird, J. M., Souslova, V., Wood, J. N., & Cervero, F. (2002). Deficits in visceral pain and referred hyperalgesia in Nav1.8 (SNS/PN3)-null mice. *Journal of Neuroscience, 22*(19), 8352–8356. Retrieved from http://www.ncbi.nlm.nih.gov/pubmed/12351708.
Le, Y., & Sauer, B. (2001). Conditional gene knockout using Cre recombinase. *Molecular Biotechnology, 17*(3), 269–275. http://dx.doi.org/10.1385/MB:17:3:269.
Lee, J. H., Park, C. K., Chen, G., Han, Q., Xie, R. G., Liu, T., ... Lee, S. Y. (2014). A monoclonal antibody that targets a NaV1.7 channel voltage sensor for pain and itch relief. *Cell, 157*(6), 1393–1404. http://dx.doi.org/10.1016/j.cell.2014.03.064.
Lees, G., & Shipton, E. (2009). Voltage-gated sodium channels in nociception and their potential as targets for new drugs in treatment of chronic neuropathic pain. *Current Anaesthesia & Critical Care, 20*(5–6), 204–208. http://dx.doi.org/10.1016/j.cacc.2009.06.002.
Leipold, E., Liebmann, L., Korenke, G. C., Heinrich, T., Giesselmann, S., Baets, J., ... Kurth, I. (2013). A de novo gain-of-function mutation in SCN11A causes loss of pain perception. *Nature Genetics, 45*(11), 1399–1404. http://dx.doi.org/10.1038/ng.2767.
Leo, S., D'Hooge, R., & Meert, T. (2010). Exploring the role of nociceptor-specific sodium channels in pain transmission using Nav1.8 and Nav1.9 knockout mice. *Behavioural Brain Research, 208*(1), 149–157. http://dx.doi.org/10.1016/j.bbr.2009.11.023.
Lindia, J. A., Kohler, M. G., Martin, W. J., & Abbadie, C. (2005). Relationship between sodium channel NaV1.3 expression and neuropathic pain behavior in rats. *Pain, 117*(1–2), 145–153. http://dx.doi.org/10.1016/j.pain.2005.05.027.
Liu, M., & Wood, J. N. (2011). The roles of sodium channels in nociception: Implications for mechanisms of neuropathic pain. *Pain Medicine, 12*(Suppl. 3), S93–S99. http://dx.doi.org/10.1111/j.1526-4637.2011.01158.x.

Lolignier, S., Amsalem, M., Maingret, F., Padilla, F., Gabriac, M., Chapuy, E., ... Busserolles, J. (2011). Nav1.9 channel contributes to mechanical and heat pain hypersensitivity induced by subacute and chronic inflammation. *PLoS One*, *6*(8), e23083. http://dx.doi.org/10.1371/journal.pone.0023083.

Luiz, A. P., Kopach, O., Santana-Varela, S., & Wood, J. N. (2015). The role of Na1.9 channel in the development of neuropathic orofacial pain associated with trigeminal neuralgia. *Molecular Pain*, *11*(1), 72. http://dx.doi.org/10.1186/s12990-015-0076-4.

Minett, M. S., Pereira, V., Sikandar, S., Matsuyama, A., Lolignier, S., Kanellopoulos, A. H., ... Wood, J. N. (2015). Endogenous opioids contribute to insensitivity to pain in humans and mice lacking sodium channel Nav1.7. *Nature Communications*, *6*, 8967. http://dx.doi.org/10.1038/ncomms9967.

Minett, M. S., Falk, S., Santana-Varela, S., Bogdanov, Y. D., Nassar, M. A., Heegaard, A. M., & Wood, J. N. (2014). Pain without nociceptors? Nav1.7-independent pain mechanisms. *Cell Reports*, *6*(2), 301–312. http://dx.doi.org/10.1016/j.celrep.2013.12.033.

Minett, M. S., Nassar, M. A., Clark, A. K., Passmore, G., Dickenson, A. H., Wang, F., ... Wood, J. N. (2012). Distinct Nav1.7-dependent pain sensations require different sets of sensory and sympathetic neurons. *Nature Communications*, *3*, 791. http://dx.doi.org/10.1038/ncomms1795.

Nassar, M. A., Baker, M. D., Levato, A., Ingram, R., Mallucci, G., McMahon, S. B., & Wood, J. N. (2006). Nerve injury induces robust allodynia and ectopic discharges in Nav1.3 null mutant mice. *Molecular Pain*, *2*, 33. http://dx.doi.org/10.1186/1744-8069-2-33.

Nassar, M. A., Levato, A., Stirling, L. C., & Wood, J. N. (2005). Neuropathic pain develops normally in mice lacking both Na(v)1.7 and Na(v)1.8. *Molecular Pain*, *1*, 24. http://dx.doi.org/10.1186/1744-8069-1-24.

Nassar, M. A., Stirling, L. C., Forlani, G., Baker, M. D., Matthews, E. A., Dickenson, A. H., & Wood, J. N. (2004). Nociceptor-specific gene deletion reveals a major role for Nav1.7 (PN1) in acute and inflammatory pain. *Proceedings of the National Academy of Sciences of the United States of America*, *101*(34), 12706–12711. http://dx.doi.org/10.1073/pnas.0404915101.

Nelson, M., Millican-Slater, R., Forrest, L. C., & Brackenbury, W. J. (2014). The sodium channel beta1 subunit mediates outgrowth of neurite-like processes on breast cancer cells and promotes tumour growth and metastasis. *International Journal of Cancer*, *135*(10), 2338–2351. http://dx.doi.org/10.1002/ijc.28890.

Nelson, M., Yang, M., Dowle, A. A., Thomas, J. R., & Brackenbury, W. J. (2015). The sodium channel-blocking antiepileptic drug phenytoin inhibits breast tumour growth and metastasis. *Molecular Cancer*, *14*, 13. http://dx.doi.org/10.1186/s12943-014-0277-x.

Novakovic, S. D., Tzoumaka, E., McGivern, J. G., Haraguchi, M., Sangameswaran, L., Gogas, K. R., ... Hunter, J. C. (1998). Distribution of the tetrodotoxin-resistant sodium channel PN3 in rat sensory neurons in normal and neuropathic conditions. *Journal of Neuroscience*, *18*(6), 2174–2187. Retrieved from http://www.ncbi.nlm.nih.gov/pubmed/9482802.

Ogata, N., & Ohishi, Y. (2002). Molecular diversity of structure and function of the voltage-gated Na+ channels. *Japanese Journal of Pharmacology*, *88*(4), 365–377. Retrieved from http://www.ncbi.nlm.nih.gov/pubmed/12046980.

Okuse, K., Malik-Hall, M., Baker, M. D., Poon, W. Y., Kong, H., Chao, M. V., & Wood, J. N. (2002). Annexin II light chain regulates sensory neuron-specific sodium channel expression. *Nature*, *417*(6889), 653–656. http://dx.doi.org/10.1038/nature00781.

Omana-Zapata, I., Khabbaz, M. A., Hunter, J. C., Clarke, D. E., & Bley, K. R. (1997). Tetrodotoxin inhibits neuropathic ectopic activity in neuromas, dorsal root ganglia and dorsal horn neurons. *Pain*, *72*(1–2), 41–49. Retrieved from http://www.ncbi.nlm.nih.gov/pubmed/9272786.

Patel, F., & Brackenbury, W. J. (2015). Dual roles of voltage-gated sodium channels in development and cancer. *International Journal of Developmental Biology*, *59*(7–9), 357–366. http://dx.doi.org/10.1387/ijdb.150171wb.

Priest, B. T., Murphy, B. A., Lindia, J. A., Diaz, C., Abbadie, C., Ritter, A. M., … Martin, W. J. (2005). Contribution of the tetrodotoxin-resistant voltage-gated sodium channel NaV1.9 to sensory transmission and nociceptive behavior. *Proceedings of the National Academy of Sciences of the United States of America*, *102*(26), 9382–9387. http://dx.doi.org/10.1073/pnas.0501549102.

Rivara, M., & Zuliani, V. (2015). Novel sodium channel antagonists in the treatment of neuropathic pain. *Expert Opinion on Investigational Drugs*, *14*, 1–12. http://dx.doi.org/10.1517/13543784.2016.1121992.

Robinson, P. P., Boissonade, F. M., Loescher, A. R., Smith, K. G., Yates, J. M., Elcock, C., … Vora, A. R. (2004). Peripheral mechanisms for the initiation of pain following trigeminal nerve injury. *Journal of Orofacial Pain*, *18*(4), 287–292. Retrieved from http://www.ncbi.nlm.nih.gov/pubmed/15636010.

Roger, S., Besson, P., & Le Guennec, J. Y. (2003). Involvement of a novel fast inward sodium current in the invasion capacity of a breast cancer cell line. *Biochimica et Biophysica Acta*, *1616*(2), 107–111. Retrieved from http://www.ncbi.nlm.nih.gov/pubmed/14561467.

Roger, S., Gillet, L., Le Guennec, J. Y., & Besson, P. (2015). Voltage-gated sodium channels and cancer: Is excitability their primary role? *Frontiers in Pharmacology*, *6*, 152. http://dx.doi.org/10.3389/fphar.2015.00152.

Rush, A. M., Craner, M. J., Kageyama, T., Dib-Hajj, S. D., Waxman, S. G., & Ranscht, B. (2005). Contactin regulates the current density and axonal expression of tetrodotoxin-resistant but not tetrodotoxin-sensitive sodium channels in DRG neurons. *European Journal of Neuroscience*, *22*(1), 39–49. http://dx.doi.org/10.1111/j.1460-9568.2005.04186.x.

Rush, A. M., Dib-Hajj, S. D., Liu, S., Cummins, T. R., Black, J. A., & Waxman, S. G. (2006). A single sodium channel mutation produces hyper- or hypoexcitability in different types of neurons. *Proceedings of the National Academy of Sciences of the United States of America*, *103*(21), 8245–8250. http://dx.doi.org/10.1073/pnas.0602813103.

Salat, K., Kowalczyk, P., Gryzlo, B., Jakubowska, A., & Kulig, K. (2014). New investigational drugs for the treatment of neuropathic pain. *Expert Opinion on Investigational Drugs*, *23*(8), 1093–1104. http://dx.doi.org/10.1517/13543784.2014.916688.

Stirling, L. C., Forlani, G., Baker, M. D., Wood, J. N., Matthews, E. A., Dickenson, A. H., & Nassar, M. A. (2005). Nociceptor-specific gene deletion using heterozygous NaV1.8-Cre recombinase mice. *Pain*, *113*(1–2), 27–36. http://dx.doi.org/10.1016/j.pain.2004.08.015.

Stock, C., & Schwab, A. (2009). Protons make tumor cells move like clockwork. *Pflügers Archiv*, *458*(5), 981–992. http://dx.doi.org/10.1007/s00424-009-0677-8.

Tate, S., Benn, S., Hick, C., Trezise, D., John, V., Mannion, R. J., … Woolf, C. J. (1998). Two sodium channels contribute to the TTX-R sodium current in primary sensory neurons. *Nature Neuroscience*, *1*(8), 653–655. http://dx.doi.org/10.1038/3652.

Waxman, S. G., Kocsis, J. D., & Black, J. A. (1994). Type III sodium channel mRNA is expressed in embryonic but not adult spinal sensory neurons, and is reexpressed following axotomy. *Journal of Neurophysiology*, *72*(1), 466–470. Retrieved from http://www.ncbi.nlm.nih.gov/pubmed/7965028.

Waxman, S. G., Merkies, I. S., Gerrits, M. M., Dib-Hajj, S. D., Lauria, G., Cox, J. J., … Faber, C. G. (2014). Sodium channel genes in pain-related disorders: Phenotype-genotype associations and recommendations for clinical use. *Lancet Neurology*, *13*(11), 1152–1160. http://dx.doi.org/10.1016/S1474-4422(14)70150-4.

Weiss, J., Pyrski, M., Jacobi, E., Bufe, B., Willnecker, V., Schick, B., … Zufall, F. (2011). Loss-of-function mutations in sodium channel Nav1.7 cause anosmia. *Nature*, *472*(7342), 186–190. http://dx.doi.org/10.1038/nature09975.

Wickramasinghe, S. R., Alvania, R. S., Ramanan, N., Wood, J. N., Mandai, K., & Ginty, D. D. (2008). Serum response factor mediates NGF-dependent target innervation by embryonic DRG sensory neurons. *Neuron*, *58*(4), 532–545. http://dx.doi.org/10.1016/j.neuron.2008.03.006.

Wood, J. N., & Baker, M. (2001). Voltage-gated sodium channels. *Current Opinion in Pharmacology*, *1*(1), 17–21. Retrieved from http://www.ncbi.nlm.nih.gov/pubmed/11712529.

Yang, M., Kozminski, D. J., Wold, L. A., Modak, R., Calhoun, J. D., Isom, L. L., & Brackenbury, W. J. (2012). Therapeutic potential for phenytoin: Targeting Na(v)1.5 sodium channels to reduce migration and invasion in metastatic breast cancer. *Breast Cancer Research and Treatment*, *134*(2), 603–615. http://dx.doi.org/10.1007/s10549-012-2102-9.

Yang, Y., Wang, Y., Li, S., Xu, Z., Li, H., Ma, L., … Shen, Y. (2004). Mutations in SCN9A, encoding a sodium channel alpha subunit, in patients with primary erythermalgia. *Journal of Medical Genetics*, *41*(3), 171–174. Retrieved from http://www.ncbi.nlm.nih.gov/pubmed/14985375.

Zakrzewska, J. M., Palmer, J., Ettlin, D. A., Obermann, M., Giblin, G. M., Morisset, V., … Gunn, K. (2013). Novel design for a phase IIa placebo-controlled, double-blind randomized withdrawal study to evaluate the safety and efficacy of CNV1014802 in patients with trigeminal neuralgia. *Trials*, *14*, 402. http://dx.doi.org/10.1186/1745-6215-14-402.

Zhang, X. Y., Wen, J., Yang, W., Wang, C., Gao, L., Zheng, L. H., … Liu, J. Y. (2013). Gain-of-function mutations in SCN11A cause familial episodic pain. *American Journal of Human Genetics*, *93*(5), 957–966. http://dx.doi.org/10.1016/j.ajhg.2013.09.016.

Zhao, J., Nassar, M. A., Gavazzi, I., & Wood, J. N. (2006). Tamoxifen-inducible NaV1.8-CreERT2 recombinase activity in nociceptive neurons of dorsal root ganglia. *Genesis*, *44*(8), 364–371. http://dx.doi.org/10.1002/dvg.20224.

CHAPTER SEVEN

Antinociception by Sigma-1 Receptor Antagonists: Central and Peripheral Effects

Luz Romero, Manuel Merlos, José Miguel Vela[1]
Drug Discovery and Preclinical Development, ESTEVE, Parc Científic de Barcelona, Baldiri Reixac 4-8, Barcelona, Spain
[1]Corresponding author: e-mail address: jvela@esteve.es

Contents

Abstract

There is plenty of evidence supporting the modulatory role of sigma-1 receptors (σ_1Rs) in nociception, mainly based on the pain-attenuated phenotype of σ_1R knockout mice and on the antinociceptive effect exerted by σ_1R antagonists, particularly in nonacute sensitizing conditions involving sustained afferent drive, activity-dependent plasticity/sensitization, and ultimately pain hypersensitivity, as it is the case in chronic pains of different etiology. Antinociceptive effects of σ_1R antagonists both when acting alone and in combination with opioids (to enhance opioid analgesia) have been reported at both central and peripheral sites. At the central level, findings at the behavioral (animal pain models), electrophysiological (spinal wind-up recordings), neurochemical (spinal release of neurotransmitters) and molecular (NMDAR function) level supports a role for σ_1R antagonists in inhibiting augmented excitability secondary to sustained afferent input. Attenuation of activity-induced plastic changes (central sensitization) following tissue injury/inflammation or nerve damage could thus underlie the central

Advances in Pharmacology, Volume 75
ISSN 1054-3589
http://dx.doi.org/10.1016/bs.apha.2015.11.003

inhibitory effect of σ_1R antagonists. Moreover, recent pieces of information confirm the involvement of σ_1R in mechanisms regulating pain at the periphery, where σ_1Rs are highly expressed, particularly in dorsal root ganglia. Indeed, local peripheral administration of σ_1R antagonists reduces inflammatory hyperalgesia. Potentiation of opioid analgesia is also supported, particularly at supraspinal sites and at the periphery, where locally administered σ_1R antagonists unmask opioid analgesia. Altogether, whereas σ_1R activation is coupled to pain facilitation and inhibition of opioid antinociception, σ_1R antagonism inhibits pain hypersensitivity and "releases the brake" enabling opioids to exert enhanced antinociceptive effects, both at the central nervous system and at the periphery.

ABBREVIATIONS

(+)-MR200 (+)-methyl (1*R*,2*S*)-2-{[4-(4-chlorophenyl)-4-hydroxypiperidin-1-yl]methyl}-1-phenylcyclopropanecarboxylate
(−)-MRV3 (−)-methyl (1*S*,2*R*)-2-[(4-hydroxy-4-phenylpiperidin-1-yl)-methyl]-1-phenylcyclopropanecarboxylate
AMPA α-amino-3-hydroxyl-5-methyl-4-isoxazole-propionate glutamate receptors
BD-1047 *N*′-[2-(3,4-dichlorophenyl)ethyl]-*N*,*N*,*N*′-trimethylethane-1,2-diamine
BD-1063 1-[2-(3,4-dichlorophenyl)ethyl]-4-methylpiperazine
B_{max} maximum amount of drug or radioligand which binds specifically to the receptors. It is used to measure the density of the receptor site in a particular preparation.
CaM Ca^{2+}-binding protein calmodulin
CCI chronic constriction injury
CNS central nervous system
DH dorsal horn
DRG dorsal root ganglia
E-52862 4-[2-(5-methyl-1-naphthalen-2-ylpyrazol-3-yl)oxyethyl]morpholine
GABA gamma-aminobutyric acid
GluN1 *N*-methyl-D-aspartate receptor subunit 1
HINT1 histidine triad nucleotide-binding protein 1
i.c.v. intracerebroventricular
i.pl. intraplantar
i.t. intrathecal
IP_3 inositol 1,4,5-trisphosphate
LC locus coeruleus
MAM mitochondrion-associated endoplasmic reticulum membrane
MOR mu opioid receptor
NE-100 4-methoxy-3-(2-phenylethoxy)-*N*,*N*-dipropylbenzeneethanamine
NMDAR *N*-methyl-D-aspartate receptor
PAG periaqueductal gray
PKA protein kinase A
PKC protein kinase C
PRE-084 2-morpholin-4-ylethyl 1-phenylcyclohexane-1-carboxylate
RVM rostroventral medulla
s.c. subcutaneous

SA4503 1-[2-(3,4-dimethoxyphenyl)ethyl]-4-(3-phenylpropyl)piperazine
TIIP thrombus-induced ischemic pain
TRP transient receptor potential
TRPA1 transient receptor potential subfamily A member 1
TRPV1 transient receptor potential vanilloid subfamily member 1
σ_1R sigma-1 receptor

1. INTRODUCTION

Sigma (σ) receptors have been classified into two subtypes (σ_1 and σ_2Rs). The gene of the σ_1R encodes a protein of 223 amino acids, with two transmembrane domains (Hanner et al., 1996), anchored to mitochondrion-associated endoplasmic reticulum membranes (MAM; Hayashi & Su, 2003, 2007) and plasma membranes (Alonso et al., 2000; Mavlyutov, Epstein, Andersen, Ziskind-Conhaim, & Ruoho, 2010). The second transmembrane domain and the C-terminus of the σ_1R are proposed to form the ligand-binding site (Chen, Hajipour, Sievert, Arbabian, & Ruoho, 2007).

σ_1Rs were found to be unique, with no significant similarity with any other known mammalian protein receptor, and to have about 90% amino acid identity and 95% similarity across species (Hanner et al., 1996; Kekuda, Prasad, Fei, Leibach, & Ganapathy, 1996; Seth, Leibach, & Ganapathy, 1997). From a functional point of view, the σ_1R physically interacts with a variety of receptors and ion channels or elements of their transduction machinery and acts as a modulator of their activity. At the endoplasmic reticulum, the σ_1R acts as a ligand-operated molecular chaperone regulating the flow of Ca^{2+} via inositol 1,4,5-trisphosphate (IP_3) receptors (Hayashi & Su, 2007; Su, Hayashi, Maurice, Buch, & Ruoho, 2010). Via the molecular chaperone activity, the σ_1R regulates protein folding/degradation, oxidative stress, and cell survival (see Hayashi, 2015a for a review). In the plasma membrane, σ_1Rs interact with components of the plasma membrane-bound signal transduction to modulate the activity of neurotransmitter receptors and ion channels, including K^+ channels, Ca^{2+} channels, *N*-methyl-D-aspartate receptor (NMDAR), and opioid receptors (see Zamanillo, Romero, Merlos, & Vela, 2013 for a review). Interestingly, its activity can be modulated (enhanced or inhibited) by σ_1R ligands in an agonist–antagonist manner.

σ_1Rs are widely distributed in mammalian central nervous system (CNS) and peripheral systems and organs. σ_1Rs are not only highly expressed in brain and spinal cord but also in several peripheral tissues (Fig. 1), e.g., dorsal root ganglia (DRG), liver, testis, lung, kidney, endocrine organs, placenta, and heart where protection against oxidative stress is regarded as one of its major physiological functions (Pal et al., 2012). In particular, the regulation

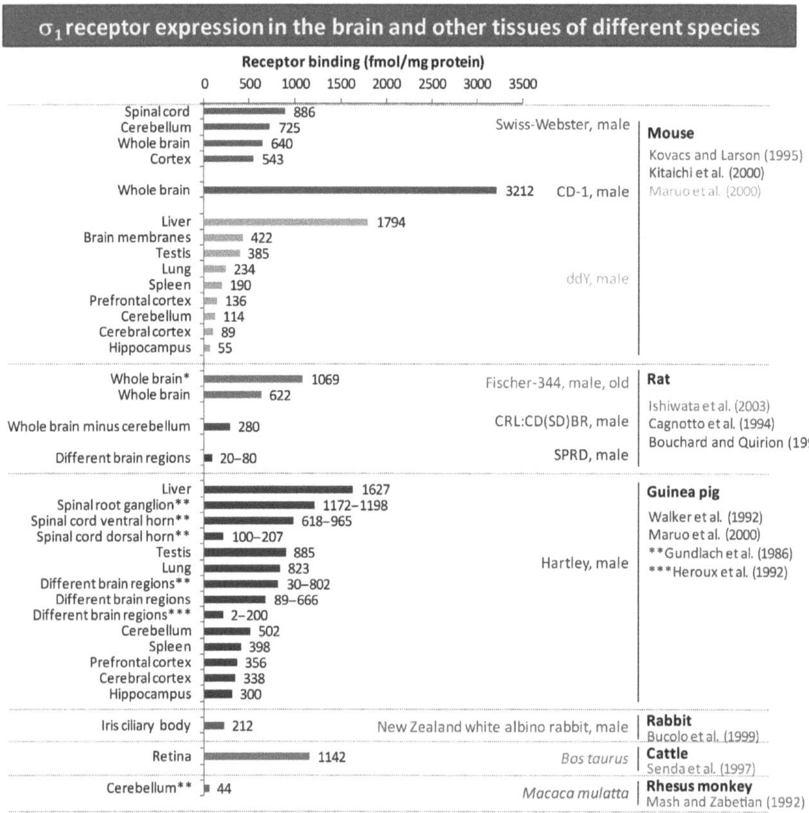

Figure 1 Quantitative *in vitro* autoradiographic and membrane homogenate studies on σ_1R binding of various radioligands in the brain and other tissues of different species. Ligands used: no label, [^{3}H](+)-pentazocine; *, [^{3}H]-SA4503; **, [^{3}H](+)-3-PPP; ***, [^{3}H]-DuP734 (Bouchard & Quirion, 1997; Bucolo, Campana, Di Toro, Cacciaguerra, & Spampinato, 1999; Cagnotto, Bastone, & Mennini, 1994; Gundlach, Largent, & Snyder, 1986; Heroux, Tam, & De Souza, 1992; Ishiwata, Kobayashi, Kawamura, & Matsuno, 2003; Kitaichi et al., 2000; Kovacs & Larson, 1995; Maruo et al., 2000; Mash & Zabetian, 1992; Senda, Matsuno, & Mita, 1997; Walker et al., 1992; see Brust, Deuther-Conrad, Lehmkuhl, Jia, & Wunsch, 2014 for a review).

of endoplasmic reticulum and mitochondrial function and their communications is suggested to contribute to the suppression of reactive oxygen species and oxidative stress (Hayashi, 2015a; Hayashi, Tsai, Mori, Fujimoto, & Su, 2011; Meunier & Hayashi, 2010; Tsai et al., 2009).

Qualitatively, the expression pattern of σ_1Rs seems to be similar in rodent and primate brain although a comprehensive and parallel quantitative analysis of σ_1Rs protein expression in the brain of different species, expected to facilitate the translation of experimental data on the imaging of σ_1Rs from *in vitro* and *in vivo* animal models into clinical application, is not yet available. Notably, intra- and inter-species as well as ligand-dependent differences exist with different receptor density, i.e., different B_{max} (maximum binding sites), being reported in different mouse strains (e.g., Swiss-Webster vs. CD-1 mice whole brain, Fig. 1) using [^{3}H]pentazocine as σ_1R-specific radioligand or in Fischer-344 rats whole brain using two different σ_1R-specific ligands [^{3}H]pentazocine and [^{3}H]SA4503 (Fig. 1). Quantitative data on the expression of σ_1Rs in human brain were not accessible (see Brust et al., 2014 for a review).

The σ_1R is expressed in areas important for pain control such as DRG neurons, dorsal spinal cord, the thalamus, the periaqueductal gray (PAG), and the rostroventral medulla (RVM) (Gundlach et al., 1986; Sánchez-Fernández et al., 2014; Fig. 2). Its expression in the spinal cord is upregulated during the induction phase of neuropathic pain following sciatic nerve constriction (Roh et al., 2008b), but it has been reported to be reduced in spinal cords following chemotherapy (oxaliplatin and paclitaxel) treatment (Tomohisa et al., 2015) and in DRGs following spinal nerve ligation (Bangaru et al., 2013). Using σ_1R knockout mice, the σ_1R was identified as a modulator of activity-induced sensitization of pain pathways (Cendán, Pujalte, Portillo-Salido, Montoliu, & Baeyens, 2005; de la Puente et al., 2009; Entrena, Cobos, Nieto, Cendan, Gris, et al., 2009; González-Cano, Merlos, Baeyens, & Cendan, 2013; Gris, Merlos, Vela, Zamanillo, & Portillo-Salido, 2014; Nieto et al., 2012, 2014; Tejada et al., 2014). These genetic as well as pharmacological findings (Vela, Merlos, & Almansa, 2015 for a review) provided evidence to consider σ_1R antagonists as an innovative and alternative approach for treating pain, especially neuropathic pain but also other sensitizing pain conditions (see Fig. 3 for a summary). In addition, preclinical evidence has pointed out their potential as an adjuvant therapy to enhance opioid analgesia, without increasing the side effects associated with the use of these narcotic pain medications (Chien & Pasternak, 1994; Sánchez-Fernández et al., 2013, 2014;

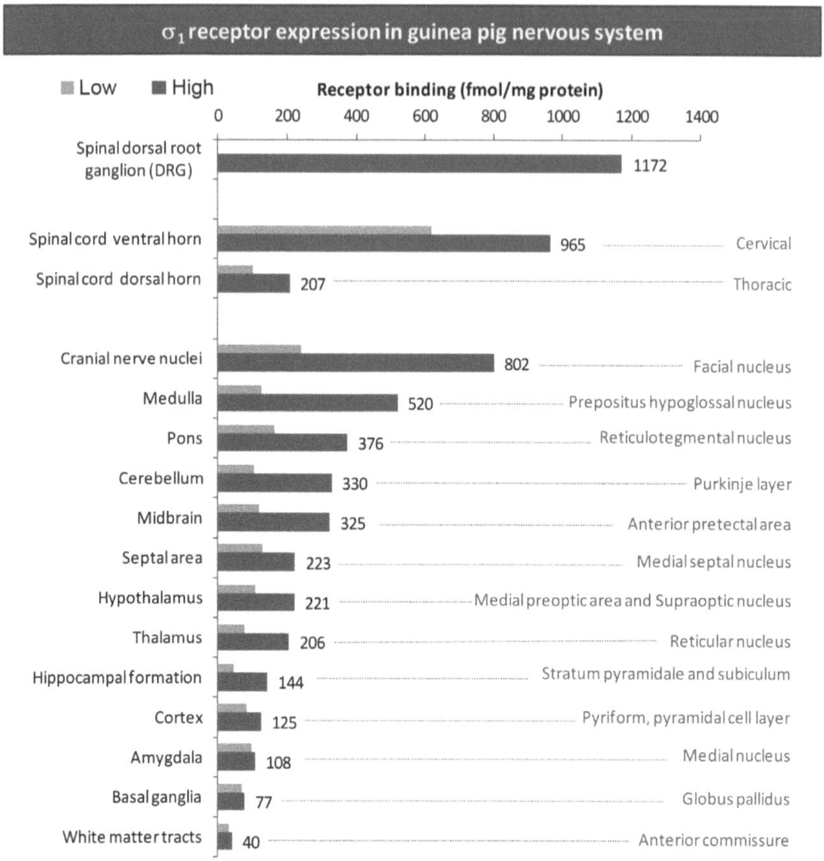

Figure 2 Regional distribution of [^{3}H](+)-3-PPP binding sites in guinea pig nervous system. Various regions, layers, or nuclei were analyzed in brain and spinal cord. For clarity, only the lower (green; light gray in the print version) and higher (blue; gray in the print version) σ_1R-binding density values found are represented in horizontal bars; and only the name of the region, layer, or nucleus with the highest receptor-binding density is noted (blue; gray in the print version). *Data from Gundlach et al. (1986).*

Vidal-Torres et al., 2013). Unlike opioids, σ_1R antagonists do not alter normal basic pain behavior as they do not exert antinociceptive effects and they do not modify the normal sensory mechanical and thermal perception in the absence of sensitizing stimuli (i.e., formalin, capsaicin, or nerve or tissue injury) (see Fig. 4 for a summary). That is, σ_1R antagonists exert anti-allodynic and antihyperalgesic effects in sensitizing conditions, enabling the reversal of diminished nociceptive thresholds back to normal values,

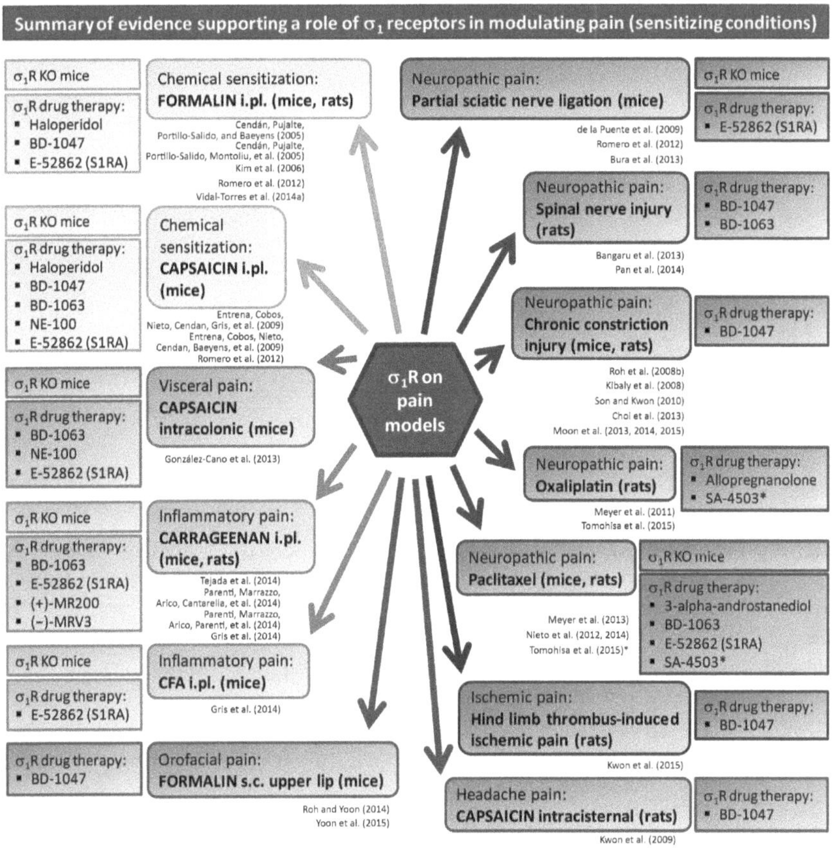

Figure 3 Preclinical evidence supporting a role of σ_1R in animal models of pain. Studies using σ_1R antagonists and σ_1R knockout (KO) mice in sensitizing conditions following tissue or nerve injury, or using chemical irritants. The asterisk indicates positive results using a σ_1R agonist (SA-4503; cutamesine).

but they do not modify normal sensory thresholds in nonsensitizing conditions (i.e., in normal conditions, in the absence of injury, or other inductors of pain hypersensitivity) (Chien & Pasternak, 1995b; Entrena, Cobos, Nieto, Cendan, Gris, et al., 2009; Kim et al., 2008; Romero et al., 2012). The σ_1R, however, modulates opioid-mediated antinociception in acute nonsensitizing models: σ_1R agonists diminish opioid antinociception whereas antagonists enhance it (Chien & Pasternak, 1993, 1994; Mei & Pasternak, 2002) (see Fig. 5 for a summary). As an example, the σ_1R antagonist E-52862 was devoid of activity in the radiant heat tail-flick test, but it

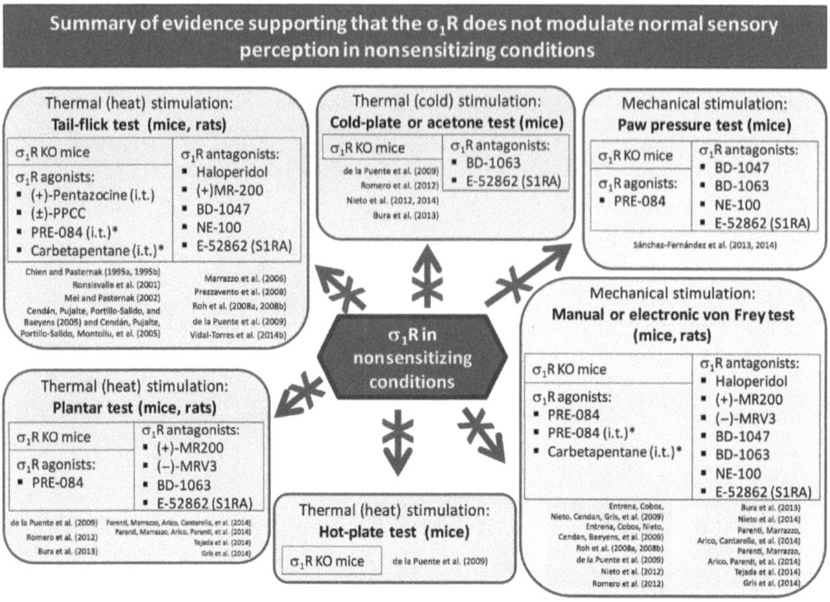

Figure 4 Preclinical evidence supporting that the σ_1R does not modulate normal sensory perception in nonsensitizing conditions (in the absence of sensitizing stimuli). Studies using σ_1R ligands and σ_1R knockout (KO) mice. σ_1R KO mice do not show differences respect to wild-type mice as it regards to their response to mechanical and thermal stimulation, and σ_1R ligands do not alter normal basic pain behavior as they do not exert antinociceptive effects and do not modify the normal sensory mechanical and thermal perception in the absence of sensitizing stimuli. The asterisks indicate a pronociceptive effect being described following i.t. administration of two σ_1R agonists.

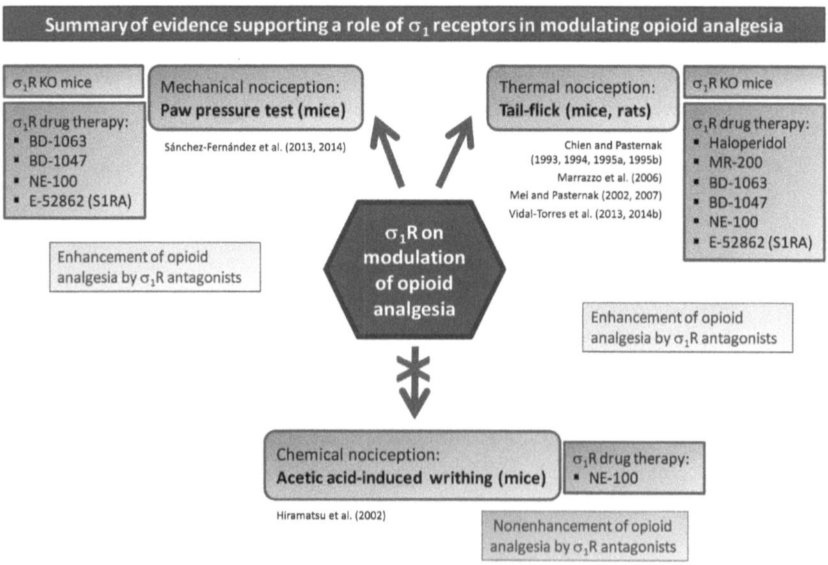

Figure 5 Preclinical evidence supporting a role of σ_1R in the modulation of opioid analgesia in animal models of pain. Studies using σ_1R antagonists and σ_1R knockout (KO) mice.

did potentiate by a factor of 2–3.3 the antinociceptive effect of several opioids, including tramadol, morphine, buprenorphine, codeine, oxycodone, and fentanyl in this acute test (Vidal-Torres et al., 2013). Moreover, E-52862 was effective in restoring antinociception of morphine once tolerance had developed (Vidal-Torres et al., 2013).

The role of σ_1R in pain has been recently reviewed and analyzed by several authors (Almansa & Vela, 2014; Cobos, Entrena, Nieto, Cendan, & Del Pozo, 2008; Davis, 2015; Gris, Cobos, Zamanillo, & Portillo-Salido, 2015; Vela et al., 2015; Zamanillo et al., 2013). In this review, we summarize the present knowledge and open questions related to the site of action (central and/or peripheral) of σ_1R antagonists on pain control, when administered alone or in combination with opioids.

2. ROLE OF CENTRAL σ_1R IN PAIN: CENTRAL ANTINOCICEPTIVE EFFECTS OF σ_1R ANTAGONISTS

2.1 Effect of σ_1R Antagonism (in the Absence of Opioid Treatment) at Central Sites: Inhibitory Effect on Central Sensitization

Central sensitization represents an enhancement in the function of neurons and circuits in central nociceptive pathways caused by increases in membrane excitability and synaptic efficacy as well as to reduced inhibition. It is a manifestation of the remarkable plasticity of the somatosensory nervous system in response to activity, inflammation, and neural injury. Central sensitization is responsible for many of the temporal, spatial, and threshold changes in pain sensibility and exemplifies the fundamental contribution of the CNS to the generation of pain hypersensitivity. Because central sensitization results from changes in the properties of neurons in the CNS, the pain is no longer coupled, as acute nociceptive pain is, to the presence, intensity, or duration of noxious peripheral stimuli. Instead, central sensitization produces pain hypersensitivity by exaggerating the sensory response elicited by nociceptive suprathreshold stimuli and by allowing the response to subthreshold stimuli, including those that usually evoke innocuous sensations. The dorsal horn (DH) of the spinal cord is the first point of integration of somatosensory information, and it is a key region where plasticity has been demonstrated (D'Mello & Dickenson, 2008; Latremoliere & Woolf, 2009; Sandkühler & Gruber-Schoffnegger, 2012; West, Bannister, Dickenson, & Bennett, 2015). Hyperexcitable spinal neurons show reduced thresholds, greater evoked responses, increased receptive field sizes, and ongoing stimulus-independent activity; changes that probably underlie allodynia, hyperalgesia, and spontaneous pain (Baron, Hans, & Dickenson, 2013; Suzuki, Kontinen, Matthews, Williams, & Dickenson, 2000). Four major neuronal components account for spinal sensitization in the DH: primary afferent inputs, DH interneurons, projection neurons of the DH, and descending modulation from the brain to the DH (D'Mello & Dickenson, 2008; Todd, 2010; West et al., 2015; Yasaka, Tiong, Hughes, Riddell, & Todd, 2010). That is, central sensitization is not only maintained by continuing input from the periphery to the DH but also modulated by intrinsic inhibitory and excitatory DH interneurons, projection DH neurons, and by descending controls, both inhibitory and facilitatory, from the midbrain and brain stem to the DH. The projections of sensitized spinal neurons to the brain, in turn, transmit altered painful messages to higher centers, which result in further plasticity in ongoing and evoked activity in some brain regions, including the amygdala (i.e., central nucleus of the amygdala), involved in the processing of emotional-affective components of pain (Gonçalves & Dickenson, 2012).

An inhibitory effect has been attributed to σ_1R antagonism on central sensitization phenomena, as supported at the behavioral, electrophysiological, neurochemical, and molecular levels.

2.1.1 Behavioral Studies: Capsaicin and Formalin Sensitization

Activation of primary afferent nociceptive fibers subsequent to intradermal injection of some chemical irritants, including capsaicin or formalin, into the plantar skin of the hind paw in rodents produces acute/immediate nociceptive behaviors followed by a delayed, secondary phase involving central sensitization (i.e., synaptic strengthening in the CNS of nociceptive transmission). σ_1R blockade by genetic (σ_1R knockout mice) and pharmacological approaches has been shown to inhibit second phase formalin and capsaicin sensitization.

Capsaicin, the main pungent ingredient in hot chili peppers, primarily acts on the transient receptor potential (TRP) vanilloid subfamily member 1 (TRPV1), a polymodal signal transducer (Tominaga et al., 1998). This receptor is a calcium channel found on key fine sensory afferent fibers (peptidergic and nonpeptidergic C-fibers and some Aδ-fibers), and so the use of capsaicin to selectively activate pain afferents has been exploited in both animal and human studies to generate central (spinal) hypersensitivity and to investigate the mechanisms behind enhanced central processing of pain

(O'Neill et al., 2012). Capsaicin injection into the plantar skin of the hind paw in rodents (or into the skin of humans) results in an immediate pain behavior followed by longer lasting secondary mechanical hypersensitivity (e.g., allodynia) that results from central sensitization (i.e., plastic changes increasing pain sensitivity at the spinal cord and/or other CNS areas due to the initial intense nociceptive discharges that follows the capsaicin injection) (Baron, 2000; Gilchrist, Allard, & Simone, 1996; Joshi et al., 2006; O'Neill et al., 2012; Sang, Gracely, Max, & Bennett, 1996; Willis, 2001). Interestingly, capsaicin was unable to induce mechanical hypersensitivity in σ_1R knockout mice, and the effect in σ_1R knockout mice was mimicked in wild-type animals treated with BD-1063, BD-1047, or NE-100, as all three σ_1R antagonists dose-dependently inhibited capsaicin-induced mechanical allodynia (Entrena, Cobos, Nieto, Cendan, Gris, et al., 2009). Other σ_1R antagonists including haloperidol and its metabolites I and II (Entrena, Cobos, Nieto, Cendan, Baeyens, et al., 2009), E-52862 (Romero et al., 2012) and some spirocyclic thiophene bioisosteres (e.g., spirocyclic thienopyran 2a) (Oberdorf et al., 2008), 1′-benzyl-3-methoxy-3*H*-spiro[[2]benzofuran-1,4′-piperidine] (Wiese et al., 2009), and a 1,3-dioxane ligand 2 (Utech et al., 2011) also produced antiallodynic effects in the capsaicin model. In addition, the σ_1R agonist PRE-084 reversed the effect of antagonists (Entrena, Cobos, Nieto, Cendan, Baeyens, et al., 2009; Entrena, Cobos, Nieto, Cendan, Gris, et al., 2009), further supporting the role played by σ_1R in capsaicin-induced central sensitization phenomena.

Formalin (formaldehyde solution) excites sensory neurons by activating transient receptor potential subfamily A member 1 (TRPA1), through a mechanism probably involving covalent modification of some residues within the TRPA1 channel protein (McNamara et al., 2007). TRPA1 is an excitatory calcium channel activated by pungent ingredients in mustard and garlic extracts that is highly expressed by a subset of C-fiber nociceptors (McNamara et al., 2007). When intradermally injected into the hind paw of a rodent, diluted (0.5–5%) formalin induces a biphasic pain response. The first phase is an initial robust phase in which paw lifting, licking, and flinching occurs during the first 10 min due to direct activation of primary afferent sensory neurons at the periphery (i.e., robust calcium influx trough TRPA1 channels on nociceptor endings). The first phase is followed by a transient decline in these nociceptive behaviors and then by a second phase of nociceptive behaviors lasting 30–60 min that reflects the amplification of the afferent input due to central sensitization (Coderre, Vaccarino, & Melzack, 1990; McNamara et al., 2007). Regarding σ_1R modulation, the first study reporting a role of σ_1R in nonacute, tonic pain conditions was done using the formalin model and σ_1R knockout mice as experimental subjects (Cendán, Pujalte, Portillo-Salido, Montoliu, et al., 2005). In this study, it was shown that both phases of formalin-induced pain were reduced by approximately 55% in mice lacking σ_1Rs in comparison to wild-type animals. Shortly after this study, the same authors reported that haloperidol and its metabolites I and II, which have affinity for σ_1R, dose-dependently inhibited formalin-induced pain in mice through a mechanism likely involving antagonism on σ_1Rs (Cendán, Pujalte, Portillo-Salido, & Baeyens, 2005). Subsequent studies using selective and prototypical σ_1R antagonists such as E-52862 (Romero et al., 2012; Vidal-Torres et al., 2014a) and BD-1047 (Kim et al., 2006; Roh and Yoon, 2014; Yoon et al., 2015), and novel σ_1R antagonists based on pyrimidine (Lan, Chen, Cao, et al., 2014) or 3,4-dihydro-2(1*H*)-quinolinone (Lan, Chen, Xu, et al., 2014) scaffolds corroborated these initial findings and pointed to the spinal cord and supraspinal CNS regions as sites for the σ_1R-mediated modulation of formalin sensitization (Kim et al., 2006; Vidal-Torres et al., 2014a). The spinal cord was first pointed out in the study by Kim et al. (2006) in mice, where intrathecal (i.t.) pretreatment with the σ_1R antagonist BD-1047 dose-dependently reduced formalin-induced pain behaviors in second phase, but not first phase, of the formalin test, concomitant with reduced formalin-evoked Fos expression in spinal DH neurons. In addition to the spinal cord, supraspinal sites were supported by the finding in rats that i.t. pretreatment with E-52862 attenuated the formalin-induced flinching behavior, but not lifting/licking behaviors, whereas E-52862 also attenuated lifting/licking when intracerebroventricularly (i.c.v.) injected (Vidal-Torres et al., 2014a). In this way, it is interesting to note that flinching is a spinal response whereas lifting/licking behaviors are supraspinal responses, and that both spinal and supraspinal descending modulation of central neural plasticity occur in formalin-induced pain (Coderre et al., 1990; Vaccarino & Chorney, 1994). Therefore, it is concluded that σ_1R acts in the CNS at both spinal and supraspinal sites to modulate pain sensitization following sustained peripheral activation of nociceptors by formalin (Figs. 6 and 7).

2.1.2 Electrophysiological Studies: Wind-Up

As discussed above, formalin and capsaicin injection trigger an initial and intense C-fiber activity but the subsequent increased pain sensitivity (i.e., phase II-formalin-induced pain and capsaicin-induced mechanical hypersensitivity) is thought to be underpinned by central mechanisms such

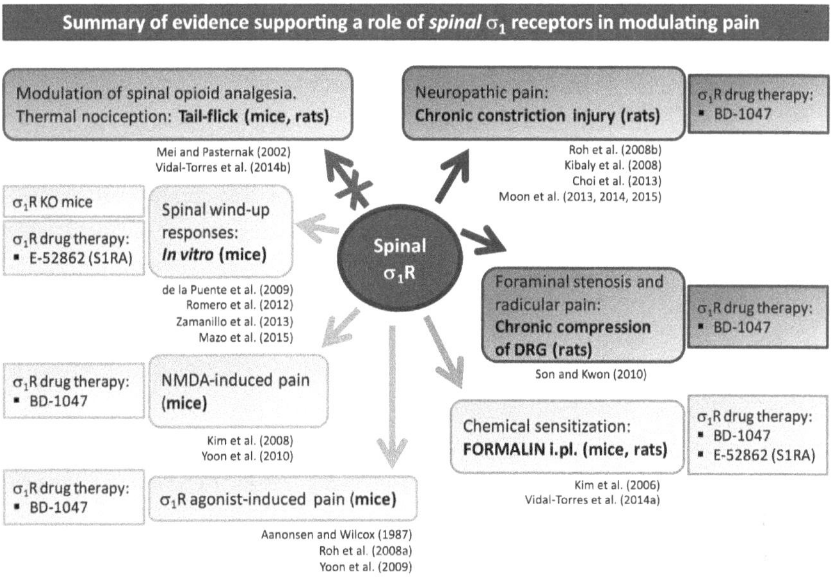

Figure 6 Preclinical evidence supporting a role of spinal σ_1R in the modulation of pain and opioid analgesia in animal models of pain. Studies using σ_1R antagonists and σ_1R knockout (KO) mice.

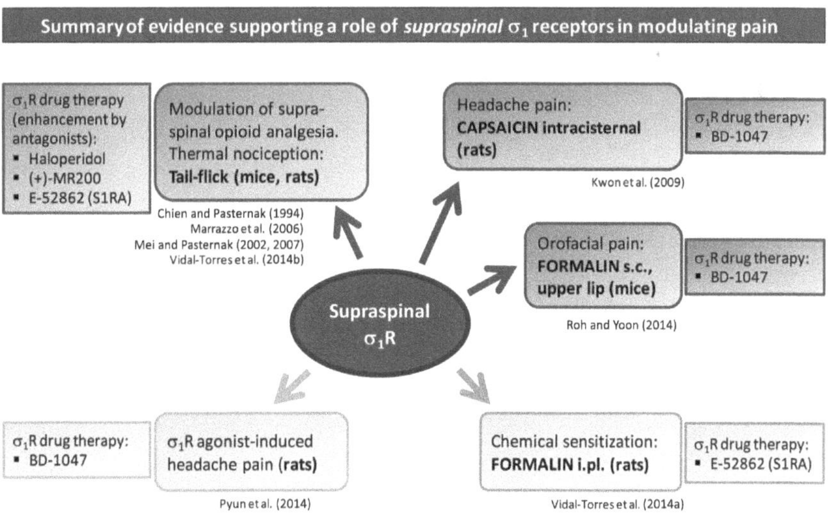

Figure 7 Preclinical evidence supporting a role of supraspinal σ_1R in the modulation of pain and opioid analgesia in animal models of pain. Studies using σ_1R antagonists and σ_1R knockout (KO) mice.

as an increased excitability of DH neurons. The modulation by σ_1Rs of the amplified response of spinal cord neurons to afferent stimulation has been investigated at the electrophysiological level in isolated spinal cords.

Repetitive stimulation of the dorsal root at stimulus intensities activating nociceptive fibers (but not nonnociceptive sensory fibers) produces a typical amplification of the nociceptive signals in the spinal cord (wind-up response). Wind-up is a short-term, frequency-dependent, amplification mechanism distinct from long-term potentiation, central sensitization, and pain hypersensitivity/hyperalgesia, but it is a form of homosynaptic central facilitation of nociceptive messages and a physiological correlate of such phenomena (Dickenson & Sullivan, 1987; Herrero, Laird, & Lopez-Garcia, 2000; Li, Simone, & Larson, 1999). To investigate if pharmacological antagonism of σ_1Rs actually modulates spinal excitability, isolated mice spinal cords were superfused with E-52862 and responses to electrical stimulation of the lumbar dorsal root were recorded. E-52862 did not modify the Aβ-fiber-mediated nonnociceptive signaling and the response to single stimuli at C-fiber intensity, which is consistent with the behavioral observation that σ_1R antagonists did not alter the normal perception of sensory subthreshold and nociceptive suprathreshold inputs in nonsensitizing conditions (Cendán, Pujalte, Portillo-Salido, Montoliu, et al., 2005; Entrena, Cobos, Nieto, Cendan, Gris, et al., 2009; Romero et al., 2012). However, σ_1R antagonists (i.e., E-52862) dose-dependently inhibited the spinal wind-up phenomenon when trains of nociceptive stimuli (repetitive stimulation of nociceptive afferent C-fibers) were applied (Mazo et al., 2015; Romero et al., 2012). Accordingly, spinal wind-up amplification of the nociceptive signals was highly reduced in spinal cords from σ_1R knockout compared to wild-type mice (de la Puente et al., 2009). Hence, electrophysiological data point to a modulatory role of σ_1R on spinal excitability, whereby pharmacological antagonism or the absence of the receptor in knockout mice, inhibits the amplified spinal response that would normally arise from repetitive nociceptor stimulation. As sustained, repetitive afferent drive comes to the spinal cord following injection of some chemical irritants, tissue injury/inflammation, or nerve damage, inhibition of spinal hyperexcitability could underlie the effects exerted by σ_1R antagonists on a wide variety of pain conditions (Fig. 3).

2.1.3 Neurochemical Studies: Modulation of Spinal Neurotransmitters

To explore underlying mechanisms, modulation by σ_1Rs of formalin-evoked changes in neurotransmitter levels in the spinal DH was investigated using concentric microdialysis in the ipsilateral DH of awake, freely moving rats (Vidal-Torres et al., 2014a). Levels of three key neurotransmitters were measured as a neurochemical correlate of three major neuronal components regulating DH neurons and accounting for spinal sensitization: glutamate for primary activating afferent inputs to the DH, gamma-aminobutyric acid (GABA) for local inhibitory DH interneurons, and noradrenaline for supraspinal descending inhibitory modulation of the DH. Formalin-induced nociception took place along with an enhancement of glutamate levels in the DH spinal cord, which is coherent with the activation of afferent glutamatergic nociceptive fibers following paw formalin injection. Systemic administration of the σ_1R antagonist E-52862 exerted antinociceptive effects on formalin-induced pain concomitantly with attenuation of formalin-evoked glutamate release and enhancement of noradrenaline levels in the spinal DH. GABA levels were not modified. These data suggest that pharmacological blockade of σ_1R reduces peripheral activating glutamatergic nociceptive inputs and enhances noradrenergic descending inhibitory inputs to the DH, but it does not modify the activity of GABAergic inhibitory DH interneurons. Interestingly, i.t. pretreatment with idazoxan (alpha 2(α_2)-adrenergic receptor antagonist) prevented the systemic antinociceptive effect of E-52862, suggesting that antinociception elicited by σ_1R blockade depends on the activation of descending inhibitory pathways, which results in enhancement of noradrenaline release into the spinal cord and activation of spinal α_2-adrenoceptors. Noradrenaline could act on presynaptic α_2-adrenoceptors on central projections of formalin-sensitive DRGs to inhibit glutamate release to the superficial DH laminae.

Glutamate is released into the DH spinal cord following activation of sensory afferents and its sustained release following sustained stimulation of nociceptors promotes plastic changes leading to spinal amplification of nociceptive messages. Thus, this excitatory amino acid plays a major role in central (spinal) sensitization phenomena, including wind-up, and the behavioral manifestations of pain sensitization/hypersensitivity (D'Mello & Dickenson, 2008; Herrero et al., 2000; Latremoliere & Woolf, 2009; Willis, 2001; Woolf & Thompson, 1991). Noradrenaline plays a major role in descending pathways that influence nociceptive signaling in the DH of the spinal cord. Descending inhibition largely involves the release of noradrenaline in the spinal cord from brain stem nuclei such as the locus coeruleus (LC), acting predominantly at the α_2-adrenoceptors, and inhibiting transmitter release from primary afferent terminals and suppressing firing of projection neurons in the DH (D'Mello & Dickenson, 2008; Millan, 2002;

West et al., 2015). The descending noradrenergic pathways from the brain stem to the DH may also undergo plastic changes in chronic pain states, which results in an increased inhibitory drive that has been suggested to be a homeostatic mechanism counteracting the increased spinal excitability (D'Mello & Dickenson, 2008; West et al., 2015). Accordingly, the finding that E-52862 inhibited formalin-evoked glutamate but enhanced noradrenaline release in the DH (Vidal-Torres et al., 2014a) is in agreement with a modulatory role of σ_1R antagonists in activity-dependent plastic changes, by promoting plasticity of descending inhibitory pathways and stopping down the plastic excitatory synaptic strengthening in the DH.

2.1.4 Molecular Studies: Modulation of the NMDAR Signaling

Among glutamate receptors, the glutamatergic NMDAR is a key mediator of activity-dependent plasticity, central sensitization, and pain hypersensitivity (Dickenson & Sullivan, 1987; D'Mello & Dickenson, 2008; Latremoliere & Woolf, 2009; Woolf & Thompson, 1991). Depolarization through glutamate acting on AMPA, kainite, and mGlu Type I, and through neuropeptides such as substance P, calcitonin gene related peptide (CGRP), and brain-derived neurotrophic factor (BDNF), removes Mg^{2+} blockade allowing glutamate to activate NMDAR, which results in an increased input of cations into the DH neuron. In particular, the NMDAR-mediated rise in intracellular Ca^{2+} is considered a key trigger for subsequent plasticity of synapses within the DH as Ca^{2+} ions results activate a number of second messenger systems, including several protein kinases that phosphorylate a variety of target proteins, including NMDARs. Phosphorylations result in increased synaptic and cellular responses to inputs and are believed to underlie, at least in part, the hypersensitivity seen in different pain states (Latremoliere & Woolf, 2009; Sandkühler, 2009).

Modulation of NMDAR function by σ_1R ligands is well documented (Bergeron, de Montigny, & Debonnel, 1996; Hayashi et al., 1995; Martina, Turcotte, Halman, & Bergeron, 2007; Monnet, Debonnel, & de Montigny, 1992, Monnet, Debonnel, Junien, & de Montigny, 1990; Yamamoto et al., 1995). σ_1R agonists increase and σ_1R antagonists decrease NMDAR currents and Ca^{2+} flow through the channel, and their respective effects are blocked when combined with each other. Accordingly, NMDA-activated current is reduced in σ_1R knockout respect to wild-type mice (Sha et al., 2013). Several mechanisms, both direct (involving physical interaction with σ_1R) and indirect (involving other elements of the transduction machinery) have been described to account for the regulation of NMDAR function by σ_1R.

The σ_1R interacts with and is functionally coupled to NMDAR. It binds to the NMDAR by interacting with the *N*-methyl-D-aspartate receptor subunit 1 (GluN1) subunit (Balasuriya, Stewart, & Edwardson, 2013; Rodríguez-Muñoz, Sánchez-Blázquez, et al., 2015; Sánchez-Blázquez et al., 2014), and this interaction accounts for at least some of the modulatory effects of σ_1R ligands on the NMDAR. The physical interaction between the σ_1R and NMDAR has been recently investigated (Rodríguez-Muñoz, Sánchez-Blázquez, et al., 2015) and summarized below. The binding of σ_1R (complete, long isoform) to the GluN1 subunit is Ca^{2+}-dependent and occurs in competition with other regulators of NMDAR activity that also bind to GluN1 such as the histidine triad nucleotide-binding protein 1 (HINT1) and the Ca^{2+}-binding protein calmodulin (CaM). The interaction of Ca^{2+}–CaM with the C-terminal GluN1 is weaker as compared to that of σ_1R, suggesting that Ca^{2+}–CaM that acts as a negative regulator of NMDAR (reducing its open rate and mean open time) when binds to GluN1 (Ataman, Gakhar, Sorensen, Hell, & Shea, 2007; Ehlers, Zhang, Bernhadt, & Huganir, 1996), cannot bind and exert its function, if the site is occupied by σ_1R. Thus, the presence of σ_1R bound to the GluN1 subunit hinders the activity-dependent feedback inhibition exerted by CaM on NMDAR activity following Ca^{2+} influx. Similarly, the binding of the σ_1R to the GluN1 subunit is an obstacle for the binding of HINT1, which is also a negative regulator of NMDAR function (Vicente-Sánchez, Sánchez-Blázquez, Rodríguez-Muñoz, & Garzón, 2013). Therefore, in the context of pain, glutamate released from nociceptive afferents induces the permeation of Ca^{2+} ions through the NMDAR pore, which promotes the binding of σ_1R to the GluN1 subunit in a Ca^{2+}-dependent manner (activity-dependent modulation), blocking the interaction of Ca^{2+}–CaM and also weakening that of HINT1 proteins with GluN1, which result in the release of the negative control and enhancement of NMDAR responsiveness. This would likely account for central sensitization phenomena and hypersensitivity in chronic pain states as the system becomes more sensitive to glutamate and thus to subsequent, sustained glutamatergic nociceptive inputs. Ligands acting on σ_1R regulate the activity of NMDARs by affecting the interaction of σ_1Rs with GluN1 subunits. Differential alteration of the tridimensional structure upon binding of ligands has been suggested to modulate (agonists enhance and antagonists diminish) the affinity of σ_1R for GluN1 binding. In this way, it has been demonstrated that the antagonists E-52862, BD-1047, and progesterone transitorily remove the binding of σ_1R to GluN1 subunits and made the NMDAR subunit available for binding the negative regulators Ca^{2+}–CaM or HINT1 (Rodríguez-Muñoz,

Sánchez-Blázquez, et al., 2015), thus suggesting that σ_1R antagonists ultimately promote the binding of negative regulators of NMDAR activity. This molecular mechanism explains how σ_1R antagonists downregulate NMDAR function and could thus also explain the antinociceptive effect exerted by σ_1R antagonists on pain sensitizing conditions (i.e., inhibition of activity-dependent plasticity, central sensitization phenomena, and ultimately pain hypersensitivity).

As previously stated, phosphorylation is a fundamental mechanism that alter channel properties of NMDARs to result in different forms of synaptic plasticity (Chen & Roche, 2007; Lee, 2006). In most cases, phosphorylation of NMDAR subunits potentiates NMDAR function. Interestingly, the σ_1R regulates phosphorylation of NMDARs. Activation of σ_1R at the spinal cord DH has been shown to increase the phosphorylation of the NMDAR GluN1 subunit, which results in the potentiation of NMDAR function and correlates with pain facilitation. In contrast, σ_1R antagonists have been shown to inhibit phosphorylation of NMDAR subunits and hence NMDAR activity and pain. In rats with chronic constriction injury (CCI) of the sciatic nerve, i.t. administration of the σ_1R antagonist BD-1047 on postoperative days 0–5 blocked the CCI-induced increase in NMDAR GluN1 subunit expression and phosphorylation, and significantly attenuated mechanical allodynia. This suppression was blocked by i.t. administration of the σ_1R agonist PRE-084 (Roh et al., 2008b). In mice, i.t. pretreatment with the selective σ_1R antagonist BD-1047 dose-dependently reduced the second phase of formalin-induced pain concomitant with a reduction of phosphorylation of GluN1 at protein kinase C (PKC)- and protein kinase A (PKA)-dependent sites in spinal DH (Kim et al., 2006). In contrast, activation of spinal σ_1R by i.t. injection of the σ_1R agonists PRE-084, carbetapentane or dehydroepiandrosterone sulfate facilitated nociception, enhanced NMDA-induced pain behavior, and promoted the phosphorylation of GluN1 (via PKC- and PKA-dependent phosphorylation) in the DH (Kim et al., 2008; Roh et al., 2008a, 2010; Yoon et al., 2009, 2010). Both the phosphorylation of the NMDAR GluN1 subunit and the pain facilitation were significantly reduced by pretreatment with the σ_1R antagonist BD-1047. Results in these studies indicate that activation of spinal σ_1R mediates pain facilitation via phosphorylation of the NMDAR GluN1 subunit, and that σ_1R antagonists downregulate its phosphorylation to reduce NMDAR function and associated NMDAR-dependent pain transmission and sensitization. However, no direct evidence is available supporting a direct interaction between the σ_1R and protein kinases to explain its modulatory effect. On the contrary, data point to an indirect upstream effect on signaling cascades leading to kinases activation, likely via receptor- and store-operated Ca^{2+} channels (e.g., modulation of plasma membrane NMDA and endoplasmic reticulum IP_3 receptors/channels leading to cytoplasmic Ca^{2+} raises).

Altogether, glutamatergic NMDAR-mediated overactivity plays a key role in central activity-dependent plasticity/sensitization, and σ_1R acts as a positive modulator of NMDAR function, which substantiates the efficacy of σ_1R antagonists in pain. In contrast to classical NMDAR antagonists, σ_1R antagonists do not block NMDAR activity but inhibit NMDAR overactivity by allowing feedback negative regulation (e.g., Ca^{2+}–CaM binding to GluN1) and ultimately precluding NMDAR sensitization (e.g., Ca^{2+}-dependent kinase activation and subsequent phosphorylation of GluN1). σ_1R antagonists could thus provide a better tolerated strategy, acting specifically to reduce NMDAR overactivity following sustained afferent glutamate release, and ultimately to reduce sensory hypersensitivity in chronic pain conditions.

2.2 Effect of σ_1R Antagonism in Combination with Opioid Treatment at Central Sites: Supraspinal Potentiation of Opioid Analgesia

σ_1Rs are known to interact with mu opioid receptors (MORs) and modulate opioid activity (Kim et al., 2010; Rodríguez-Muñoz, Sánchez-Blázquez, et al., 2015; Fig. 5). Several studies support modulation of not only mu but also kappa and delta opioid analgesia by a σ_1R system: σ_1R agonists diminish whereas σ_1R antagonists and antisense treatments enhance opioid antinociception. The modulatory effect occurs when σ_1R ligands are systemically administered and also when injected supraspinally (e.g., i.c.v. administration) (Fig. 7), but not at the spinal level (Fig. 6). When given supraspinally, the σ_1R agonist (+)pentazocine diminished systemic mu, delta, kappa1, and kappa3 opioid analgesia, as determined using the radiant heat tail-flick test in CD-1 mice. Spinal morphine analgesia was unaffected by (+)pentazocine given either spinally or supraspinally (Mei & Pasternak, 2002). Accordingly, downregulation of supraspinal σ_1R-binding sites using an antisense approach potentiated mu, delta, kappa1, and kappa3 analgesia in CD-1 mice (Mei & Pasternak, 2002); and σ_1R antagonists potentiated the antinociceptive effect of opioids by acting supraspinally. In the radiant heat tail-flick test in rats, systemic administration of (+)-MR200 increased the antinociceptive effect of i.c.v. administered mu and delta, but not kappa, opioid receptor agonists (Marrazzo et al., 2006), and E-52862 administered i.c.v., but not i.t., enhanced the antinociceptive effect of systemic morphine (Vidal-Torres et al., 2014b). In mice, using the warm water tail-flick test, i.c.v. administration of E-52862, BD-1047, NE-100, and progesterone also enhanced the analgesic activity of i.c.v. administered morphine (Rodríguez-Muñoz, Sánchez-Blázquez, et al., 2015). The agonist PRE-084 did not affect morphine analgesia but prevented E-52862 from enhancing opioid antinociception when administered i.c.v. (Rodríguez-Muñoz, Sánchez-Blázquez, et al., 2015).

Some brain stem regions, particularly the PAG, the RVM, and the LC have been identified as supraspinal sites for σ_1R ligands to exert their modulatory effects on opioid analgesia in the tail-flick test (Mei & Pasternak, 2007). In a microinjection study in rats, morphine was a potent analgesic in all three regions and coadministration of the σ_1R agonist (+)pentazocine diminished the analgesic actions of morphine in all three regions, although the PAG was far less sensitive than the other two. Blockade of the σ_1R with haloperidol in the RVM markedly enhanced the analgesic actions of coadministered morphine, even if morphine was microinjected into the PAG. This effect was mimicked by downregulation of RVM σ_1Rs using an antisense approach. In contrast, haloperidol failed to enhance morphine antinociception when coadministered in either the LC or the PAG suggesting a major involvement of the RVM (Mei & Pasternak, 2007).

A recent study has linked the physical and functional association between σ_1R and MOR with NMDAR, within a specialized protein assembly that facilitates functional cross-regulation (Rodríguez-Muñoz, Cortés-Montero, Pozo-Rodrigálvarez, Sánchez-Blázquez, & Garzón-Niño, 2015; Rodríguez-Muñoz, Sánchez-Blázquez, et al., 2015). Activation of MOR with morphine promotes the phosphorylation of NMDAR subunits and enhances NMDAR conductance, which is critical for synaptic plasticity (Lisman, Yasuda, & Raghavachari, 2012; Mao, Jin, Xue, Chu, & Wang, 2014). In turn, activation of NMDAR increases MOR phosphorylation, reduces the association of the MOR with G-proteins, and diminishes the antinociceptive capacity of morphine (Garzón, Rodríguez-Muñoz, & Sánchez-Blázquez, 2012). Thus, a functional cross-regulation occurs, whereby activation of MORs by morphine results in enhancement of NMDAR function, which in turn exerts a negative feedback effect on MOR signaling to ultimately decrease opioid analgesia. Mechanistically, both the HINT1 and the σ_1R protein bind to MOR and to the GluN1 subunit of the NMDAR and work together to regulate the cross talk between MORs and NMDARs. In the case of the σ_1R, the binding to MOR and NMDAR increases in the presence of Ca^{2+}. σ_1R agonists keep HINT1 at the MOR and stimulate MOR–NMDAR cross talk, whereas σ_1R antagonists allow the transfer of HINT1 to GluN1 subunits and disengage both receptors (i.e., the activation of MORs does not recruit NMDAR activity, and that of the NMDAR does not impair MOR-mediated effects). Accordingly, it has been proposed that the σ_1R binds to the NMDAR GluN1 subunit when Ca^{2+} raises as a consequence of increased NMDAR activity and that σ_1R antagonists diminish the affinity of σ_1R by GluN1 (prevent the binding of σ_1R to the GluN1 subunit), keep the σ_1R bound to the MOR, and weaken the interaction of HINT1 with MOR, making it possible for HINT1 to exit the MOR and bind to the GluN1 subunit, which altogether result in disruption of the "deleterious" cross talk between MORs and NMDARs (Rodríguez-Muñoz, Sánchez-Blázquez, et al., 2015; Rodríguez-Muñoz, Cortés-Montero, et al., 2015; Fig. 8).

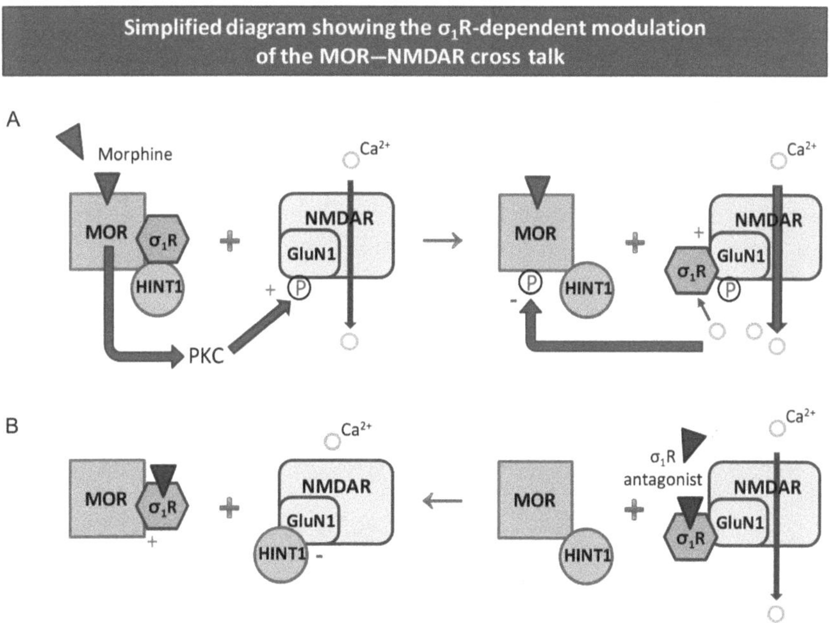

Figure 8 Simplified diagram showing the σ_1R-dependent modulation of the MOR–NMDAR cross talk. (A) Activation of MOR brings about the activation of PKC that phosphorylates NMDAR and enhance its function. The enhanced NMDAR function increases calcium levels in its environment, which promotes the transfer of the σ_1R from the MOR toward the activated NMDAR GluN1 subunit. In addition, NMDAR activity exerts a negative feedback effect on MOR signaling to ultimately decrease opioid analgesia. (B) σ_1R antagonists keep the σ_1R bound to the MOR, weakening the MOR–HINT1 interaction while preventing σ_1R binding to the GluN1 subunit; both simultaneous actions make it possible for HINT1 to exit the MOR toward the GluN1 subunit. In contrast, σ_1R agonists stabilize MOR–HINT1 and promote σ_1R binding to the GluN1 subunit, thus increasing the recruitment of NMDAR activity by MORs (not shown; Rodríguez-Muñoz, Cortés-Montero, et al., 2015; Rodríguez-Muñoz, Sánchez-Blázquez, et al., 2015).

3. ROLE OF PERIPHERAL σ_1R IN PAIN: PERIPHERAL ANTINOCICEPTIVE EFFECTS OF σ_1R ANTAGONISTS

Increasing evidence suggests that activity from the periphery is essential, not only to initiate but also to maintain pain symptoms (Richards & McMahon, 2013). Experience from clinical studies using lidocaine and capsaicin patches, local steroids, regional anesthesia, among others clearly demonstrates that blocking the peripheral nociceptive input is an effective strategy to relieve chronic pain. Interestingly, an inhibitory effect has been attributed to σ_1R antagonism at the periphery (Fig. 9), both when administered alone or in combination with opioids. Studies focused on the peripheral approach merit further efforts, as targeting the periphery could be a good approach to overcome the typical side effects related to CNS actions of current analgesic agents.

3.1 Effect of σ_1R Antagonism (in the Absence of Opioid Treatment) at Peripheral Sites: Inhibitory Effect on Peripheral Sensitization and Neuroprotection?

Several studies have shown that inhibition of σ_1R leads to decreased amplification of pain signaling within the CNS (Figs. 6 and 7). Indeed,

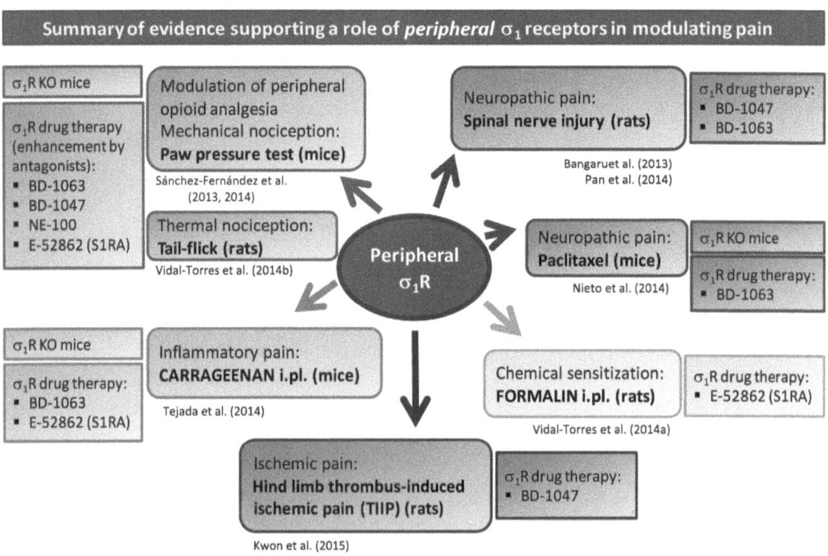

Figure 9 Preclinical evidence supporting a role of peripheral σ_1R in the modulation of pain and opioid analgesia in animal models of pain. Studies using σ_1R antagonists and σ_1R knockout (KO) mice.

σ_1R is expressed in several areas of the CNS specialized in nociceptive signaling processing (Alonso et al., 2000; Figs. 1 and 2), but σ_1R is also expressed in peripheral tissues including DRG neurons (Bangaru et al., 2013; Figs. 1 and 2). Importantly, its high density in DRGs, in which σ_1R expression is roughly an order of magnitude higher than in several CNS areas involved in pain signaling, including basolateral amygdala, RVM, PAG, and dorsal spinal cord, points to a functional role of peripheral σ_1R in pain modulation (Sánchez-Fernández et al., 2014). It is expressed by both sensory neurons and satellite cells in rat DRGs and its expression is downregulated in axotomized neurons and accompanying satellite glial cells (Bangaru et al., 2013). Therefore, regulation of σ_1R expression in neuropathic pain does not provide a direct explanation for pain relief after σ_1R blockade but could instead represent an adaptive counteracting mechanism.

Although the role of peripheral σ_1R on pain has not been extensively studied (Tejada et al., 2014), recent pieces of information are actually confirming their involvement in mechanisms regulating pain. Systemic administration of the selective σ_1R antagonist E-52862 produced an attenuation of the flinching and lifting/licking behaviors in the formalin test in rats, which was concomitant with an enhancement of noradrenaline levels and a reduction of formalin-evoked glutamate release in the spinal DH. Although a supraspinal effect was confirmed by the local (i.c.v) administration of E-52862, a peripheral contribution was also shown. In fact, intraplantar (i.pl.) administration of E-52862 in the ipsilateral paw (but not in the contralateral) reduced lifting/licking behaviors in phase I and II of the formalin test (Vidal-Torres et al., 2014a).

Recent studies have also evaluated the role of σ_1R in inflammatory pain (Gris et al., 2014; Parenti, Marrazzo, Arico, Cantarella, et al., 2014; Tejada et al., 2014; for review, see Gris et al., 2015; Figs. 3 and 9). Systemic administration of several σ_1R antagonists were effective in the carrageenan- and complete Freund's adjuvant-induced pain models. Particularly, the study by Tejada and colleagues (2014) described the importance of peripheral σ_1R in the carrageenan-induced pain model in mice. They used a behavioral approach in which the local (i.pl.) administration of the σ_1R agonist PRE-084 abolished the systemic antihypersensitive effect of the σ_1R antagonists BD-1063 and E-52862. Moreover, the i.pl. administration of the σ_1R antagonist E-52862 in the inflamed paw was sufficient to completely reverse inflammatory hyperalgesia. The antihyperalgesic effect of locally administered E-52862 was reverted by the i.pl. administration of the σ_1R agonist

PRE-084 and was absent in σ_1R knockout mice, thus confirming that the peripheral antihyperalgesic effect of E-52862 was mediated through σ_1R (Tejada et al., 2014). As a conclusion, authors open the possibility of targeting peripheral σ_1R to ameliorate inflammatory hyperalgesia.

A peripheral σ_1R-related mechanism might be more relevant in the modulation of inflammatory pain than in pain evoked by other etiologies because this type of pain is characterized by a pronounced enhancement of nociceptor responsiveness (peripheral sensitization) in response to the inflammatory mediators released at the inflammation site (Xu & Yaksh, 2011). Due to the σ_1R pleiotropic chaperoning nature it could, by acting downstream to the activation of different receptors and channels, modulate the intracellular signaling of a variety of algesic mediators released at the inflamed site. Bradykinin and nitric oxide (NO) are key mediators released during inflammation that contributes to peripheral sensitization (Chuang et al., 2001; Meller & Gebhart, 1993), and σ_1R activation enhances both bradykinin-induced Ca^{2+} signaling in neuronal-like cell cultures (Hayashi, Maurice, & Su, 2000; Hong, Nuwayhid, & Werling, 2004) and NO signaling (Roh et al., 2011). In addition, pain sensitization after peripheral inflammation involves plastic changes mediated by an increase in spinal excitatory neurotransmission together with activation of kinases, including ERK1/2, which are known to be modulated by σ_1R (de la Puente et al., 2009; Galán, López-García, Cervero, & Laird, 2002; Ji, Befort, Brenner, & Woolf, 2002).

In addition to inflammatory pain, the contribution of peripheral σ_1R to ischemic pain has been recently demonstrated in a rat model of hind limb thrombus-induced mechanical allodynia (Kwon et al., 2015). σ_1R expression significantly increased in skin, sciatic nerve, and DRG at 3 days post-thrombus-induced ischemic pain in rats. Authors also suggested a facilitatory effect of σ_1R on acid-sensing ion channels (ASICs) and purinergic P2X receptors, as i.pl. injection of the σ_1R antagonist BD-1047 reduced mechanical allodynia synergistically with the ASIC blocker amiloride and the P2X antagonist TNP-ATP (Kwon et al., 2015). Regarding neuropathic pain, σ_1R antagonism has been shown to restore injury-induced decrease of voltage-gated Ca^{2+} current in dissociated rat DRG neurons following spinal nerve ligation, but had no effect on control and noninjured DRGs, which is discussed as an antinociceptive mechanism as inward calcium currents are required for natural suppression of repetitive firing via opening of Ca^{2+}-activated K^+ channels (Pan, Guo, Kwok, Hogan, & Wu, 2014).

Neuroprotective but also neurotoxic roles have been attributed to σ_1R in the CNS by mechanisms involving modulation of cellular Ca^{2+} homeostasis, excitotoxicity, oxidative and nitrosative damage, and endoplasmic reticulum and mitochondrial stress. Indeed, both σ_1R agonists (DeCoster, Klette, Knight, & Tortella, 1995; Griesmaier et al., 2012; Katnik, Guerrero, Pennypacker, Herrera, & Cuevas, 2006; Mancuso et al., 2012; Shimazu et al., 2000; Vagnerova, Hurn, Bhardwaj, & Kirsch, 2006) and antagonists (Bhide et al., 2013; DeCoster et al., 1995; Luedtke et al., 2012; Schetz et al., 2007; Shimazu et al., 2000) have been reported to exert protective effects on neurons using different *in vitro* and/or *in vivo* experimental approaches. In the context of pain, it has been reported that antagonism on the σ_1R exerts a preventive effect against peripheral neuropathy. In particular, genetic inactivation (σ_1R knockout mice) and pharmacological blockade of σ_1Rs have been shown to prevent paclitaxel-induced sensory nerve mitochondrial abnormalities, concomitant with the prevention of paclitaxel-induced pain hypersensitivity (cold and mechanical allodynia) (Nieto et al., 2014). In contrast, in another study, the σ_1R agonist SA4503, but not the σ_1R antagonist NE-100, was found to produce antinociceptive effects against chemotherapeutic-induced neuropathic pain in rats (Tomohisa et al., 2015). Mitochondrial function/dysfunction has been suggested as a causal or contributory mechanism of normal sensory processing and chronic pain not only in painful peripheral neuropathies evoked by chemotherapy but also in diabetes and human immunodeficiency virus (HIV) (Flatters, 2015); and σ_1Rs at the endoplasmic reticulum–mitochondrion contact (MAM) are known to regulate mitochondrial function, including intramitochondrial Ca^{2+} homeostasis, oxidative stress, and cellular bioenergetics (Hayashi, 2015b; Su et al., 2010). Unfortunately, the role played by σ_1Rs in regulating pain-related mitochondrial dysfunction has not yet been addressed from a mechanistic point of view.

3.2 Effect of σ_1R Antagonism in Combination with Opioid Treatment at Peripheral Sites: Local Potentiation of Opioid Analgesia

It has been recently reported that the inhibition of peripheral σ_1R potentiates opioid antinociception (Sánchez-Fernández et al., 2013, 2014). In nonsensitizing conditions, systemic (subcutaneous, s.c.) or local i.pl. administrations of several σ_1R antagonists (i.e., BD-1063, BD-1047, NE-100, and E-52862) were devoid of effect in an acute model of mechanical nociception in mice (paw pressure test). Local i.pl. administration of morphine was also devoid of antinociceptive effects against mechanical stimulation in wild type but not in σ_1R knockout mice. This effect was limited to the injected paw. Interestingly, enhancement of peripheral morphine antinociception was replicated in wild-type mice locally coadministered with σ_1R antagonists and the opioid (Sánchez-Fernández, 2013). In a following paper, the same authors extended their findings to other opioids (fentanyl, oxycodone, buprenorphine, loperamide, tramadol) and confirmed the peripheral nature of the MOR agonist-σ_1R antagonist interaction: (a) the enhanced antinociceptive effect of the combination occurs when both the opioid agonist and the σ_1R antagonist were administered i.pl.; (b) the enhanced antinociception was reversed with the peripherally restricted opioid antagonist naloxone methiodide; and (c) the peripherally restricted opioid agonist loperamide, which was totally ineffective when given alone, showed a clear antinociceptive effect when combined with s.c. or i.pl. administered E-52862. The selective effect on σ_1Rs was confirmed by reversion with the σ_1R agonist PRE-084 and the lack of effect of σ_1R antagonists when administered to σ_1R knockout mice. The authors conclude that a tonic inhibition of opioid analgesia by σ_1R is present at the periphery at least in mechanical nociceptive pain (Sánchez-Fernández et al., 2014). Interestingly, opioid-induced side effects, such as hyperlocomotion and fentanyl- or loperamide-induced inhibition of gastrointestinal transit, were not potentiated in σ_1R knockout mice or by σ_1R antagonist coadministration. The enhancement of opioid antinociception has also been reported to include a peripheral component (in addition to a supraspinal one) using thermal nociceptive stimuli (radiant heat tail-flick test) in rats (Vidal-Torres et al., 2014a). In this study, the systemic administration of peripheral opioid agonist loperamide was devoid of antinociceptive effect when given alone but produced antinociception when combined with E-52862. The antinociceptive effect of the combination was abolished by the systemic administration of the peripheral opioid antagonist naloxone methiodide, thus confirming the peripheral nature of the interaction. Therefore, it seems that, like in the CNS but perhaps more pronounced as opiods are essentially devoid of antinociceptive activity when acting solely at the periphery, the σ_1R exerts an inhibitory role precluding opioid-induced peripheral antinociception and that σ_1R antagonism "releases the brake" enabling opioids to exert clear cut antinociceptive effects.

CONFLICT OF INTEREST

The authors are full-time employees of ESTEVE. The authors have no other relevant affiliation or financial involvement, have received no payment in preparation of this manuscript or have any conflict with the subject matter or materials discussed in the manuscript apart from those disclosed.

REFERENCES

Aanonsen, L. M., & Wilcox, G. L. (1987). Nociceptive action of excitatory amino acids in the mouse: Effects of spinally administered opioids, phencyclidine and sigma agonists. *The Journal of Pharmacology and Experimental Therapeutics*, *243*(1), 9–19. Retrieved from PM:2822907.

Almansa, C., & Vela, J. M. (2014). Selective sigma-1 receptor antagonists for the treatment of pain. *Future Medicinal Chemistry*, *6*(10), 1179–1199. Retrieved from PM:25078137.

Alonso, G., Phan, V., Guillemain, I., Saunier, M., Legrand, A., Anoal, M., et al. (2000). Immunocytochemical localization of the sigma(1) receptor in the adult rat central nervous system. *Neuroscience*, *97*(1), 155–170. Retrieved from PM:10771347.

Ataman, Z. A., Gakhar, L., Sorensen, B. R., Hell, J. W., & Shea, M. A. (2007). The NMDA receptor NR1 C1 region bound to calmodulin: Structural insights into functional differences between homologous domains. *Structure*, *15*(12), 1603–1617. Retrieved from PM:18073110.

Balasuriya, D., Stewart, A. P., & Edwardson, J. M. (2013). The sigma-1 receptor interacts directly with GluN1 but not GluN2A in the GluN1/GluN2A NMDA receptor. *The Journal of Neuroscience*, *33*(46), 18219–18224. Retrieved from PM:24227730.

Bangaru, M. L., Weihrauch, D., Tang, Q. B., Zoga, V., Hogan, Q., & Wu, H. E. (2013). Sigma-1 receptor expression in sensory neurons and the effect of painful peripheral nerve injury. *Molecular Pain*, *9*, 47. Retrieved from PM:24015960.

Baron, R. (2000). Capsaicin and nociception: From basic mechanisms to novel drugs. *Lancet*, *356*(9232), 785–787. Retrieved from PM:11022922.

Baron, R., Hans, G., & Dickenson, A. H. (2013). Peripheral input and its importance for central sensitization. *Annals of Neurology*, *74*(5), 630–636. Retrieved from PM:24018757.

Bergeron, R., de Montigny, C., & Debonnel, G. (1996). Potentiation of neuronal NMDA response induced by dehydroepiandrosterone and its suppression by progesterone: Effects mediated via sigma receptors. *The Journal of Neuroscience*, *16*(3), 1193–1202. Retrieved from PM:8558248.

Bhide, N., Lindenbach, D., Surrena, M. A., Goldenberg, A. A., Bishop, C., Berger, S. P., et al. (2013). The effects of BMY-14802 against L-DOPA- and dopamine agonist-induced dyskinesia in the hemiparkinsonian rat. *Psychopharmacology*, *227*(3), 533–544. Retrieved from PM:23389756.

Bouchard, P., & Quirion, R. (1997). [3H]1,3-di(2-tolyl)guanidine and [3H](+)pentazocine binding sites in the rat brain: Autoradiographic visualization of the putative sigma1 and sigma2 receptor subtypes. *Neuroscience*, *76*(2), 467–477. Retrieved from PM:9015331.

Brust, P., Deuther-Conrad, W., Lehmkuhl, K., Jia, H., & Wunsch, B. (2014). Molecular imaging of sigma1 receptors in vivo: Current status and perspectives. *Current Medicinal Chemistry*, *21*(1), 35–69. Retrieved from PM:23992342.

Bucolo, C., Campana, G., Di Toro, R., Cacciaguerra, S., & Spampinato, S. (1999). Sigma1 recognition sites in rabbit iris-ciliary body: Topical sigma1-site agonists lower intraocular pressure. *The Journal of Pharmacology and Experimental Therapeutics*, *289*(3), 1362–1369. Retrieved from PM:10336527.

Bura, A. S., Guegan, T., Zamanillo, D., Vela, J. M., & Maldonado, R. (2013). Operant self-administration of a sigma ligand improves nociceptive and emotional manifestations of neuropathic pain. *European Journal of Pain, 17*(6), 832–843. Retrieved from PM:23172791.

Cagnotto, A., Bastone, A., & Mennini, T. (1994). [3H](+)-pentazocine binding to rat brain sigma 1 receptors. *European Journal of Pharmacology, 266*(2), 131–138. Retrieved from PM:8157067.

Cendán, C. M., Pujalte, J. M., Portillo-Salido, E., & Baeyens, J. M. (2005a). Antinociceptive effects of haloperidol and its metabolites in the formalin test in mice. *Psychopharmacology, 182*(4), 485–493. Retrieved from PM:16075285.

Cendán, C. M., Pujalte, J. M., Portillo-Salido, E., Montoliu, L., & Baeyens, J. M. (2005b). Formalin-induced pain is reduced in sigma(1) receptor knockout mice. *European Journal of Pharmacology, 511*(1), 73–74. Retrieved from PM:15777781.

Chen, Y., Hajipour, A. R., Sievert, M. K., Arbabian, M., & Ruoho, A. E. (2007). Characterization of the cocaine binding site on the sigma-1 receptor. *Biochemistry, 46*(11), 3532–3542. Retrieved from PM:17315983.

Chen, B. S., & Roche, K. W. (2007). Regulation of NMDA receptors by phosphorylation. *Neuropharmacology, 53*(3), 362–368. Retrieved from PM:17644144.

Chien, C. C., & Pasternak, G. W. (1993). Functional antagonism of morphine analgesia by (+)-pentazocine: Evidence for an anti-opioid sigma 1 system. *European Journal of Pharmacology, 250*(1), R7–R8. Retrieved from PM:8119306.

Chien, C. C., & Pasternak, G. W. (1994). Selective antagonism of opioid analgesia by a sigma system. *The Journal of Pharmacology and Experimental Therapeutics, 271*(3), 1583–1590. Retrieved from PM:7996472.

Chien, C. C., & Pasternak, G. W. (1995a). (−)-Pentazocine analgesia in mice: Interactions with a sigma receptor system. *European Journal of Pharmacology, 294*(1), 303–308. Retrieved from PM:8788445.

Chien, C. C., & Pasternak, G. W. (1995b). Sigma antagonists potentiate opioid analgesia in rats. *Neuroscience Letters, 190*(2), 137–139. Retrieved from PM:7644123.

Choi, S. R., Roh, D. H., Yoon, S. Y., Kang, S. Y., Moon, J. Y., Kwon, S. G., et al. (2013). Spinal sigma-1 receptors activate NADPH oxidase 2 leading to the induction of pain hypersensitivity in mice and mechanical allodynia in neuropathic rats. *Pharmacological Research, 74*, 56–67. Retrieved from PM:23732704.

Chuang, H. H., Prescott, E. D., Kong, H., Shields, S., Jordt, S. E., Basbaum, A. I., et al. (2001). Bradykinin and nerve growth factor release the capsaicin receptor from PtdIns(4,5)P2-mediated inhibition. *Nature, 411*(6840), 957–962. Retrieved from PM:11418861.

Cobos, E. J., Entrena, J. M., Nieto, F. R., Cendan, C. M., & Del Pozo, E. (2008). Pharmacology and therapeutic potential of sigma(1) receptor ligands. *Current Neuropharmacology, 6*(4), 344–366. Retrieved from PM:19587856.

Coderre, T. J., Vaccarino, A. L., & Melzack, R. (1990). Central nervous system plasticity in the tonic pain response to subcutaneous formalin injection. *Brain Research, 535*(1), 155–158. Retrieved from PM:2292020.

Davis, M. P. (2015). Sigma-1 receptors and animal studies centered on pain and analgesia. *Expert. Opin. Drug Discov, 10*(8), 885–900. Retrieved from PM:26037105.

de la Puente, B., Nadal, X., Portillo-Salido, E., Sanchez-Arroyos, R., Ovalle, S., Palacios, G., et al. (2009). Sigma-1 receptors regulate activity-induced spinal sensitization and neuropathic pain after peripheral nerve injury. *Pain, 145*(3), 294–303. Retrieved from PM:19505761.

DeCoster, M. A., Klette, K. L., Knight, E. S., & Tortella, F. C. (1995). Sigma receptor-mediated neuroprotection against glutamatetoxicity in primary rat neuronal cultures. *Brain Research, 671*(1), 45–53. Retrieved from PM:7728532.

Dickenson, A. H., & Sullivan, A. F. (1987). Evidence for a role of the NMDA receptor in the frequency dependent potentiation of deep rat dorsal horn nociceptive neurones

following C fibre stimulation. *Neuropharmacology*, *26*(8), 1235–1238. Retrieved from PM:2821443.
D'Mello, R., & Dickenson, A. H. (2008). Spinal cord mechanisms of pain. *British Journal of Anaesthesia*, *101*(1), 8–16. Retrieved from PM:18417503.
Ehlers, M. D., Zhang, S., Bernhadt, J. P., & Huganir, R. L. (1996). Inactivation of NMDA receptors by direct interaction of calmodulin with the NR1 subunit. *Cell*, *84*(5), 745–755. Retrieved from PM:8625412.
Entrena, J. M., Cobos, E. J., Nieto, F. R., Cendan, C. M., Baeyens, J. M., & Del Pozo, E. (2009a). Antagonism by haloperidol and its metabolites of mechanical hypersensitivity induced by intraplantar capsaicin in mice: Role of sigma-1 receptors. *Psychopharmacology*, *205*(1), 21–33. Retrieved from PM:19326101.
Entrena, J. M., Cobos, E. J., Nieto, F. R., Cendan, C. M., Gris, G., Del Pozo, E., et al. (2009b). Sigma-1 receptors are essential for capsaicin-induced mechanical hypersensitivity: Studies with selective sigma-1 ligands and sigma-1 knockout mice. *Pain*, *143*(3), 252–261. Retrieved from PM:19375855.
Flatters, S. J. (2015). The contribution of mitochondria to sensory processing and pain. *Progress in Molecular Biology and Translational Science*, *131*, 119–146. Retrieved from PM:25744672.
Galán, A., López-García, J. A., Cervero, F., & Laird, J. M. (2002). Activation of spinal extracellular signaling-regulated kinase-1 and -2 by intraplantar carrageenan in rodents. *Neuroscience Letters*, *322*(1), 37–40. Retrieved from PM:11958838.
Garzón, J., Rodríguez-Muñoz, M., & Sánchez-Blázquez, P. (2012). Direct association of Mu-opioid and NMDA glutamate receptors supports their cross-regulation: Molecular implications for opioid tolerance. *Current Drug Abuse Reviews*, *5*(3), 199–226. Retrieved from PM:22920535.
Gilchrist, H. D., Allard, B. L., & Simone, D. A. (1996). Enhanced withdrawal responses to heat and mechanical stimuli following intraplantar injection of capsaicin in rats. *Pain*, *67*(1), 179–188. Retrieved from PM:8895246.
Gonçalves, L., & Dickenson, A. H. (2012). Asymmetric time-dependent activation of right central amygdala neurones in rats with peripheral neuropathy and pregabalin modulation. *The European Journal of Neuroscience*, *36*(9), 3204–3213. Retrieved from PM:22861166.
González-Cano, R., Merlos, M., Baeyens, J. M., & Cendan, C. M. (2013). σ1 Receptors are involved in the visceral pain induced by intracolonic administration of capsaicin in mice. *Anesthesiology*, *118*(3), 691–700. Retrieved from PM:23299362.
Griesmaier, E., Posod, A., Gross, M., Neubauer, V., Wegleiter, K., Hermann, M., et al. (2012). Neuroprotective effects of the sigma-1 receptor ligand PRE-084 against excitotoxic perinatal brain injury in newborn mice. *Experimental Neurology*, *237*(2), 388–395. Retrieved from PM:22771763.
Gris, G., Cobos, E. J., Zamanillo, D., & Portillo-Salido, E. (2015). Sigma-1 receptor and inflammatory pain. *Inflammation Research*, *64*(6), 377–381. Retrieved from PM:25902777.
Gris, G., Merlos, M., Vela, J. M., Zamanillo, D., & Portillo-Salido, E. (2014). S1RA, a selective sigma-1 receptor antagonist, inhibits inflammatory pain in the carrageenan and complete Freund's adjuvant models in mice. *Behavioural Pharmacology*, *25*(3), 226–235. Retrieved from PM:24776490.
Gundlach, A. L., Largent, B. L., & Snyder, S. H. (1986). Autoradiographic localization of sigma receptor binding sites in guinea pig and rat central nervous system with (+)3H-3-(3-hydroxyphenyl)-N-(1-propyl)piperidine. *The Journal of Neuroscience*, *6*(6), 1757–1770. Retrieved from PM:3012017.
Hanner, M., Moebius, F. F., Flandorfer, A., Knaus, H. G., Striessnig, J., Kempner, E., et al. (1996). Purification, molecular cloning, and expression of the mammalian sigma1-binding site. *Proceedings of the National Academy of Sciences of the United States of America*, *93*(15), 8072–8077. Retrieved from PM:8755605.

Hayashi, T. (2015a). Sigma-1 receptor: The novel intracellular target of neuropsychotherapeutic drugs. *Journal of Pharmacological Sciences*, *127*(1), 2–5. Retrieved from PM:25704011.

Hayashi, T. (2015b). Conversion of psychological stress into cellular stress response: Roles of the sigma-1 receptor in the process. *Psychiatry and Clinical Neurosciences*, *69*(4), 179–191. Retrieved from PM:25495202.

Hayashi, T., Kagaya, A., Takebayashi, M., Shimizu, M., Uchitomi, Y., Motohashi, N., et al. (1995). Modulation by sigma ligands of intracellular free Ca++ mobilization by N-methyl-D-aspartate in primary culture of rat frontal cortical neurons. *The Journal of Pharmacology and Experimental Therapeutics*, *275*(1), 207–214. Retrieved from PM:7562551.

Hayashi, T., Maurice, T., & Su, T. P. (2000). Ca(2+) signaling via sigma(1)-receptors: Novel regulatory mechanism affecting intracellular Ca(2+) concentration. *The Journal of Pharmacology and Experimental Therapeutics*, *293*(3), 788–798. Retrieved from PM:10869377.

Hayashi, T., & Su, T. P. (2003). Sigma-1 receptors (sigma(1) binding sites) form raft-like microdomains and target lipid droplets on the endoplasmic reticulum: Roles in endoplasmic reticulum lipid compartmentalization and export. *The Journal of Pharmacology and Experimental Therapeutics*, *306*(2), 718–725. Retrieved from PM:12730355.

Hayashi, T., & Su, T. P. (2007). Sigma-1 receptor chaperones at the ER-mitochondrion interface regulate Ca(2+) signaling and cell survival. *Cell*, *131*(3), 596–610. Retrieved from PM:17981125.

Hayashi, T., Tsai, S. Y., Mori, T., Fujimoto, M., & Su, T. P. (2011). Targeting ligand-operated chaperone sigma-1 receptors in the treatment of neuropsychiatric disorders. *Expert Opinion on Therapeutic Targets*, *15*(5), 557–577. Retrieved from PM:21375464.

Heroux, J. A., Tam, S. W., & De Souza, E. B. (1992). Autoradiographic identification and characterization of sigma receptors in guinea pig brain using [3H]1(cyclopropylmethyl)-4-(2′-(4″-fluorophenyl)-2′-oxoethyl) piperidine ([3H]DuP 734), a novel sigma receptor ligand. *Brain Research*, *598*(1–2), 76–86. Retrieved from PM:1486505.

Herrero, J. F., Laird, J. M., & Lopez-Garcia, J. A. (2000). Wind-up of spinal cord neurones and pain sensation: Much ado about something? *Progress in Neurobiology*, *61*(2), 169–203. Retrieved from PM:10704997.

Hiramatsu, M., Hoshino, T., Kameyama, T., & Nabeshima, T. (2002). Involvement of kappa-opioid and sigma receptors in short-term memory in mice. *European Journal of Pharmacology*, *453*(1), 91–98. Retrieved from PM:12393064.

Hong, W., Nuwayhid, S. J., & Werling, L. L. (2004). Modulation of bradykinin-induced calcium changes in SH-SY5Y cells by neurosteroids and sigma receptor ligands via a shared mechanism. *Synapse*, *54*(2), 102–110. Retrieved from PM:15352135.

Ishiwata, K., Kobayashi, T., Kawamura, K., & Matsuno, K. (2003). Age-related changes of the binding of [3H]SA4503 to sigma1 receptors in the rat brain. *Annals of Nuclear Medicine*, *17*(1), 73–77. Retrieved from PM:12691135.

Ji, R. R., Befort, K., Brenner, G. J., & Woolf, C. J. (2002). ERK MAP kinase activation in superficial spinal cord neurons induces prodynorphin and NK-1 upregulation and contributes to persistent inflammatory pain hypersensitivity. *The Journal of Neuroscience*, *22*(2), 478–485. Retrieved from PM:11784793.

Joshi, S. K., Hernandez, G., Mikusa, J. P., Zhu, C. Z., Zhong, C., Salyers, A., et al. (2006). Comparison of antinociceptive actions of standard analgesics in attenuating capsaicin and nerve-injury-induced mechanical hypersensitivity. *Neuroscience*, *143*(2), 587–596. Retrieved from PM:16962719.

Katnik, C., Guerrero, W. R., Pennypacker, K. R., Herrera, Y., & Cuevas, J. (2006). Sigma-1 receptor activation prevents intracellular calcium dysregulation in cortical neurons during in vitro ischemia. *The Journal of Pharmacology and Experimental Therapeutics*, *319*(3), 1355–1365. Retrieved from PM:16988055.

Kekuda, R., Prasad, P. D., Fei, Y. J., Leibach, F. H., & Ganapathy, V. (1996). Cloning and functional expression of the human type 1 sigma receptor (hSigmaR1). *Biochemical and Biophysical Research Communications*, *229*(2), 553–558. Retrieved from PM:8954936.

Kibaly, C., Meyer, L., Patte-Mensah, C., & Mensah-Nyagan, A. G. (2008). Biochemical and functional evidence for the control of pain mechanisms by dehydroepiandrosterone endogenously synthesized in the spinal cord. *The FASEB Journal*, *22*(1), 93–104. Retrieved from PM:17720801.

Kim, F. J., Kovalyshyn, I., Burgman, M., Neilan, C., Chien, C. C., & Pasternak, G. W. (2010). Sigma 1 receptor modulation of G-protein-coupled receptor signaling: Potentiation of opioid transduction independent from receptor binding. *Molecular Pharmacology*, 77(4), 695–703. Retrieved from PM:20089882.

Kim, H. W., Kwon, Y. B., Roh, D. H., Yoon, S. Y., Han, H. J., Kim, K. W., et al. (2006). Intrathecal treatment with sigma1 receptor antagonists reduces formalin-induced phosphorylation of NMDA receptor subunit 1 and the second phase of formalin test in mice. *British Journal of Pharmacology*, *148*(4), 490–498. Retrieved from PM:16682960.

Kim, H. W., Roh, D. H., Yoon, S. Y., Seo, H. S., Kwon, Y. B., Han, H. J., et al. (2008). Activation of the spinal sigma-1 receptor enhances NMDA-induced pain via PKC- and PKA-dependent phosphorylation of the NR1 subunit in mice. *British Journal of Pharmacology*, *154*(5), 1125–1134. Retrieved from PM:18493253.

Kitaichi, K., Chabot, J. G., Moebius, F. F., Flandorfer, A., Glossmann, H., & Quirion, R. (2000). Expression of the purported sigma(1) (sigma(1)) receptor in the mammalian brain and its possible relevance in deficits induced by antagonism of the NMDA receptor complex as revealed using an antisense strategy. *Journal of Chemical Neuroanatomy*, *20*(3–4), 375–387. Retrieved from PM:11207432.

Kovacs, K. J., & Larson, A. A. (1995). Discrepancies in characterization of sigma sites in the mouse central nervous system. *European Journal of Pharmacology*, *285*(2), 127–134. Retrieved from PM:8566130.

Kwon, Y. B., Jeong, Y. C., Kwon, J. K., Son, J. S., & Kim, K. W. (2009). The antinociceptive effect of sigma-1 receptor antagonist, BD1047, in a capsaicin induced headache model in rats. *Korean Journal of Physiology & Pharmacology*, *13*(6), 425–429. Retrieved from PM:20054487.

Kwon, S. G., Roh, D. H., Yoon, S. Y., Choi, S. R., Choi, H. S., Moon, J. Y., et al. (2015). Role of peripheral sigma-1 receptors in ischaemic pain: Potential interactions with ASIC and P2X receptors. *European Journal of Pain*. http://dx.doi.org/10.1002/ejp.774. [Epub ahead of print].

Lan, Y., Chen, Y., Cao, X., Zhang, J., Wang, J., Xu, X., et al. (2014a). Synthesis and biological evaluation of novel sigma-1 receptor antagonists based on pyrimidine scaffold as agents for treating neuropathic pain. *Journal of Medicinal Chemistry*, *57*(24), 10404–10423. Retrieved from PM:25420090.

Lan, Y., Chen, Y., Xu, X., Qiu, Y., Liu, S., Liu, X., et al. (2014b). Synthesis and biological evaluation of a novel sigma-1 receptor antagonist based on 3,4-dihydro-2(1H)-quinolinone scaffold as a potential analgesic. *European Journal of Medicinal Chemistry*, *79*, 216–230. Retrieved from PM:24735647.

Latremoliere, A., & Woolf, C. J. (2009). Central sensitization: A generator of pain hypersensitivity by central neural plasticity. *The Journal of Pain*, *10*(9), 895–926. Retrieved from PM:19712899.

Lee, H. K. (2006). Synaptic plasticity and phosphorylation. *Pharmacology & Therapeutics*, *112*(3), 810–832. Retrieved from PM:16904750.

Li, J., Simone, D. A., & Larson, A. A. (1999). Windup leads to characteristics of central sensitization. *Pain*, *79*(1), 75–82. Retrieved from PM:9928779.

Lisman, J., Yasuda, R., & Raghavachari, S. (2012). Mechanisms of CaMKII action in long-term potentiation. *Nature Reviews Neuroscience*, *13*(3), 169–182. Retrieved from PM:22334212.

Luedtke, R. R., Perez, E., Yang, S. H., Liu, R., Vangveravong, S., Tu, Z., et al. (2012). Neuroprotective effects of high affinity sigma-1 receptor selective compounds. *Brain Research, 1441*, 17–26. Retrieved from PM:22285434.

Mancuso, R., Oliván, S., Rando, A., Casas, C., Osta, R., & Navarro, X. (2012). Sigma-1R agonist improves motor function and motoneuron survival in ALS mice. *Neurotherapeutics, 9*(4), 814–826. Retrieved from PM:22935988.

Mao, L. M., Jin, D. Z., Xue, B., Chu, X. P., & Wang, J. Q. (2014). Phosphorylation and regulation of glutamate receptors by CaMKII. *Sheng Li Xue Bao, 66*(3), 365–372. Retrieved from PM:24964855.

Marrazzo, A., Parenti, C., Scavo, V., Ronsisvalle, S., Scoto, G. M., & Ronsisvalle, G. (2006). In vivo evaluation of (+)-MR200 as a new selective sigma ligand modulating MOP, DOP and KOP supraspinal analgesia. *Life Sciences, 78*(21), 2449–2453. Retrieved from PM:16324720.

Martina, M., Turcotte, M. E., Halman, S., & Bergeron, R. (2007). The sigma-1 receptor modulates NMDA receptor synaptic transmission and plasticity via SK channels in rat hippocampus. *The Journal of Physiology, 578*(Pt. 1), 143–157. Retrieved from PM:17068104.

Maruo, J., Yoshida, A., Shimohira, I., Matsuno, K., Mita, S., & Ueda, H. (2000). Binding of [35S]GTPgammaS stimulated by (+)-pentazocine sigma receptor agonist, is abundant in the guinea pig spleen. *Life Sciences, 67*(5), 599–603. Retrieved from PM:10993125.

Mash, D. C., & Zabetian, C. P. (1992). Sigma receptors are associated with cortical limbic areas in the primate brain. *Synapse, 12*(3), 195–205. Retrieved from PM:1481139.

Mavlyutov, T. A., Epstein, M. L., Andersen, K. A., Ziskind-Conhaim, L., & Ruoho, A. E. (2010). The sigma-1 receptor is enriched in postsynaptic sites of C-terminals in mouse motoneurons. An anatomical and behavioral study. *Neuroscience, 167*(2), 247–255. Retrieved from PM:20167253.

Mazo, I., Roza, C., Zamanillo, D., Merlos, M., Vela, J. M., & Lopez-Garcia, J. A. (2015). Effects of centrally acting analgesics on spinal segmental reflexes and wind-up. *European Journal of Pain, 19*(7), 1012–1020. Retrieved from PM:25469831.

McNamara, C. R., Mandel-Brehm, J., Bautista, D. M., Siemens, J., Deranian, K. L., Zhao, M., et al. (2007). TRPA1 mediates formalin-induced pain. *Proceedings of the National Academy of Sciences of the United States of America, 104*(33), 13525–13530. Retrieved from PM:17686976.

Mei, J., & Pasternak, G. W. (2002). Sigma1 receptor modulation of opioid analgesia in the mouse. *The Journal of Pharmacology and Experimental Therapeutics, 300*(3), 1070–1074. Retrieved from PM:11861817.

Mei, J., & Pasternak, G. W. (2007). Modulation of brainstem opiate analgesia in the rat by sigma 1 receptors: A microinjection study. *The Journal of Pharmacology and Experimental Therapeutics, 322*(3), 1278–1285. Retrieved from PM:17545312.

Meller, S. T., & Gebhart, G. F. (1993). Nitric oxide (NO) and nociceptive processing in the spinal cord. *Pain, 52*(2), 127–136. Retrieved from PM:8455960.

Meunier, J., & Hayashi, T. (2010). Sigma-1 receptors regulate Bcl-2 expression by reactive oxygen species-dependent transcriptional regulation of nuclear factor kappaB. *The Journal of Pharmacology and Experimental Therapeutics, 332*(2), 388–397. Retrieved from PM:19855099.

Meyer, L., Patte-Mensah, C., Taleb, O., & Mensah-Nyagan, A. G. (2011). Allopregnanolone prevents and suppresses oxaliplatin-evoked painful neuropathy: Multi-parametric assessment and direct evidence. *Pain, 152*(1), 170–181. Retrieved from PM:21071147.

Meyer, L., Patte-Mensah, C., Taleb, O., & Mensah-Nyagan, A. G. (2013). Neurosteroid 3alpha-androstanediol efficiently counteracts paclitaxel-induced peripheral neuropathy and painful symptoms. *PLoS One, 8*(11), e80915. Retrieved from PM:24260511.

Millan, M. J. (2002). Descending control of pain. *Progress in Neurobiology, 66*(6), 355–474. Retrieved from PM:12034378.

Monnet, F. P., Debonnel, G., & de Montigny, C. (1992). In vivo electrophysiological evidence for a selective modulation of N-methyl-D-aspartate-induced neuronal activation in rat CA3 dorsal hippocampus by sigma ligands. *The Journal of Pharmacology and Experimental Therapeutics, 261*(1), 123–130. Retrieved from PM:1532832.

Monnet, F. P., Debonnel, G., Junien, J. L., & de Montigny, C. (1990). N-methyl-D-aspartate-induced neuronal activation is selectively modulated by sigma receptors. *European Journal of Pharmacology, 179*(3), 441–445. Retrieved from PM:2163857.

Moon, J. Y., Choi, S. R., Roh, D. H., Yoon, S. Y., Kwon, S. G., Choi, H. S., et al. (2015). Spinal sigma-1 receptor activation increases the production of d-serine in astrocytes which contributes to the development of mechanical allodynia in a mouse model of neuropathic pain. *Pharmacological Research, 100*, 353–364. Retrieved from PM:26316425.

Moon, J. Y., Roh, D. H., Yoon, S. Y., Choi, S. R., Kwon, S. G., Choi, H. S., et al. (2014). σ1 receptors activate astrocytes via p38 MAPK phosphorylation leading to the development of mechanical allodynia in a mouse model of neuropathic pain. *British Journal of Pharmacology, 171*(24), 5881–5897. Retrieved from PM:25158784.

Moon, J. Y., Roh, D. H., Yoon, S. Y., Kang, S. Y., Choi, S. R., Kwon, S. G., et al. (2013). Sigma-1 receptor-mediated increase in spinal p38 MAPK phosphorylation leads to the induction of mechanical allodynia in mice and neuropathic rats. *Experimental Neurology, 247*, 383–391. Retrieved from PM:23333567.

Nieto, F. R., Cendan, C. M., Canizares, F. J., Cubero, M. A., Vela, J. M., Fernandez-Segura, E., et al. (2014). Genetic inactivation and pharmacological blockade of sigma-1 receptors prevent paclitaxel-induced sensory-nerve mitochondrial abnormalities and neuropathic pain in mice. *Molecular Pain, 10*, 11. Retrieved from PM:24517272.

Nieto, F. R., Cendan, C. M., Sánchez-Fernáandez, C., Cobos, E. J., Entrena, J. M., Tejada, M. A., et al. (2012). Role of sigma-1 receptors in paclitaxel-induced neuropathic pain in mice. *The Journal of Pain, 13*(11), 1107–1121. Retrieved from PM:23063344.

Oberdorf, C., Schepmann, D., Vela, J. M., Diaz, J. L., Holenz, J., & Wunsch, B. (2008). Thiophenebioisosteres of spirocyclic sigma receptor ligands. 1. N-substituted spiro [piperidine-4,4′-thieno[3,2-c]pyrans]. *Journal of Medicinal Chemistry, 51*(20), 6531–6537. Retrieved from PM:18816044.

O'Neill, J., Brock, C., Olesen, A. E., Andresen, T., Nilsson, M., & Dickenson, A. H. (2012). Unravelling the mystery of capsaicin: A tool to understand and treat pain. *Pharmacological Reviews, 64*(4), 939–971. Retrieved from PM:23023032.

Pal, A., Fontanilla, D., Gopalakrishnan, A., Chae, Y. K., Markley, J. L., & Ruoho, A. E. (2012). The sigma-1 receptor protects against cellular oxidative stress and activates antioxidant response elements. *European Journal of Pharmacology, 682*(1–3), 12–20. Retrieved from PM:22381068.

Pan, B., Guo, Y., Kwok, W. M., Hogan, Q., & Wu, H. E. (2014). Sigma-1 receptor antagonism restores injury-induced decrease of voltage-gated Ca2+ current in sensory neurons. *The Journal of Pharmacology and Experimental Therapeutics, 350*(2), 290–300. Retrieved from PM:24891452.

Parenti, C., Marrazzo, A., Arico, G., Cantarella, G., Prezzavento, O., Ronsisvalle, S., et al. (2014). Effects of a selective sigma 1 antagonist compound on inflammatory pain. *Inflammation, 37*(1), 261–266. Retrieved from PM:24049016.

Parenti, C., Marrazzo, A., Arico, G., Parenti, R., Pasquinucci, L., Ronsisvalle, S., et al. (2014). The antagonistic effect of the sigma 1 receptor ligand (+)-MR200 on persistent pain induced by inflammation. *Inflammation Research, 63*(3), 231–237. Retrieved from PM:24316864.

Prezzavento, O., Parenti, C., Marrazzo, A., Ronsisvalle, S., Vittorio, F., Aricò, G., et al. (2008). A new sigma ligand, (+/−)-PPCC, antagonizes kappa opioid receptor-mediated antinociceptive effect. *Life Sciences*, *82*(11–12), 549–553. Retrieved from PM:18261749.

Pyun, K., Son, J. S., & Kwon, Y. B. (2014). Chronic activation of sigma-1 receptor evokes nociceptive activation of trigeminal nucleus caudalis in rats. *Pharmacology, Biochemistry, and Behavior*, *124*, 278–283. Retrieved from PM:24992726.

Richards, N., & McMahon, S. B. (2013). Targeting novel peripheral mediators for the treatment of chronic pain. *British Journal of Anaesthesia*, *111*(1), 46–51. Retrieved from PM:23794644.

Rodríguez-Muñoz, M., Cortés-Montero, E., Pozo-Rodrigálvarez, A., Sánchez-Blázquez, P., & Garzón-Niño, J. (2015). The ON:OFF switch, σ1R-HINT1 protein, controls GPCR-NMDA receptor cross-regulation: Implications in neurological disorders. *Oncotarget*, *6*(43), 35458–35477. Retrieved from PM:26461475.

Rodríguez-Muñoz, M., Sánchez-Blázquez, P., Herrero-Labrador, R., Martínez-Murillo, R., Merlos, M., Vela, J. M., et al. (2015). The sigma1 receptor engages the redox-regulated HINT1 protein to bring opioid analgesia under NMDA receptor negative control. *Antioxidants & Redox Signaling*, *22*(10), 799–818. Retrieved from PM:25557043.

Roh, D. H., Choi, S. R., Yoon, S. Y., Kang, S. Y., Moon, J. Y., Kwon, S. G., et al. (2011). Spinal neuronal NOS activation mediates sigma-1 receptor-induced mechanical and thermal hypersensitivity in mice: Involvement of PKC-dependent GluN1 phosphorylation. *British Journal of Pharmacology*, *163*(8), 1707–1720. Retrieved from PM:21391983.

Roh, D. H., Kim, H. W., Yoon, S. Y., Seo, H. S., Kwon, Y. B., Kim, K. W., et al. (2008a). Intrathecal administration of sigma-1 receptor agonists facilitates nociception: Involvement of a protein kinase C-dependent pathway. *Journal of Neuroscience Research*, *86*(16), 3644–3654. Retrieved from PM:18655205.

Roh, D. H., Kim, H. W., Yoon, S. Y., Seo, H. S., Kwon, Y. B., Kim, K. W., et al. (2008b). Intrathecal injection of the sigma(1) receptor antagonist BD1047 blocks both mechanical allodynia and increases in spinal NR1 expression during the induction phase of rodent neuropathic pain. *Anesthesiology*, *109*(5), 879–889. Retrieved from PM:18946301.

Roh, D. H., & Yoon, S. Y. (2014). Sigma-1 receptor antagonist, BD1047 reduces nociceptive responses and phosphorylation of p38 MAPK in mice orofacial formalin model. *Biological & Pharmaceutical Bulletin*, *37*(1), 145–151. Retrieved from PM:24152609.

Roh, D. H., Yoon, S. Y., Seo, H. S., Kang, S. Y., Moon, J. Y., Song, S., et al. (2010). Sigma-1 receptor-induced increase in murine spinal NR1 phosphorylation is mediated by the PKCalpha and epsilon, but not the PKCzeta, isoforms. *Neuroscience Letters*, *477*(2), 95–99. Retrieved from PM:20417251.

Romero, L., Zamanillo, D., Nadal, X., Sanchez-Arroyos, R., Rivera-Arconada, I., Dordal, A., et al. (2012). Pharmacological properties of S1RA, a new sigma-1 receptor antagonist that inhibits neuropathic pain and activity-induced spinal sensitization. *British Journal of Pharmacology*, *166*(8), 2289–2306. Retrieved from PM:22404321.

Ronsisvalle, G., Marrazzo, A., Prezzavento, O., Cagnotto, A., Tiziana, Mennini T., Parenti, C., et al. (2001). Opioid and sigma receptor studies. New developments in the design of selective sigma ligands (Plenary lecture presented at the Hungarian–German–Italian–Polish Joint Meeting on Medicinal Chemistry, Budapest, Hungary, 2–6 September 2001). *Pure and Applied Chemistry*, *73*(9), 1499–1509.

Sánchez-Blázquez, P., Rodriguez-Munoz, M., Herrero-Labrador, R., Burgueno, J., Zamanillo, D., & Garzon, J. (2014). The calcium-sensitive sigma-1 receptor prevents cannabinoids from provoking glutamate NMDA receptor hypofunction: Implications in antinociception and psychotic diseases. *The International Journal of Neuropsychopharmacology*, *17*(12), 1943–1955. Retrieved from PM:24485144.

Sánchez-Fernández, C., Montilla-Garcia, A., Gonzalez-Cano, R., Nieto, F. R., Romero, L., Artacho-Cordon, A., et al. (2014). Modulation of peripheral mu-opioid analgesia by sigma1 receptors. *The Journal of Pharmacology and Experimental Therapeutics*, *348*(1), 32–45. Retrieved from PM:24155346.

Sánchez-Fernández, C., Nieto, F. R., Gonzalez-Cano, R., Artacho-Cordon, A., Romero, L., Montilla-Garcia, A., et al. (2013). Potentiation of morphine-induced mechanical antinociception by sigma(1) receptor inhibition: Role of peripheral sigma (1) receptors. *Neuropharmacology*, *70*, 348–358. Retrieved from PM:23524304.

Sandkühler, J. (2009). Models and mechanisms of hyperalgesia and allodynia. *Physiological Reviews*, *89*(2), 707–758. Retrieved from PM:19342617.

Sandkühler, J., & Gruber-Schoffnegger, D. (2012). Hyperalgesia by synaptic long-term potentiation (LTP): An update. *Current Opinion in Pharmacology*, *12*(1), 18–27. Retrieved from PM:22078436.

Sang, C. N., Gracely, R. H., Max, M. B., & Bennett, G. J. (1996). Capsaicin-evoked mechanical allodynia and hyperalgesia cross nerve territories. Evidence for a central mechanism. *Anesthesiology*, *85*(3), 491–496. Retrieved from PM:8853078.

Schetz, J. A., Perez, E., Liu, R., Chen, S., Lee, I., & Simpkins, J. W. (2007). A prototypical sigma-1 receptor antagonist protects against brain ischemia. *Brain Research*, *1181*, 1–9Retrieved from PM:17919467.

Senda, T., Matsuno, K., & Mita, S. (1997). The presence of sigma receptor subtypes in bovine retinal membranes. *Experimental Eye Research*, *64*(5), 857–860. Retrieved from PM:9245918.

Seth, P., Leibach, F. H., & Ganapathy, V. (1997). Cloning and structural analysis of the cDNA and the gene encoding the murine type 1 sigma receptor. *Biochemical and Biophysical Research Communications*, *241*(2), 535–540. Retrieved from PM:9425306.

Sha, S., Qu, W. J., Li, L., Lu, Z. H., Chen, L., Yu, W. F., et al. (2013). Sigma-1 receptor knockout impairs neurogenesis in dentate gyrus of adult hippocampus via down-regulation of NMDA receptors. *CNS Neuroscience & Therapeutics*, *19*(9), 705–713. Retrieved from PM:23745740.

Shimazu, S., Katsuki, H., Takenaka, C., Tomita, M., Kume, T., & Kaneko, S. (2000). Sigma receptor ligands attenuate N-methyl-D-aspartate cytotoxicity in dopaminergic neurons of mesencephalic slice cultures. *European Journal of Pharmacology*, *388*(2), 139–146. Retrieved from PM:10666505.

Son, J. S., & Kwon, Y. B. (2010). Sigma-1 receptor antagonist BD1047 reduces allodynia and spinal ERK phosphorylation following chronic compression of dorsal root ganglion in rats. *Korean Journal of Physiology & Pharmacology*, *14*(6), 359–364. Retrieved from PM:21311675.

Su, T. P., Hayashi, T., Maurice, T., Buch, S., & Ruoho, A. E. (2010). The sigma-1 receptor chaperone as an inter-organelle signaling modulator. *Trends in Pharmacological Sciences*, *31*(12), 557–566. Retrieved from PM:20869780.

Suzuki, R., Kontinen, V. K., Matthews, E., Williams, E., & Dickenson, A. H. (2000). Enlargement of the receptive field size to low intensity mechanical stimulation in the rat spinal nerve ligation model of neuropathy. *Experimental Neurology*, *163*(2), 408–413. Retrieved from PM:10833315.

Tejada, M. A., Montilla-Garcia, A., Sánchez-Fernández, C., Entrena, J. M., Perazzoli, G., Baeyens, J. M., et al. (2014). Sigma-1 receptor inhibition reverses acute inflammatory hyperalgesia in mice: Role of peripheral sigma-1 receptors. *Psychopharmacology*, *231*(19), 3855–3869. Retrieved from PM:24639046.

Todd, A. J. (2010). Neuronal circuitry for pain processing in the dorsal horn. *Nature Reviews. Neuroscience*, *11*(12), 823–836. Retrieved from PM:21068766.

Tominaga, M., Caterina, M. J., Malmberg, A. B., Rosen, T. A., Gilbert, H., Skinner, K., et al. (1998). The cloned capsaicin receptor integrates multiple pain-producing stimuli. *Neuron*, *21*(3), 531–543. Retrieved from PM:9768840.

Tomohisa, M., Junpei, O., Aki, M., Masato, H., Mika, F., Kazumi, Y., et al. (2015). Possible involvement of the sigma-1 receptor chaperone in chemotherapeutic-induced neuropathic pain. *Synapse, 69*(11), 526–532. Retrieved from PM:26234785.

Tsai, S. Y., Hayashi, T., Harvey, B. K., Wang, Y., Wu, W. W., Shen, R. F., et al. (2009). Sigma-1 receptors regulate hippocampal dendritic spine formation via a free radical-sensitive mechanism involving Rac1xGTP pathway. *Proceedings of the National Academy of Sciences of the United States of America, 106*(52), 22468–22473. Retrieved from PM:20018732.

Utech, T., Kohler, J., Buschmann, H., Holenz, J., Vela, J. M., & Wunsch, B. (2011). Synthesis and pharmacological evaluation of a potent and selective sigma1 receptor antagonist with high antiallodynic activity. *Arch der Pharmazie (Weinheim, Germany), 344*(7), 415–421. Retrieved from PM:21598296.

Vaccarino, A. L., & Chorney, D. A. (1994). Descending modulation of central neural plasticity in the formalin pain test. *Brain Research, 666*(1), 104–108. Retrieved from PM:7889357.

Vagnerova, K., Hurn, P. D., Bhardwaj, A., & Kirsch, J. R. (2006). Sigma 1 receptor agonists act as neuroprotective drugs through inhibition of inducible nitric oxide synthase. *Anesthesia and Analgesia, 103*(2), 430–434. Retrieved from PM:16861428.

Vela, J. M., Merlos, M., & Almansa, C. (2015). Investigational sigma-1 receptor antagonists for the treatment of pain. *Expert Opinion on Investigational Drugs, 24*(7), 883–896. Retrieved from PM:26037209.

Vicente-Sánchez, A., Sánchez-Blázquez, P., Rodríguez-Muñoz, M., & Garzón, J. (2013). HINT1 protein cooperates with cannabinoid 1 receptor to negatively regulate glutamate NMDA receptor activity. *Molecular Brain, 6*, 42. Retrieved from PM:24093505.

Vidal-Torres, A., de la Puente, B., Rocasalbas, M., Tourino, C., Bura, S. A., Fernandez-Pastor, B., et al. (2013). Sigma-1 receptor antagonism as opioid adjuvant strategy: Enhancement of opioid antinociception without increasing adverse effects. *European Journal of Pharmacology, 711*(1–3), 63–72. Retrieved from PM:23632394.

Vidal-Torres, A., Fernandez-Pastor, B., Carceller, A., Vela, J. M., Merlos, M., & Zamanillo, D. (2014). Effects of the selective sigma-1 receptor antagonist S1RA on formalin-induced pain behavior and neurotransmitter release in the spinal cord in rats. *Journal of Neurochemistry, 129*(3), 484–494. Retrieved from PM:24384038.

Vidal-Torres, A., Fernández-Pastor, B., Carceller, A., Vela, J. M., Merlos, M., & Zamanillo, D. (2014). Supraspinal and peripheral but not intrathecal sigma-1 receptor blockade by the selective sigma-1 receptor antagonist E-52862 enhances morphine antinociception. In *15th World Congress on Pain.*

Walker, J. M., Bowen, W. D., Goldstein, S. R., Roberts, A. H., Patrick, S. L., Hohmann, A. G., et al. (1992). Autoradiographic distribution of [3H](+)-pentazocine and [3H]1,3-di-o-tolylguanidine (DTG) binding sites in guinea pig brain: A comparative study. *Brain Research, 581*(1), 33–38. Retrieved from PM:1323368.

West, S. J., Bannister, K., Dickenson, A. H., & Bennett, D. L. (2015). Circuitry and plasticity of the dorsal horn—Toward a better understanding of neuropathic pain. *Neuroscience, 300*, 254–275. Retrieved from PM:25987204.

Wiese, C., Grosse, M. E., Schepmann, D., Vela, J. M., Holenz, J., Buschmann, H., et al. (2009). Pharmacological and metabolic characterisation of the potent sigma1 receptor ligand 1′-benzyl-3-methoxy-3H-spiro[[2]benzofuran-1,4′-piperidine]. *The Journal of Pharmacy and Pharmacology, 61*(5), 631–640. Retrieved from PM:19406002.

Willis, W. D. (2001). Role of neurotransmitters in sensitization of pain responses. *Annals of the New York Academy of Sciences, 933*, 142–156. Retrieved from PM:12000017.

Woolf, C. J., & Thompson, S. W. (1991). The induction and maintenance of central sensitization is dependent on N-methyl-D-aspartic acid receptor activation; implications for the treatment of post-injury pain hypersensitivity states. *Pain*, *44*(3), 293–299. Retrieved from PM:1828878.

Xu, Q., & Yaksh, T. L. (2011). A brief comparison of the pathophysiology of inflammatory versus neuropathic pain. *Current Opinion in Anaesthesiology*, *24*(4), 400–407. Retrieved from PM:21659872.

Yamamoto, H., Yamamoto, T., Sagi, N., Klenerova, V., Goji, K., Kawai, N., et al. (1995). Sigma ligands indirectly modulate the NMDA receptor-ion channel complex on intact neuronal cells via sigma 1 site. *The Journal of Neuroscience*, *15*(1 Pt. 2), 731–736. Retrieved from PM:7529831.

Yasaka, T., Tiong, S. Y., Hughes, D. I., Riddell, J. S., & Todd, A. J. (2010). Populations of inhibitory and excitatory interneurons in lamina II of the adult rat spinal dorsal horn revealed by a combined electrophysiological and anatomical approach. *Pain*, *151*(2), 475–488. Retrieved from PM:20817353.

Yoon, S. Y., Kang, S. Y., Kim, H. W., Kim, H. C., & Roh, D. H. (2015). Clonidine reduces nociceptive responses in mouse orofacial formalin model: Potentiation by sigma-1 receptor antagonist BD1047 without impaired motor coordination. *Biological & Pharmaceutical Bulletin*, *38*(9), 1320–1327. Retrieved from PM:26328487.

Yoon, S. Y., Roh, D. H., Seo, H. S., Kang, S. Y., Han, H. J., Beitz, A. J., et al. (2009). Intrathecal injection of the neurosteroid, DHEAS, produces mechanical allodynia in mice: Involvement of spinal sigma-1 and GABA receptors. *British Journal of Pharmacology*, *157*(4), 666–673. Retrieved from PM:19422393.

Yoon, S. Y., Roh, D. H., Seo, H. S., Kang, S. Y., Moon, J. Y., Song, S., et al. (2010). An increase in spinal dehydroepiandrosteronesulfate (DHEAS) enhances NMDA-induced pain via phosphorylation of the NR1 subunit in mice: Involvement of the sigma-1 receptor. *Neuropharmacology*, *59*(6), 460–467. Retrieved from PM:20600171.

Zamanillo, D., Romero, L., Merlos, M., & Vela, J. M. (2013). Sigma 1 receptor: A new therapeutic target for pain. *European Journal of Pharmacology*, *716*(1–3), 78–93. Retrieved from PM:23500210.

CHAPTER EIGHT

Central N/OFQ-NOP Receptor System in Pain Modulation

Norikazu Kiguchi, Huiping Ding, Mei-Chuan Ko[1]
Department of Physiology and Pharmacology, Wake Forest University School of Medicine, Winston-Salem, North Carolina, USA
[1]Corresponding author: e-mail address: mko@wakehealth.edu

Contents

Abstract

Two decades have passed since the peptide, nociceptin/orphanin FQ (N/OFQ), and its cognate (NOP) receptor were discovered. Although NOP receptor activation causes a similar pattern of intracellular actions as mu-opioid (MOP) receptors, NOP receptor-mediated pain modulation in rodents are more complicated than MOP receptor

Advances in Pharmacology, Volume 75
ISSN 1054-3589
http://dx.doi.org/10.1016/bs.apha.2015.10.001

activation. This review highlights the functional evidence of spinal, supraspinal, and systemic actions of NOP receptor agonists for regulating pain. In rodents, effects of the N/OFQ-NOP receptor system in spinal and supraspinal sites for modulating pain are bidirectional depending on the doses, assays, and pain modalities. The net effect of systemically administered NOP receptor agonists may depend on relative contribution of spinal and supraspinal actions of the N/OFQ-NOP receptor signaling in rodents under different pain states. In stark contrast, NOP receptor agonists produce only antinociception and antihypersensitivity in spinal and supraspinal regions of nonhuman primates regardless of doses and assays. More importantly, NOP receptor agonists and a few bifunctional NOP/MOP receptor agonists do not exhibit reinforcing effects (abuse liability), respiratory depression, itch pruritus, nor do they delay the gastrointestinal transit function (constipation) in nonhuman primates. Depending upon their intrinsic efficacies for activating NOP and MOP receptors, bifunctional NOP/MOP receptor agonists warrant additional investigation in primates regarding their side effect profiles. Nevertheless, NOP receptor-related agonists display a much wider therapeutic window as compared to that of MOP receptor agonists in primates. Both selective NOP receptor agonists and bifunctional NOP/MOP receptor agonists hold great potential as effective and safe analgesics without typical opioid-associated side effects in humans.

ABBREVIATIONS

BU08028 (2*S*)-2-[(5*R*,6*R*,7*R*,14*S*)-*N*-cyclopropylmethyl-4,5-epoxy-6,14-ethano-3-hydroxy-6-methoxymorphinan-7-yl]-3,3-dimethylpentan-2-ol
CCI chronic constriction injury
CFA complete Freund's adjuvant
CNS central nervous system
DOP delta-opioid peptide
GABA gamma aminobutyric acid
GTPγS guanosine 5′-*O*-(3-thio)triphosphate
i.c.v. intracerebroventricular
KOP kappa-opioid peptide
MOP mu-opioid peptide
N/OFQ nociceptin/orphanin FQ
NOP N/OFQ peptide
ORL1 opioid receptor like 1
PAG periaqueductal gray
ppN/OFQ prepro-N/OFQ
PWT peptide welding technology
Ro64-6198 (1*S*,3*aS*)-8-(2,3,3*a*,4,5,6-hexahydro-1*H*-phenalen-1-yl)-1-phenyl-1,3,8-triaza-spiro[4.5]decan-4-one
Ro65-6570 8-acenaphthen-1-yl-phenyl-1,3,8-triaza-spiro[4,5]decan-4-one
RVM rostral ventromedial medulla
SCH 221510 8-[bis(2-methylphenyl)-methyl]-3-phenyl-8-azabicyclo[3.2.1]octan-3-ol
SNL spinal nerve ligation
SR14150 1-(1-cyclooctylpiperidin-4-yl)-indolin-2-one
SR16435 1-(1-(bicyclo[3.3.1]nonan-9-yl)piperidin-4-yl)indolin-2-one
SR16835 1-(1-(2,3,3*a*,4,5,6-hexahydro-1*H*-phenalen-1-yl)piperidinl-4-yl)-indolin-2-one

UFP-101 [Nphe^{1}, Arg^{14}, Lys^{15}]N/OFQ-NH_2
UFP-112 [(pF)Phe^{4},Aib^{7},Arg^{14},Lys^{15}]N/OFQ-NH_2
vlPAG ventrolateral PAG

1. INTRODUCTION

After the cloning of delta- (Evans, Keith, Morrison, Magendzo, & Edwards, 1992; Kieffer, Befort, Gaveriaux-Ruff, & Hirth, 1992), kappa- (Yasuda et al., 1993), and mu- (Chen, Mestek, Liu, Hurley, & Yu, 1993) opioid receptors (DOP, KOP, and MOP receptors, respectively), several groups of scientists in 1994 identified a G-protein coupled receptor with high homology to opioid receptors and this receptor was named opioid receptor like 1 (ORL1) (Bunzow et al., 1994; Fukuda et al., 1994; Mollereau et al., 1994; Nishi, Takeshima, Mori, Nakagawara, & Takeuchi, 1994; Wang et al., 1994). Subsequently, an endogenous haptadecapeptide (FGGFTGARKSARKLANQ) selective for ORL1 was discovered independently by two groups. This peptide was named "nociceptin" by one group based on its ability to elicit hyperalgesia following supraspinal administration in mice (Meunier et al., 1995). The other group named this same peptide as "orphanin FQ" based on the recognition of ORL1 and its first and last amino acid residues (Reinscheid et al., 1995). After the identification of nociceptin/orphanin FQ (N/OFQ), the ORL1 was renamed N/OFQ peptide (NOP) receptor based on the nomenclature guidelines recommended by the International Union of Basic and Clinical Pharmacology (Cox, Christie, Devi, Toll, & Traynor, 2015).

1.1 Characteristics of N/OFQ and the NOP Receptor

N/OFQ is derived from a precursor prepro-N/OFQ (ppN/OFQ), which is encoded on chromosome 8p21 in humans (Mollereau et al., 1996), and the sequence of ppN/OFQ gene has similar structural features to precursors of classical opioid peptides, such as prepro-enkephalin, -dynorphin, and -opiomelanocortin (Sundstrom, Dreborg, & Larhammar, 2010). The amino acid sequence of ppN/OFQ is highly conserved across several animal species, and ppN/OFQ and N/OFQ are widely distributed in the peripheral and central nervous system (CNS) of both rodents and primates. In particular, N/OFQ is provided by interneurons in numerous areas of the brain (Neal et al., 1999b; Peluso et al., 1998; Witta, Palkovits, Rosenberger, & Cox, 2004), suggesting its multiple effects on brain function. N/OFQ is also expressed in the dorsal horn and ventral horn of the spinal cord which integrate sensory processing (Neal et al., 1999b).

On the other hand, NOP receptor gene is encoded on chromosome 20 in humans (Lambert, 2008; Sundstrom et al., 2010), and its primary structure is also highly conserved across mammalians (Calo & Guerrini, 2013). According to several biochemical studies and three-dimensional crystal structure analysis, positions of amino acid residues configuring the binding pocket of NOP receptor differ from those of DOP, KOP, and MOP receptors (Granier et al., 2012; Manglik et al., 2012; Thompson et al., 2012; Wu et al., 2012). Consequentially, the hydrophobic and hydrophilic parts of the binding pockets of the NOP receptor and other opioid receptors are different. These atomic details of ligand–receptor recognition explain marked differences in the binding selectivity of corresponding ligands in spite of high sequence homology between the NOP receptor and classical opioid receptors (Calo & Guerrini, 2013; Calo, Guerrini, Rizzi, Salvadori, & Regoli, 2000; Schröder, Lambert, Ko, & Koch, 2014). Like N/OFQ, the NOP receptor is abundant in multiple brain areas and spinal cord (Berthele et al., 2003; Neal et al., 1999a), indicating that the N/OFQ-NOP receptor system plays a fundamental role in regulating several functions including pain.

1.2 Cellular Actions of the N/OFQ-NOP Receptor System

Similar to classical opioid receptors (i.e., DOP, KOP, and MOP receptors), NOP receptor is coupled to pertussis toxin-sensitive Gi/o proteins, which inhibit adenylate cyclase and voltage-gated calcium channels and activate inward potassium channels (Hawes, Graziano, & Lambert, 2000; Ma et al., 1997; Margas, Sedeek, & Ruiz-Velasco, 2008). These cellular events following NOP receptor activation reduce synaptic transmission, by either reducing neurotransmitter release via presynaptically located NOP receptors or inhibiting neuronal excitability via postsynaptically located NOP receptors (Connor, Vaughan, Chieng, & Christie, 1996; Connor, Yeo, & Henderson, 1996; Knoflach, Reinscheid, Civelli, & Kemp, 1996). Indeed, NOP receptor activation has been shown to inhibit the release of a variety of neurotransmitters (e.g., glutamate, gamma aminobutyric acid (GABA), substance P, and noradrenaline) in the CNS (Nicol et al., 1998; Nicol, Lambert, Rowbotham, Smart, & McKnight, 1996; Schlicker & Morari, 2000). Although NOP receptor activation induces a similar pattern of intracellular events as MOP, DOP, and KOP receptors, NOP receptor-mediated effects on pain modulation are more complicated than MOP receptor activation. Depending on the administration routes and animal species, NOP receptor activation could potentially lead to either pronociceptive or antinociceptive effect (Schröder et al., 2014). In this review, we highlight the functional evidence of central N/OFQ-NOP receptor system for regulating pain processing. In specific, we discuss the pharmacological evidence of spinal and supraspinal NOP receptor activation and integrated outcomes from systemic administration of NOP receptor-related ligands between rodents and nonhuman primates. Accumulated evidence strongly supports the therapeutic potential of NOP receptor-related agonists as effective and safe analgesics in primates.

2. SPINAL ACTIONS OF THE N/OFQ-NOP RECEPTOR SYSTEM

2.1 Spinal Actions of NOP Receptor Agonists in Rodent Models of Acute Pain

Since the NOP receptor is present at central pain-processing pathways (Anton et al., 1996; Mollereau & Mouledous, 2000; Neal et al., 1999a), several groups of researchers have investigated the function of spinal N/OFQ-NOP receptor system in pain modulation. In rodents, several lines of evidence demonstrate that intrathecal administration of N/OFQ at nanomole doses produced antinociceptive effects in the rodent tail flick test (King, Rossi, Chang, Williams, & Pasternak, 1997; Xu, Hao, & Wiesenfeld-Hallin, 1996). Intrathecal N/OFQ also had antinociceptive effects in the formalin-induced pain behaviors (Erb et al., 1997; Yamamoto, Nozaki-Taguchi, & Kimura, 1997a) and potentiated morphine-induced antinociception (Tian et al., 1997). Through chemical modifications of N/OFQ by increasing its agonist potency and decreasing its peptidase sensitivity, a NOP receptor agonist, UFP-112 (Arduin et al., 2007), exhibited antinociceptive effects with higher potency and longer duration than N/OFQ in mice (Calo et al., 2011; Rizzi et al., 2007). Nevertheless, lower femtomole doses of intrathecal N/OFQ caused pain-like behaviors in mice, suggesting biphasic actions of N/OFQ (Inoue et al., 1999; Sakurada et al., 1999). Except for lower doses, higher doses of intrathecal N/OFQ might inhibit the excitatory glutamatergic transmission via presynaptic and postsynaptic NOP receptor activation, leading to spinal analgesia (Le Cudennec, Suaudeau, & Costentin, 2002). Additionally, N/OFQ inhibited action potentials in cultured spinal cord based on the firing of both C- and A-fibers (Faber,

Chambers, Evans, & Henderson, 1996), and C-fiber-evoked excitation of dorsal horn neurons (Stanfa, Chapman, Kerr, & Dickenson, 1996).

2.2 Spinal Actions of NOP Receptor Agonists in Rodent Models of Chronic Pain

Spinal NOP receptor activation exerted potent and efficacious anti-hyperalgesic and antiallodynic effects in rodents under chronic pain. For example, intrathecal N/OFQ inhibited carrageenan- and complete Freund's adjuvant (CFA)-induced thermal hyperalgesia in rats (Chen & Sommer, 2007; Hao, Xu, Wiesenfeld-Hallin, & Xu, 1998; Yamamoto, Nozaki-Taguchi, & Kimura, 1997b). In addition, intrathecal N/OFQ attenuated thermal hyperalgesia and mechanical allodynia in rats under neuropathic pain caused by chronic constriction injury (CCI) or spinal nerve ligation (SNL) (Corradini, Briscini, Ongini, & Bertorelli, 2001; Courteix et al., 2004; Yamamoto & Nozaki-Taguchi, 1997). Interestingly, preemptive administration of N/OFQ delayed the development of chronic pain induced by CCI (Yamamoto, Ohtori, & Chiba, 2000). Similar to N/OFQ, a selective nonpeptidic NOP receptor agonist, Ro64-6198, inhibited mechanical and cold allodynia derived from CCI, without affecting pain threshold in naïve rats (Obara, Przewlocki, & Przewlocka, 2005). Furthermore, intrathecal N/OFQ attenuated mechanical hyperalgesia in diabetic rats and was more potent in producing antinociceptive effects in diabetic mice as compared to naive mice (Courteix et al., 2004; Kamei, Ohsawa, Kashiwazaki, & Nagase, 1999). These NOP receptor agonist-induced antihyperalgesic and antiallodynic effects might be at least in part explained by an upregulation of the NOP receptors in the spinal cord under these painful conditions. In fact, expression of N/OFQ and the NOP receptor were upregulated in the dorsal horn of rats under carrageenan- and CFA-induced inflammation, respectively (Jia, Linden, Serie, & Seybold, 1998; Rosen, Lundeberg, Bytner, & Nylander, 2000). Importantly, the NOP receptor was also upregulated in the dorsal horn of rats with CCI (Briscini, Corradini, Ongini, & Bertorelli, 2002) and the inhibitory effect of N/OFQ on spinal wide dynamic range neurons was enhanced in rats under neuropathic pain (Sotgiu, Bellomi, & Biella, 2004).

2.3 Spinal Actions of NOP Receptor Agonists in Primate Pain Models

According to the radioligand binding assay, the NOP receptor is widely distributed in the spinal cord of nonhuman primates (Bridge, Wainwright,

Reilly, & Oliver, 2003). Unlike findings in rodents, intrathecal administration of N/OFQ over a wide range from femtomole to nanomole doses only produced antinociceptive effects without eliciting pronociceptive responses in a monkey thermal nociceptive assay, and these effects can be reversed by a NOP receptor antagonist (Ko & Naughton, 2009; Ko, Wei, Woods, & Kennedy, 2006). Although NOP receptors are expressed in neural substrates involved in pain processing in rodents and primates (Berthele et al., 2003; Bridge et al., 2003; Neal et al., 1999a), there is no anatomical study to directly compare the distribution of NOP receptors in different populations of neurons. It is important to further investigate the nature of nociceptive neurons expressing NOP receptors and determine if they have different properties for releasing pain-inhibiting and -eliciting neuropeptides between rodents and primates. Using an innovative chemical approach, peptide welding technology (PWT), different tetrabranched derivatives of N/OFQ has been generated and PWT-N/OFQ derivatives behaved as high-affinity, potent, and selective full NOP receptor agonists (Rizzi et al., 2014). In particular, PWT2-N/OFQ was 40-fold more potent and produced an extremely long-lasting inhibitory effect than the natural peptide N/OFQ in mice (Rizzi et al., 2014). More importantly, this largely increased potency and improved duration of action exhibited by PWT2-N/OFQ can be translated from rodents to primates. Intrathecal administration of PWT2-N/OFQ potently produced full antinociceptive effects lasted for more than 24 h in monkeys (Rizzi et al., 2015). Under similar experimental conditions, PWT2-N/OFQ (0.3–3 nmol) is approximately 30-fold more potent than N/OFQ (10–100 nmol) and the duration of antinociceptive action of PWT2-N/OFQ (~24 h) is 10-fold longer than that of N/OFQ (~2.5 h) in primates (Ding, Hayashida, et al., 2015; Ko et al., 2006; Rizzi et al., 2015). It is worth noting that among all agonists selective for opioid receptor subtypes, NOP receptor agonists are the only class of drugs that are able to change the nociceptive threshold of primates without side effects commonly caused by MOP receptor agonists (Lin & Ko, 2013).

Although the analgesic efficacy of spinal NOP receptor agonists in patients under neuropathic pain is unknown, intrathecal UFP-112 was 10 times more potent than morphine in attenuating acute pain and capsaicin-induced thermal allodynia in monkeys (Hu, Calo, Guerrini, & Ko, 2010). Capsaicin evokes pain by activating the transient receptor potential vanilloid type 1, which has been implicated in the transduction of diverse pain modalities including diabetic neuropathy (Aykanat et al., 2012; Szolcsanyi & Sandor, 2012). It has been used in both humans and nonhuman primates to investigate pain mechanisms and explore novel pharmacological interventions (Butelman, Harris, & Kreek, 2004; Eisenach, Hood, Curry, & Tong, 1997; Park, Max, Robinovitz, Gracely, & Bennett, 1995). Given full antiallodynic effects of intrathecal UFP-112 in primates, NOP receptor agonists hold a great potential for clinical use as strong analgesics. In addition, carrageenan-induced thermal hyperalgesia has been developed as an inflammatory pain model in nonhuman primates to assess the analgesic efficacy of opioids and nonsteroidal anti-inflammatory drugs (Sukhtankar, Lee, Rice, & Ko, 2014). Unlike classical opioid peptides such as β-endorphin and enkephalins, intrathecal N/OFQ completely inhibited carrageenan-induced hyperalgesia without eliciting itch scratching in monkeys (Lee & Ko, 2015). These findings collectively demonstrate that spinal NOP receptor activation produces antinociceptive and antihypersensitive effects across different pain modalities in nonhuman primates. The promising therapeutic profile of NOP receptor agonists in primates encourages further development of this class of drugs as spinal analgesics.

3. SUPRASPINAL ACTIONS OF THE N/OFQ-NOP RECEPTOR SYSTEM

3.1 Supraspinal Actions of NOP Receptor Agonists in Rodent Models of Acute Pain

The NOP receptor is abundant in supraspinal areas, such as thalamus, hypothalamus, locus coeruleus, periaqueductal gray (PAG), and rostral ventromedial medulla (RVM), which modulate ascending and descending pain pathways (Civelli, 2008; Heinricher, McGaraughty, & Grandy, 1997; Mollereau & Mouledous, 2000; Neal et al., 1999a). Supraspinal actions of the N/OFQ-NOP receptor system are complicated, as supraspinal NOP receptor activation produces opposite effects on pain processing depending on the pain state and species. Initial studies reported that intracerebroventricular (i.c.v.) administration of N/OFQ produced hyperalgesia in the mouse hot plate and tail flick tests (Meunier et al., 1995; Reinscheid et al., 1995) and i.c.v. N/OFQ counteracted morphine-induced antinociception in the rodent tail flick test (King, Chang, & Pasternak, 1998; Tian et al., 1997). In addition, a peptidic analog of N/OFQ, [$Phe^1\psi(CH_2\text{-}NH)Gly^2$]N/OFQ-(1–13)-$NH_2$ (Butour, Moisand, Mollereau, & Meunier, 1998; Grisel, Farrier, Wilson, & Mogil, 1998), also elicited pronociceptive effects after i.c.v. administration in mice and rats, and inhibited morphine-induced antinociception in the mouse tail withdrawal assay (Calo et al., 1998; Wang, Zhu, Cao, & Wu, 1999b). Although exact mechanisms of NOP receptor agonist-induced pronociceptive effects are unclear, it is hypothesized that two types of neurons (ON cells and OFF cells) in the RVM, which regulate descending inhibition of pain, might be differentially regulated by the NOP receptor. Firing of ON cells induces enhanced and prolonged nociception, whereas excitation of OFF cells leads to antinociception. ON cells are normally dominant through tonic inhibition of OFF cells via GABA-dependent mechanisms (Fields, 2004). Analgesia is produced by MOP receptor-dependent inhibition of ON cells, followed by excitation of OFF cells (Heinricher, Morgan, Tortorici, & Fields, 1994). In contrast, supraspinal NOP receptor ligands may directly inhibit OFF cells and induce antiopioid action and subsequent pronociceptive effects (Heinricher et al., 1997). On the other hand, i.c.v. administration of a highly selective peptidic NOP receptor antagonist, [Nphe^1, Arg^{14}, Lys^{15}]N/OFQ-NH^2 (UFP-101) (Calo et al., 2005; McDonald, Calo, Guerrini, & Lambert, 2003), exerted antinociceptive effects in the mouse formalin test (Rizzi et al., 2006). These findings suggest that supraspinal N/OFQ-NOP receptor system might be constitutively pronociceptive in rodent models of acute pain.

3.2 Supraspinal Actions of NOP Receptor Agonists in Rodent Models of Chronic Pain

Based on the limited literature, supraspinal actions of NOP receptor agonists in rodents under chronic pain have mixed results depending on pain modalities. Following i.c.v. administration, a NOP receptor agonist, [Phe$^1\psi$(CH_2-NH)Gly^2]N/OFQ-(1–13)-NH_2, caused hyperalgesia and inhibited morphine-induced antihyperalgesia in rats with CFA-induced inflammation (Bertorelli et al., 1999). Conversely, microinjection of a NOP receptor antagonist, UFP-101, into ventrolateral PAG (vlPAG) reversed carrageenan-induced mechanical allodynia in rats (Scoto, Arico, Iemolo, Ronsisvalle, & Parenti, 2009). Therefore, in rodent models of inflammatory pain, supraspinal N/OFQ-NOP receptor system seems to elicit pronociceptive effects.

After i.c.v. administration, highly selective nonpeptidic NOP receptor agonists, GRT-TA2210 and Ro65-6570 (Hashiba et al., 2001; Linz, Christoph, Schiene, Koch, & Englberger, 2013), attenuated CCI-induced allodynia (Linz et al., 2013; Schiene, Christoph, Kogel, & Tzschentke, 2013). In contrast, microinjection of a NOP receptor antagonist UFP-101 into vlPAG attenuated CCI-induced tactile allodynia in rats (Scoto et al., 2009). It is currently unknown how NOP receptor agonists and antagonists, administered at different neuroanatomical sites in brain can result in similar antiallodynic effects. It is plausible to detect different drug actions derived from a brain subregion (e.g., vlPAG) versus an integrated outcome from the entire supraspinal region following i.c.v. administration. Clearly, additional antagonist studies using the supraspinal, not microinjection, delivery route will provide a general functional profile of supraspinal N/OFQ-NOP receptor system in rodents under neuropathic pain.

Although some reports demonstrate that upregulation of either N/OFQ or the NOP receptor under chronic pain conditions, their correlations with functional evidence of NOP receptor ligands has not been fully characterized. For example, NOP receptor positive cells in the PAG and RVM were increased, while N/OFQ was increased in cingulate cortex, but not PAG and RVM, in rats under CCI (Ma, Xie, Dong, Wang, & Wu, 2005; Rosen et al., 2000). Furthermore, N/OFQ expression was upregulated in the PAG at a later period in SNL rats (Sun, Wang, Zhao, Chang, & Han, 2001). The direction of pain modulation via supraspinal N/OFQ-NOP receptor system might be changed along with temporal upregulation and functional plasticity of the NOP receptor henceforth (Schröder et al., 2014). Influence of chronic pain state (e.g., inflammatory vs. neuropathic pain) on the function of descending inhibitory pathways in supraspinal areas warrants further investigation with region-specific and i.c.v. administration of NOP receptor agonists and antagonists. It is noteworthy that actual analgesic profile and relative therapeutic index in humans will likely be related to the integrated effect of either intrathecal/epidural or oral/systemic administration, since local brain or i.c.v. administration is not widely used in clinical practice.

3.3 Supraspinal Actions of N/OFQ in a Primate Model of Acute Pain

With improved surgical techniques, a recent study has established an intrathecal catheterization procedure by placing the catheter tip in the cisterna magna of rhesus monkeys, thus allowing practical supraspinal administration (Ding, Hayashida, et al., 2015). Unlike supraspinal N/OFQ-induced pronociception in rodents, intracisternal administration of N/OFQ dose dependently produced antinociceptive effects which were reversed by a NOP receptor antagonist J-113397 in monkeys (Ding, Hayashida, et al., 2015). For comparison, intracisternal substance P and morphine produced hyperalgesia and antinociception, respectively, in the same group of monkeys. Furthermore, intracisternal N/OFQ did not produce anti-morphine actions in these nonhuman primates (Ding, Hayashida, et al., 2015). These findings provide distinct functional profiles of supraspinal N/OFQ-NOP receptor system between rodents and primates. More importantly, this intrathecal catheter implantation not only documents the functional role of central N/OFQ-NOP receptor system for pain inhibition, but also illustrates how we can study supraspinal neuropeptides' pain-eliciting or pain-inhibiting effects in awake, behaving primates.

4. SYSTEMIC ACTIONS OF THE N/OFQ-NOP RECEPTOR SYSTEM

4.1 Systemic Actions of NOP Receptor Agonists in Rodent Models of Acute Pain

As mentioned above, the involvement of N/OFQ-NOP receptor system in nociceptive processing is multimodal depending upon pain modalities and routes of administration in rodents. Effects of systemically administered NOP receptor agonists depend on the integration of peripheral, spinal, and supraspinal sties of action. Early studies show that systemic administration of a nonpeptidic NOP receptor agonist Ro64-6198 did not produce antinociceptive effects in the mouse and rat tail flick tests, nor in the mouse tail immersion test (Dautzenberg et al., 2001; Jenck et al., 2000; Kotlinska et al., 2003). This net effect of systemic Ro64-6198 could be integrated from spinal antinociceptive action and supraspinal pronociceptive action of the N/OFQ-NOP receptor signaling. There is only one study showing that systemic Ro64-6198 produced antinociceptive effects in the mouse hot plate test (Reiss, Wichmann, Tekeshima, Kieffer, & Ouagazzal, 2008). However, systemic Ro64-6198 increased pain sensitivity in the mouse tail flick test by supraspinally inhibiting stress-induced analgesia (Reiss et al., 2008). Overall, systemic administration of selective NOP receptor agonists does not produce a robust analgesic profile in rodent acute pain models.

4.2 Systemic Actions of NOP Receptor Agonists in Rodent Models of Chronic Pain

Unlike their analgesic efficacy against acute pain, systemic administration of NOP receptor agonists exhibited antihyperalgesic effects in rodents under inflammatory pain. Systemic GRT-TA2210 and Ro65-6570 attenuated CFA-induced inflammatory pain in rats without disrupting locomotor activity (Linz et al., 2013; Schiene et al., 2013). Moreover, a nonpeptidic

NOP receptor agonist, SCH 221510 (Varty et al., 2008), produced anti-hypersensitive effects on trinitrobenzene sulfonic acid-induced inflammatory pain (Sobczak et al., 2014; Sobczak, Salaga, Storr, & Fichna, 2013). These pharmacological findings agree with the functional studies from either ppN/OFQ or NOP receptor knockout mice that displayed normal sensitivity to acute pain, but showed increased inflammatory hyperalgesia (Depner, Reinscheid, Takeshima, Brune, & Zeilhofer, 2003). In addition, systemic Ro65-6570 also produced antihyperalgesic and antiallodynic effects in both mice and rats under neuropathic pain without locomotor side effects (Schiene et al., 2013). These findings collectively support the therapeutic potential of systemic NOP receptor agonists as analgesics in rodent models of chronic pain. The analgesic efficacy of systemic NOP receptor agonists in rodents under chronic pain may depend on the functional plasticity of the N/OFQ-NOP receptor system across spinal and supraspinal regions (Schröder et al., 2014).

4.3 Systemic Actions of NOP Receptor Agonists in Primate Pain Models

Contrary to their pain modality-dependent efficacy in rodent models, systemic administration of NOP receptor agonists has generally produced analgesic effects across different nonhuman primate models. Following subcutaneous administration, Ro64-6198 dose dependently produced antinociceptive effects against an acute thermal nociceptive stimulus in monkeys (Ko et al., 2009; Lin & Ko, 2013). As mentioned above, capsaicin-induced allodynia has been used in both nonhuman primates and humans to distinguish strong analgesics (Butelman et al., 2004; Eisenach et al., 1997; Park et al., 1995). Crucially, systemic Ro64-6198 potently inhibited capsaicin-induced thermal allodynia in monkeys (Ko et al., 2009). In addition, systemic Ro64-6198 potently attenuated carrageenan-induced hyperalgesia in the monkey inflammatory pain model (Sukhtankar et al., 2014). Importantly, just like Ro64-6198, another NOP receptor agonist with different chemical structure, SCH 221510 (Varty et al., 2008), produced antinociceptive and antihypersensitive efficacy against acute pain, capsaicin-induced allodynia and carrageenan-induced hyperalgesia in monkeys following systemic administration (Cremeans, Gruley, Kyle, & Ko, 2012; Wladischkin et al., 2012). These findings strongly indicate that NOP receptor agonists may be effective for treating pain derived from different nociceptive origins in humans.

5. THERAPEUTIC POTENTIAL OF NOP RECEPTOR-RELATED AGONISTS AS ANALGESICS

5.1 Development of Bifunctional NOP/MOP Receptor Agonists

In the early stage of developing NOP receptor-related ligands as analgesics, the effort was mainly focused on NOP receptor antagonists due to central NOP receptor-mediated pronociception and antiopioid actions, and NOP receptor antagonist-induced antihyperalgesia in rodent pain models (Lutfy et al., 2003; Meunier et al., 1995; Mogil et al., 1996; Reinscheid et al., 1995). For example, pretreatment with a NOP receptor antagonist J-113397 potentiated antinociceptive effects of buprenorphine in mice, indicating that NOP receptor activation compromised buprenorphine-induced antinociception (Lutfy et al., 2003). However, J-113397 did not enhance buprenorphine-induced antinociception in monkeys. Instead, NOP receptor agonists, Ro64-6198 and SCH 221510, produced synergistic antinociception with buprenorphine without eliciting other side effects in monkeys (Cremeans et al., 2012). This antinociceptive synergism by coactivation of both NOP and MOP receptors not only occurs following systemic administration but also exists in the spinal cord (Courteix et al., 2004; Hu et al., 2010; Ko & Naughton, 2009). Mounting evidence in the past few years indicates that central N/OFQ-NOP receptor signaling does not function opposing the effects of MOP receptor agonists, especially in primates (Ding, Hayashida, et al., 2015; Ko & Naughton, 2009). More importantly, ligands with agonist actions on both NOP and MOP receptors (i.e., *bifunctional NOP/MOP receptor agonists*) may represent effective and safe analgesics as they have a wider therapeutic window and a slower development of tolerance to analgesic efficacy (Lin & Ko, 2013).

Medicinal chemists have developed several series of NOP receptor-related ligands with different efficacies on NOP and MOP receptors for distinct therapeutic applications (Calo & Guerrini, 2013; Husbands, 2013; Journigan, Polgar, Khroyan, & Zaveri, 2014; Kumar et al., 2014; Schunk et al., 2014; Toll, 2013; Zaveri, Jiang, Olsen, Polgar, & Toll, 2013). Table 1 highlights several mixed NOP/MOP receptor agonists, [Dmt^1] N/OFQ(1–13)-NH_2 (Molinari et al., 2013), SR14150 (Spagnolo et al., 2008), SR16435 (Khroyan et al., 2009), SR16835 (Toll et al., 2009), and BU08028 (Khroyan, Polgar, Cami-Kobeci, et al., 2011), in terms of their antinociceptive and antihypersensitive actions. Generally, systemic

Table 1 Multiple Effects of NOP Receptor-Related Ligands on Regulating Pain Processing

NOP Receptor-Related Ligands	Findings in Rodents	Findings in Primates
NOP receptor agonists (peptides)		
N/OFQ	Spinal, acute pain ↓ (Erb et al., 1997; King et al., 1997; Xu et al., 1996; Yamamoto et al., 1997a)	Spinal, acute pain ↓ (Ko & Naughton, 2009; Ko et al., 2006)
	Spinal, acute pain ↑ (Inoue et al., 1999; Sakurada et al., 1999)	
	Spinal, inflammatory pain ↓ (Chen & Sommer, 2007; Hao et al., 1998; Yamamoto et al., 1997b)	
	Spinal, neuropathic pain ↓ (Corradini et al., 2001; Courteix et al., 2004; Yamamoto & Nozaki-Taguchi, 1997)	
	Supraspinal, acute pain ↑ (Meunier et al., 1995; Reinscheid et al., 1995)	Supraspinal, acute pain ↓ (Ding, Hayashida, et al., 2015)
	Supraspinal, inflammatory pain ↑ (Wang, Zhu, Cao, & Wu, 1999a; Zhu, Cao, Xu, & Wu, 1997)	
[Phe[1]ψ(CH_2-NH)Gly[2]] N/OFQ-(1–13)-NH_2	Supraspinal, acute pain ↑ (Calo et al., 1998; Wang et al., 1999b)	
	Supraspinal, inflammatory pain ↑ (Bertorelli et al., 1999)	
UFP-112	Spinal, acute pain ↓ (Calo et al., 2011; Rizzi et al., 2007)	Spinal, acute pain ↓ (Hu et al., 2010)
		Spinal, capsaicin-induced allodynia ↓ (Hu et al., 2010)
PWT2-N/OFQ	Spinal, acute pain ↓ (Rizzi et al., 2015)	Spinal, acute pain ↓ (Rizzi et al., 2015)
	Spinal, neuropathic pain ↓ (Rizzi et al., 2015)	
NOP receptor agonists (nonpeptides)		
Ro64-6198	Spinal, neuropathic pain ↓ (Obara et al., 2005)	
	Systemic, acute pain ↓ (Reiss et al., 2008)	Systemic, acute pain ↓ (Ko et al., 2009)

Table 1 Multiple Effects of NOP Receptor-Related Ligands on Regulating Pain Processing—cont'd

NOP Receptor-Related Ligands	Findings in Rodents	Findings in Primates
	Systemic, acute pain ↑ (Reiss et al., 2008)	Systemic, inflammatory pain ↓ (Sukhtankar et al., 2014) Systemic, capsaicin-induced allodynia ↓ (Ko et al., 2009)
Ro65-6570	Supraspinal, neuropathic pain ↓ (Schiene et al., 2013) Systemic, inflammatory pain ↓ (Schiene et al., 2013) Systemic, neuropathic pain ↓ (Schiene et al., 2013)	
GRT-TA2210	Supraspinal, neuropathic pain ↓ (Linz et al., 2013) Systemic, inflammatory pain ↓ (Linz et al., 2013)	
SCH 221510	Systemic, inflammatory pain ↓ (Sobczak et al., 2013, 2014)	Systemic, acute pain ↓ (Cremeans et al., 2012) Systemic, inflammatory pain ↓ (Wladischkin et al., 2012) Systemic, capsaicin-induced allodynia ↓ (Wladischkin et al., 2012)
NOP receptor antagonist		
UFP-101	Supraspinal, acute pain ↓ (Rizzi et al., 2006) Supraspinal, inflammatory pain ↓ (Scoto et al., 2009) Supraspinal, neuropathic pain ↓ (Scoto et al., 2009)	
Mixed NOP/MOP receptor agonists		
[Dmt[1]]N/OFQ (1–13)-NH_2	Spinal, acute pain ↓ (Calo et al., 2012)	Spinal, acute pain ↓ (Molinari et al., 2013)
SR16435	Spinal, inflammatory pain ↓ (Sukhtankar, Zaveri, Husbands, & Ko, 2013)	

Continued

Table 1 Multiple Effects of NOP Receptor-Related Ligands on Regulating Pain Processing—cont'd

NOP Receptor-Related Ligands	Findings in Rodents	Findings in Primates
	Spinal, neuropathic pain ↓ (Sukhtankar et al., 2013) Systemic, acute pain ↓ (Khroyan, Polgar, Jiang, Zaveri, & Toll, 2009)	
SR14150	Systemic, neuropathic pain ↓ (Khroyan, Polgar, Orduna, et al., 2011)	
SR16835	Systemic, neuropathic pain ↓ (Khroyan, Polgar, Orduna, et al., 2011)	
BU08028	Spinal, inflammatory pain ↓ (Sukhtankar et al., 2013) Spinal, neuropathic pain ↓ (Sukhtankar et al., 2013) Systemic, acute pain ↓ (Khroyan, Polgar, Cami-Kobeci, et al., 2011)	Systemic, acute pain ↓ (Ding, Czoty, et al., 2015) Systemic, capsaicin-induced allodynia ↓ (Ding, Czoty, et al., 2015)
Cebranopadol	Systemic, acute pain ↓ (Linz et al., 2014) Systemic, inflammatory pain ↓ (Linz et al., 2014) Systemic, neuropathic pain ↓ (Linz et al., 2014)	

↓, Antinociception or antihypersensitivity; ↑, pronociception or hypersensitivity.

administration of these mixed NOP/MOP receptor agonists effectively blocked hyperalgesia and allodynia in rodent models of chronic pain. However, antagonist studies do not elucidate the contribution of spinal versus supraspinal NOP and MOP receptors in these antihypersensitive effects by systemic NOP/MOP receptor agonists. On the other hand, intrathecal administration of mixed NOP/MOP receptor agonists, SR16435 and BU08028, attenuated nerve injury-induced tactile allodynia and inflammation-associated thermal hyperalgesia more potently than selective NOP or MOP receptor agonists in mice (Sukhtankar et al., 2013). In addition, repeated intrathecal administration of SR16435 showed a delayed development of tolerance to antiallodynic effects as compared to a MOP receptor agonist (Sukhtankar et al., 2013). This delayed tolerance development could be attributed to the consequence of repeated coactivation of NOP and MOP receptors, i.e., a synergistic action with a larger reservoir for both receptor populations (Lin & Ko, 2013).

It is worth noting that cebranopadol, the first NOP and opioid receptor agonist, is currently in clinical development for the treatment of severe chronic pain (Salat, Jakubowska, & Kulig, 2015). Cebranopadol binds with nanomolar affinity to the NOP receptor and classical opioid receptors, and it has nearly full agonist activity at human NOP, MOP, and DOP receptors and partial agonist activity at the KOP receptor, based on the $[^{35}S]GTP\gamma S$ binding assay (Linz et al., 2014). Across diverse rodent models of acute and chronic pain, cebranopadol displayed highly potent (i.e., ED50 values: 0.5–5 μg/kg by intravenous route) and efficacious antinociceptive and antihypersensitive effects. Interestingly, antihypersensitive effects of cebranopadol could be partially blocked by either the NOP receptor antagonist J-113397 or the MOP receptor-preferring antagonist naloxone (Linz et al., 2014). More importantly, at equianalgesic doses, cebranopadol showed a delayed development of analgesic tolerance as compared to morphine, and its analgesic doses did not disrupt motor coordination in rats (Linz et al., 2014). Cebranopadol has been registered for several clinical trials and both scientific and medical care communities are earnestly waiting for the outcomes of these trials.

5.2 Lack of Major Side Effects Commonly Associated with MOP Receptor Agonists

Based on the current literature, selective NOP receptor agonists display a much wider therapeutic window as compared to that of MOP receptor agonists in primates (Lin & Ko, 2013). Only at a dose that is approximately 100-fold higher than its antihyperalgesic dose, systemic Ro64-6198 produced sedative effects in monkeys (Podlesnik et al., 2011; Sukhtankar et al., 2014). Across a wide analgesic dose range, NOP receptor agonists do not produce reinforcing effects (abuse liability), respiratory depression, itch pruritus, nor do they delay the gastrointestinal transit function (constipation potential) (Cremeans et al., 2012; Ko et al., 2009; Sukhtankar et al., 2014; Wladischkin et al., 2012). These side effects are commonly associated with clinically used opioid analgesics. In the past few decades, research on classical opioid receptors, i.e., MOP, DOP, and KOP receptors, has expanded our understanding of how opioid drugs act, but could not shed light on the discovering of a new generation of opioid analgesics without MOP receptor agonist-associated side effects (Corbett, Henderson, McKnight, & Paterson, 2006). Research on selective NOP receptor agonists in primates in the past 10 years has opened a new avenue for developing effective and safe analgesics with fewer side effects (Lin & Ko, 2013; Schröder et al., 2014).

Emerging evidence indicates that mixed NOP/MOP receptor agonists also display a promising therapeutic profile as analgesics in primates. As mentioned above, such agonists exhibited improved potency and delayed development of analgesic tolerance (Linz et al., 2014; Sukhtankar et al., 2013). For instance, BU08028 is a recently developed buprenorphine analog which has binding affinity (i.e., Ki: 1–10 nM) for the NOP and classical opioid receptors. However, this ligand only has detectable efficacy on both NOP and MOP receptors, i.e., 20–40% stimulation by the $[^{35}S]GTP\gamma S$ binding assay (Khroyan, Polgar, Cami-Kobeci, et al., 2011). This mixed NOP/MOP receptor agonist produced morphine-comparable maximal antinociception which was reversed equally by both NOP and MOP receptor antagonists in the monkey thermal nociceptive assays (Ding, Czoty, et al., 2015). More importantly, unlike buprenorphine, BU08028 did not produce reinforcing effects in the monkey drug self-administration assay. At doses within and 10-fold higher than the antinociceptive dose range, BU08028 did not compromise physiological functions including respiratory and cardiovascular activities in monkeys (Ding, Czoty, et al., 2015). These recent findings strongly support the therapeutic potential of bifunctional NOP/MOP receptor agonists as innovative analgesics in primates.

Among newly developed NOP receptor-related agonists, there are differential intrinsic efficacies (i.e., from low, mid, to full efficacy) for activating both NOP and MOP receptors (Calo & Guerrini, 2013; Husbands, 2013; Journigan et al., 2014; Khroyan, Polgar, Cami-Kobeci, et al., 2011; Schunk et al., 2014). Some ligands may produce reinforcing effects and/or respiratory depression if their efficacy on the MOP receptor is not low enough. Given the species differences in the pharmacological profiles of NOP and MOP receptor-related ligands between rodents and primates (Lin & Ko, 2013; Schröder et al., 2014), it is important to study the side effect profiles (e.g., abuse liability, respiratory depression, and physical dependence) of these ligands in awake, behaving monkeys. Such studies will validate the therapeutic profiles of systemic bifunctional NOP/MOP receptor agonists and help identify candidate ligands as a translational bridge for their therapeutic applications in humans.

6. CONCLUSION

Taken together, functional profiles of central NOP receptor activation are different between rodents and primates. In rodents, antinociceptive and antihypersensitive actions of the N/OFQ-NOP receptor system in spinal and supraspinal areas are bidirectional depending on the doses, assays, and pain modalities. In stark contrast, NOP receptor-related ligands, i.e., both selective NOP receptor agonists and mixed NOP/MOP receptor agonists, produced only antinociception and antihypersensitivity in primates regardless of doses and assays applied. Most importantly, spinal administration of NOP receptor-related agonists exhibited analgesic efficacy across different rodent and primate pain models. Depending upon their intrinsic efficacies for activating NOP and MOP receptors, mixed NOP/MOP receptor agonists warrant additional investigation in primates regarding their side effect profiles. Effects of acute and chronic administration of such ligands will determine their tolerability and facilitate the development of candidate ligands as a new generation of analgesics in humans.

CONFLICT OF INTEREST

N.K. and H.D. declare that there is no conflict of interest. M.C.K. received research contracts from Grünenthal GmbH and Purdue Pharma L.P.

ACKNOWLEDGMENTS

The U.S. National Institutes of Health, National Institute on Drug Abuse (DA032568, DA035359, and DA040104), National Institute of Arthritis and Musculoskeletal and Skin Diseases (AR059193 and AR064456), and the U.S. Department of Defense (W81XWH-13-2-0045) supported this work.

REFERENCES

Anton, B., Fein, J., To, T., Li, X., Silberstein, L., & Evans, C. J. (1996). Immunohistochemical localization of ORL-1 in the central nervous system of the rat. *The Journal of Comparative Neurology*, *368*(2), 229–251.

Arduin, M., Spagnolo, B., Calo, G., Guerrini, R., Carra, G., Fischetti, C., et al. (2007). Synthesis and biological activity of nociceptin/orphanin FQ analogues substituted in position 7 or 11 with Calpha, alpha-dialkylated amino acids. *Bioorganic & Medicinal Chemistry*, *15*(13), 4434–4443.

Aykanat, V., Gentgall, M., Briggs, N., Williams, D., Yap, S., & Rolan, P. (2012). Intradermal capsaicin as a neuropathic pain model in patients with unilateral sciatica. *British Journal of Clinical Pharmacology, 73*(1), 37–45.

Berthele, A., Platzer, S., Dworzak, D., Schadrack, J., Mahal, B., Buttner, A., et al. (2003). [3H]-nociceptin ligand-binding and nociceptin opioid receptor mRNA expression in the human brain. *Neuroscience, 121*(3), 629–640.

Bertorelli, R., Corradini, L., Rafiq, K., Tupper, J., Calo, G., & Ongini, E. (1999). Nociceptin and the ORL-1 ligand [Phe1psi (CH2-NH)Gly2]nociceptin(1-13)NH2 exert anti-opioid effects in the Freund's adjuvant-induced arthritic rat model of chronic pain. *British Journal of Pharmacology, 128*(6), 1252–1258.

Bridge, K. E., Wainwright, A., Reilly, K., & Oliver, K. R. (2003). Autoradiographic localization of (125)i[Tyr(14)] nociceptin/orphanin FQ binding sites in macaque primate CNS. *Neuroscience, 118*(2), 513–523.

Briscini, L., Corradini, L., Ongini, E., & Bertorelli, R. (2002). Up-regulation of ORL-1 receptors in spinal tissue of allodynic rats after sciatic nerve injury. *European Journal of Pharmacology, 447*(1), 59–65.

Bunzow, J. R., Saez, C., Mortrud, M., Bouvier, C., Williams, J. T., Low, M., et al. (1994). Molecular cloning and tissue distribution of a putative member of the rat opioid receptor gene family that is not a mu, delta or kappa opioid receptor type. *FEBS Letters, 347*(2-3), 284–288.

Butelman, E. R., Harris, T. J., & Kreek, M. J. (2004). Antiallodynic effects of loperamide and fentanyl against topical capsaicin-induced allodynia in unanesthetized primates. *The Journal of Pharmacology and Experimental Therapeutics, 311*(1), 155–163.

Butour, J. L., Moisand, C., Mollereau, C., & Meunier, J. C. (1998). [Phe1psi(CH2-NH)-Gly2]nociceptin-(1-13)-NH2 is an agonist of the nociceptin (ORL1) receptor. *European Journal of Pharmacology, 349*(1), R5–R6.

Calo, G., & Guerrini, R. (2013). Medicinal chemistry, pharmacology, and biological actions of peptide ligands selective for the nociceptin/orphanin FQ receptor. In M. C. Ko & S. M. Husbands (Eds.), *ACS symposium series: Vol. 1131. Research and development of opioid-related ligands* (pp. 275–325). Washington, DC: American Chemical Society.

Calo, G., Guerrini, R., Rizzi, A., Salvadori, S., Burmeister, M., Kapusta, D. R., et al. (2005). UFP-101, a peptide antagonist selective for the nociceptin/orphanin FQ receptor. *CNS Drug Reviews, 11*(2), 97–112.

Calo, G., Guerrini, R., Rizzi, A., Salvadori, S., & Regoli, D. (2000). Pharmacology of nociceptin and its receptor: A novel therapeutic target. *British Journal of Pharmacology, 129*(7), 1261–1283.

Calo, G., Molinari, S., Camarda, V., Rizzi, A., Marzola, G., Salvadori, S., et al. (2012). [Dmt1]N/OFQ(1-13)-NH2, a potent NOP/MOP receptor mixed agonist. *The FASEB Journal, 26*(Suppl.), 836.1.

Calo, G., Rizzi, A., Cifani, C., Micioni Di Bonaventura, M. V., Regoli, D., Massi, M., et al. (2011). UFP-112 a potent and long-lasting agonist selective for the nociceptin/orphanin FQ receptor. *CNS Neuroscience & Therapeutics, 17*(3), 178–198.

Calo, G., Rizzi, A., Marzola, G., Guerrini, R., Salvadori, S., Beani, L., et al. (1998). Pharmacological characterization of the nociceptin receptor mediating hyperalgesia in the mouse tail withdrawal assay. *British Journal of Pharmacology, 125*(2), 373–378.

Chen, Y., Mestek, A., Liu, J., Hurley, J. A., & Yu, L. (1993). Molecular cloning and functional expression of a mu-opioid receptor from rat brain. *Molecular Pharmacology, 44*(1), 8–12.

Chen, Y., & Sommer, C. (2007). Activation of the nociceptin opioid system in rat sensory neurons produces antinociceptive effects in inflammatory pain: Involvement of inflammatory mediators. *Journal of Neuroscience Research, 85*(7), 1478–1488.

Civelli, O. (2008). The orphanin FQ/nociceptin (OFQ/N) system. *Results and Problems in Cell Differentiation*, *46*, 1–25.

Connor, M., Vaughan, C. W., Chieng, B., & Christie, M. J. (1996). Nociceptin receptor coupling to a potassium conductance in rat locus coeruleus neurones in vitro. *British Journal of Pharmacology*, *119*(8), 1614–1618.

Connor, M., Yeo, A., & Henderson, G. (1996). The effect of nociceptin on Ca2+ channel current and intracellular Ca2+ in the SH-SY5Y human neuroblastoma cell line. *British Journal of Pharmacology*, *118*(2), 205–207.

Corbett, A. D., Henderson, G., McKnight, A. T., & Paterson, S. J. (2006). 75 years of opioid research: The exciting but vain quest for the Holy Grail. *British Journal of Pharmacology*, *147*(Suppl. 1), S153–S162.

Corradini, L., Briscini, L., Ongini, E., & Bertorelli, R. (2001). The putative OP(4) antagonist, [Nphe(1)]nociceptin(1-13)NH(2), prevents the effects of nociceptin in neuropathic rats. *Brain Research*, *905*(1-2), 127–133.

Courteix, C., Coudore-Civiale, M. A., Privat, A. M., Pelissier, T., Eschalier, A., & Fialip, J. (2004). Evidence for an exclusive antinociceptive effect of nociceptin/orphanin FQ, an endogenous ligand for the ORL1 receptor, in two animal models of neuropathic pain. *Pain*, *110*(1–2), 236–245.

Cox, B. M., Christie, M. J., Devi, L., Toll, L., & Traynor, J. R. (2015). Challenges for opioid receptor nomenclature: IUPHAR review 9. *British Journal of Pharmacology*, *172*(2), 317–323.

Cremeans, C. M., Gruley, E., Kyle, D. J., & Ko, M. C. (2012). Roles of mu-opioid receptors and nociceptin/orphanin FQ peptide receptors in buprenorphine-induced physiological responses in primates. *The Journal of Pharmacology and Experimental Therapeutics*, *343*(1), 72–81.

Dautzenberg, F. M., Wichmann, J., Higelin, J., Py-Lang, G., Kratzeisen, C., Malherbe, P., et al. (2001). Pharmacological characterization of the novel nonpeptide orphanin FQ/nociceptin receptor agonist Ro 64-6198: Rapid and reversible desensitization of the ORL1 receptor in vitro and lack of tolerance in vivo. *The Journal of Pharmacology and Experimental Therapeutics*, *298*(2), 812–819.

Depner, U. B., Reinscheid, R. K., Takeshima, H., Brune, K., & Zeilhofer, H. U. (2003). Normal sensitivity to acute pain, but increased inflammatory hyperalgesia in mice lacking the nociceptin precursor polypeptide or the nociceptin receptor. *The European Journal of Neuroscience*, *17*(11), 2381–2387.

Ding, H., Czoty, P., Cami-Kobeci, G., Sukhtankar, D., Nader, M., Husbands, S., et al. (2015). BU08028 displays a promising therapeutic profile as an analgesic in monkeys. *The FASEB Journal*, *29*(Suppl.), 616.2.

Ding, H., Hayashida, K., Suto, T., Sukhtankar, D. D., Kimura, M., Mendenhall, V., et al. (2015). Supraspinal actions of nociceptin/orphanin FQ, morphine and substance P in regulating pain and itch in non-human primates. *British Journal of Pharmacology*, *172*(13), 3302–3312.

Eisenach, J. C., Hood, D. D., Curry, R., & Tong, C. (1997). Alfentanil, but not amitriptyline, reduces pain, hyperalgesia, and allodynia from intradermal injection of capsaicin in humans. *Anesthesiology*, *86*(6), 1279–1287.

Erb, K., Liebel, J. T., Tegeder, I., Zeilhofer, H. U., Brune, K., & Geisslinger, G. (1997). Spinally delivered nociceptin/orphanin FQ reduces flinching behaviour in the rat formalin test. *Neuroreport*, *8*(8), 1967–1970.

Evans, C. J., Keith, D. E., Jr., Morrison, H., Magendzo, K., & Edwards, R. H. (1992). Cloning of a delta opioid receptor by functional expression. *Science*, *258*(5090), 1952–1955.

Faber, E. S., Chambers, J. P., Evans, R. H., & Henderson, G. (1996). Depression of glutamatergic transmission by nociceptin in the neonatal rat hemisected spinal cord preparation in vitro. *British Journal of Pharmacology*, *119*(2), 189–190.

Fields, H. (2004). State-dependent opioid control of pain. *Nature Reviews. Neuroscience*, *5*(7), 565–575.

Fukuda, K., Kato, S., Mori, K., Nishi, M., Takeshima, H., Iwabe, N., et al. (1994). cDNA cloning and regional distribution of a novel member of the opioid receptor family. *FEBS Letters*, *343*(1), 42–46.

Granier, S., Manglik, A., Kruse, A. C., Kobilka, T. S., Thian, F. S., Weis, W. I., et al. (2012). Structure of the delta-opioid receptor bound to naltrindole. *Nature*, *485*(7398), 400–404.

Grisel, J. E., Farrier, D. E., Wilson, S. G., & Mogil, J. S. (1998). [Phe1psi(CH2-NH)Gly2] nociceptin-(1-13)-NH2 acts as an agonist of the orphanin FQ/nociceptin receptor in vivo. *European Journal of Pharmacology*, *357*(1), R1–R3.

Hao, J. X., Xu, I. S., Wiesenfeld-Hallin, Z., & Xu, X. J. (1998). Anti-hyperalgesic and anti-allodynic effects of intrathecal nociceptin/orphanin FQ in rats after spinal cord injury, peripheral nerve injury and inflammation. *Pain*, *76*(3), 385–393.

Hashiba, E., Harrison, C., Galo, G., Guerrini, R., Rowbotham, D. J., Smith, G., et al. (2001). Characterisation and comparison of novel ligands for the nociceptin/orphanin FQ receptor. *Naunyn-Schmiedeberg's Archives of Pharmacology*, *363*(1), 28–33.

Hawes, B. E., Graziano, M. P., & Lambert, D. G. (2000). Cellular actions of nociceptin: Transduction mechanisms. *Peptides*, *21*(7), 961–967.

Heinricher, M. M., McGaraughty, S., & Grandy, D. K. (1997). Circuitry underlying anti-opioid actions of orphanin FQ in the rostral ventromedial medulla. *Journal of Neurophysiology*, *78*(6), 3351–3358.

Heinricher, M. M., Morgan, M. M., Tortorici, V., & Fields, H. L. (1994). Disinhibition of off-cells and antinociception produced by an opioid action within the rostral ventromedial medulla. *Neuroscience*, *63*(1), 279–288.

Hu, E., Calo, G., Guerrini, R., & Ko, M. C. (2010). Long-lasting antinociceptive spinal effects in primates of the novel nociceptin/orphanin FQ receptor agonist UFP-112. *Pain*, *148*(1), 107–113.

Husbands, S. M. (2013). Buprenorphine and related orvinols. In M. C. Ko & S. M. Husbands (Eds.), *ACS symposium series: Vol. 1131. Research and development of opioid-related ligands* (pp. 127–144). Washington, DC: American Chemical Society.

Inoue, M., Shimohira, I., Yoshida, A., Zimmer, A., Takeshima, H., Sakurada, T., et al. (1999). Dose-related opposite modulation by nociceptin/orphanin FQ of substance P nociception in the nociceptors and spinal cord. *The Journal of Pharmacology and Experimental Therapeutics*, *291*(1), 308–313.

Jenck, F., Wichmann, J., Dautzenberg, F. M., Moreau, J. L., Ouagazzal, A. M., Martin, J. R., et al. (2000). A synthetic agonist at the orphanin FQ/nociceptin receptor ORL1: Anxiolytic profile in the rat. *Proceedings of the National Academy of Sciences of the United States of America*, *97*(9), 4938–4943.

Jia, Y., Linden, D. R., Serie, J. R., & Seybold, V. S. (1998). Nociceptin/orphanin FQ binding increases in superficial laminae of the rat spinal cord during persistent peripheral inflammation. *Neuroscience Letters*, *250*(1), 21–24.

Journigan, V. B., Polgar, W. E., Khroyan, T. V., & Zaveri, N. T. (2014). Designing bifunctional NOP receptor-mu opioid receptor ligands from NOP-receptor selective scaffolds. Part II. *Bioorganic & Medicinal Chemistry*, *22*(8), 2508–2516.

Kamei, J., Ohsawa, M., Kashiwazaki, T., & Nagase, H. (1999). Antinociceptive effects of the ORL1 receptor agonist nociceptin/orphanin FQ in diabetic mice. *European Journal of Pharmacology*, *370*(2), 109–116.

Khroyan, T. V., Polgar, W. E., Cami-Kobeci, G., Husbands, S. M., Zaveri, N. T., & Toll, L. (2011a). The first universal opioid ligand, (2S)-2-[(5R,6R,7R,14S)-N-cyclopropylmethyl-4,5-epoxy-6,14-ethano-3-hydroxy-6-meth oxymorphinan-7-yl]-3,3-dimethylpentan-2-ol (BU08028): Characterization of the in vitro profile and in vivo behavioral effects in mouse models of acute pain and cocaine-induced reward. *The Journal of Pharmacology and Experimental Therapeutics*, *336*(3), 952–961.

Khroyan, T. V., Polgar, W. E., Jiang, F., Zaveri, N. T., & Toll, L. (2009). Nociceptin/orphanin FQ receptor activation attenuates antinociception induced by mixed nociceptin/orphanin FQ/mu-opioid receptor agonists. *The Journal of Pharmacology and Experimental Therapeutics*, *331*(3), 946–953.

Khroyan, T. V., Polgar, W. E., Orduna, J., Montenegro, J., Jiang, F., Zaveri, N. T., et al. (2011b). Differential effects of nociceptin/orphanin FQ (NOP) receptor agonists in acute versus chronic pain: Studies with bifunctional NOP/mu receptor agonists in the sciatic nerve ligation chronic pain model in mice. *The Journal of Pharmacology and Experimental Therapeutics*, *339*(2), 687–693.

Kieffer, B. L., Befort, K., Gaveriaux-Ruff, C., & Hirth, C. G. (1992). The delta-opioid receptor: Isolation of a cDNA by expression cloning and pharmacological characterization. *Proceedings of the National Academy of Sciences of the United States of America*, *89*(24), 12048–12052.

King, M., Chang, A., & Pasternak, G. W. (1998). Functional blockade of opioid analgesia by orphanin FQ/nociceptin. *Biochemical Pharmacology*, *55*(9), 1537–1540.

King, M. A., Rossi, G. C., Chang, A. H., Williams, L., & Pasternak, G. W. (1997). Spinal analgesic activity of orphanin FQ/nociceptin and its fragments. *Neuroscience Letters*, *223*(2), 113–116.

Knoflach, F., Reinscheid, R. K., Civelli, O., & Kemp, J. A. (1996). Modulation of voltage-gated calcium channels by orphanin FQ in freshly dissociated hippocampal neurons. *The Journal of Neuroscience*, *16*(21), 6657–6664.

Ko, M. C., & Naughton, N. N. (2009). Antinociceptive effects of nociceptin/orphanin FQ administered intrathecally in monkeys. *The Journal of Pain*, *10*(5), 509–516.

Ko, M. C., Wei, H., Woods, J. H., & Kennedy, R. T. (2006). Effects of intrathecally administered nociceptin/orphanin FQ in monkeys: Behavioral and mass spectrometric studies. *The Journal of Pharmacology and Experimental Therapeutics*, *318*(3), 1257–1264.

Ko, M. C., Woods, J. H., Fantegrossi, W. E., Galuska, C. M., Wichmann, J., & Prinssen, E. P. (2009). Behavioral effects of a synthetic agonist selective for nociceptin/orphanin FQ peptide receptors in monkeys. *Neuropsychopharmacology*, *34*(9), 2088–2096.

Kotlinska, J., Wichmann, J., Rafalski, P., Talarek, S., Dylag, T., & Silberring, J. (2003). Non-peptidergic OP4 receptor agonist inhibits morphine antinociception but does not influence morphine dependence. *Neuroreport*, *14*(4), 601–604.

Kumar, V., Ridzwan, I. E., Grivas, K., Lewis, J. W., Clark, M. J., Meurice, C., et al. (2014). Selectively promiscuous opioid ligands: Discovery of high affinity/low efficacy opioid ligands with substantial nociceptin opioid peptide receptor affinity. *Journal of Medicinal Chemistry*, *57*(10), 4049–4057.

Lambert, D. G. (2008). The nociceptin/orphanin FQ receptor: A target with broad therapeutic potential. *Nature Reviews. Drug Discovery*, *7*(8), 694–710.

Le Cudennec, C., Suaudeau, C., & Costentin, J. (2002). Evidence for a localization of [(3)H] nociceptin binding sites on medullar primary afferent fibers. *Journal of Neuroscience Research*, *68*(4), 496–500.

Lee, H., & Ko, M. C. (2015). Distinct functions of opioid-related peptides and gastrin-releasing peptide in regulating itch and pain in the spinal cord of primates. *Scientific Reports*, *5*, 11676.

Lin, A. P., & Ko, M. C. (2013). The therapeutic potential of nociceptin/orphanin FQ receptor agonists as analgesics without abuse liability. *ACS Chemical Neuroscience*, *4*(2), 214–224.

Linz, K., Christoph, T., Schiene, K., Koch, T., & Englberger, W. (2013). GRT-TA2210, a selective NOP receptor agonist, is active in mouse models of inflammatory and neuropathic pain. In *EFIC—8th "Pain in Europe" congress 2013, Florence, Italy*. Abstract 599.

Linz, K., Christoph, T., Tzschentke, T. M., Koch, T., Schiene, K., Gautrois, M., et al. (2014). Cebranopadol: A novel potent analgesic nociceptin/orphanin FQ peptide

and opioid receptor agonist. *The Journal of Pharmacology and Experimental Therapeutics, 349*(3), 535–548.
Lutfy, K., Eitan, S., Bryant, C. D., Yang, Y. C., Saliminejad, N., Walwyn, W., et al. (2003). Buprenorphine-induced antinociception is mediated by mu-opioid receptors and compromised by concomitant activation of opioid receptor-like receptors. *The Journal of Neuroscience, 23*(32), 10331–10337.
Ma, L., Cheng, Z. J., Fan, G. H., Cai, Y. C., Jiang, L. Z., & Pei, G. (1997). Functional expression, activation and desensitization of opioid receptor-like receptor ORL1 in neuroblastoma x glioma NG108-15 hybrid cells. *FEBS Letters, 403*(1), 91–94.
Ma, F., Xie, H., Dong, Z. Q., Wang, Y. Q., & Wu, G. C. (2005). Expression of ORL1 mRNA in some brain nuclei in neuropathic pain rats. *Brain Research, 1043*(1–2), 214–217.
Manglik, A., Kruse, A. C., Kobilka, T. S., Thian, F. S., Mathiesen, J. M., Sunahara, R. K., et al. (2012). Crystal structure of the micro-opioid receptor bound to a morphinan antagonist. *Nature, 485*(7398), 321–326.
Margas, W., Sedeek, K., & Ruiz-Velasco, V. (2008). Coupling specificity of NOP opioid receptors to pertussis-toxin-sensitive Galpha proteins in adult rat stellate ganglion neurons using small interference RNA. *Journal of Neurophysiology, 100*(3), 1420–1432.
McDonald, J., Calo, G., Guerrini, R., & Lambert, D. G. (2003). UFP-101, a high affinity antagonist for the nociceptin/orphanin FQ receptor: Radioligand and GTPgamma(35)S binding studies. *Naunyn-Schmiedeberg's Archives of Pharmacology, 367*(2), 183–187.
Meunier, J. C., Mollereau, C., Toll, L., Suaudeau, C., Moisand, C., Alvinerie, P., et al. (1995). Isolation and structure of the endogenous agonist of opioid receptor-like ORL1 receptor. *Nature, 377*(6549), 532–535.
Mogil, J. S., Grisel, J. E., Reinscheid, R. K., Civelli, O., Belknap, J. K., & Grandy, D. K. (1996). Orphanin FQ is a functional anti-opioid peptide. *Neuroscience, 75*(2), 333–337.
Molinari, S., Camarda, V., Rizzi, A., Marzola, G., Salvadori, S., Marzola, E., et al. (2013). [Dmt1]N/OFQ(1-13)-NH2: A potent nociceptin/orphanin FQ and opioid receptor universal agonist. *British Journal of Pharmacology, 168*(1), 151–162.
Mollereau, C., & Mouledous, L. (2000). Tissue distribution of the opioid receptor-like (ORL1) receptor. *Peptides, 21*(7), 907–917.
Mollereau, C., Parmentier, M., Mailleux, P., Butour, J. L., Moisand, C., Chalon, P., et al. (1994). ORL1, a novel member of the opioid receptor family. Cloning, functional expression and localization. *FEBS Letters, 341*(1), 33–38.
Mollereau, C., Simons, M. J., Soularue, P., Liners, F., Vassart, G., Meunier, J. C., et al. (1996). Structure, tissue distribution, and chromosomal localization of the prepronociceptin gene. *Proceedings of the National Academy of Sciences of the United States of America, 93*(16), 8666–8670.
Neal, C. R., Jr., Mansour, A., Reinscheid, R., Nothacker, H. P., Civelli, O., Akil, H., et al. (1999a). Opioid receptor-like (ORL1) receptor distribution in the rat central nervous system: Comparison of ORL1 receptor mRNA expression with (125)I-[(14)Tyr]-orphanin FQ binding. *The Journal of Comparative Neurology, 412*(4), 563–605.
Neal, C. R., Jr., Mansour, A., Reinscheid, R., Nothacker, H. P., Civelli, O., & Watson, S. J., Jr. (1999b). Localization of orphanin FQ (nociceptin) peptide and messenger RNA in the central nervous system of the rat. *The Journal of Comparative Neurology, 406*(4), 503–547.
Nicol, B., Lambert, D. G., Rowbotham, D. J., Okuda-Ashitaka, E., Ito, S., Smart, D., et al. (1998). Nocistatin reverses nociceptin inhibition of glutamate release from rat brain slices. *European Journal of Pharmacology, 356*(2-3), R1–R3.
Nicol, B., Lambert, D. G., Rowbotham, D. J., Smart, D., & McKnight, A. T. (1996). Nociceptin induced inhibition of K+ evoked glutamate release from rat cerebrocortical slices. *British Journal of Pharmacology, 119*(6), 1081–1083.

Nishi, M., Takeshima, H., Mori, M., Nakagawara, K., & Takeuchi, T. (1994). Structure and chromosomal mapping of genes for the mouse kappa-opioid receptor and an opioid receptor homologue (MOR-C). *Biochemical and Biophysical Research Communications, 205*(2), 1353–1357.

Obara, I., Przewlocki, R., & Przewlocka, B. (2005). Spinal and local peripheral antiallodynic activity of Ro64-6198 in neuropathic pain in the rat. *Pain, 116*(1-2), 17–25.

Park, K. M., Max, M. B., Robinovitz, E., Gracely, R. H., & Bennett, G. J. (1995). Effects of intravenous ketamine, alfentanil, or placebo on pain, pinprick hyperalgesia, and allodynia produced by intradermal capsaicin in human subjects. *Pain, 63*(2), 163–172.

Peluso, J., LaForge, K. S., Matthes, H. W., Kreek, M. J., Kieffer, B. L., & Gaveriaux-Ruff, C. (1998). Distribution of nociceptin/orphanin FQ receptor transcript in human central nervous system and immune cells. *Journal of Neuroimmunology, 81*(1-2), 184–192.

Podlesnik, C. A., Ko, M. C., Winger, G., Wichmann, J., Prinssen, E. P., & Woods, J. H. (2011). The effects of nociceptin/orphanin FQ receptor agonist Ro 64-6198 and diazepam on antinociception and remifentanil self-administration in rhesus monkeys. *Psychopharmacology, 213*(1), 53–60.

Reinscheid, R. K., Nothacker, H. P., Bourson, A., Ardati, A., Henningsen, R. A., Bunzow, J. R., et al. (1995). Orphanin FQ: A neuropeptide that activates an opioidlike G protein-coupled receptor. *Science, 270*(5237), 792–794.

Reiss, D., Wichmann, J., Tekeshima, H., Kieffer, B. L., & Ouagazzal, A. M. (2008). Effects of nociceptin/orphanin FQ receptor (NOP) agonist, Ro64-6198, on reactivity to acute pain in mice: Comparison to morphine. *European Journal of Pharmacology, 579*(1-3), 141–148.

Rizzi, A., Malfacini, D., Cerlesi, M. C., Ruzza, C., Marzola, E., Bird, M. F., et al. (2014). In vitro and in vivo pharmacological characterization of nociceptin/orphanin FQ tetrabranched derivatives. *British Journal of Pharmacology, 171*(17), 4138–4153.

Rizzi, A., Nazzaro, C., Marzola, G. G., Zucchini, S., Trapella, C., Guerrini, R., et al. (2006). Endogenous nociceptin/orphanin FQ signalling produces opposite spinal antinociceptive and supraspinal pronociceptive effects in the mouse formalin test: Pharmacological and genetic evidences. *Pain, 124*(1-2), 100–108.

Rizzi, A., Spagnolo, B., Wainford, R. D., Fischetti, C., Guerrini, R., Marzola, G., et al. (2007). In vitro and in vivo studies on UFP-112, a novel potent and long lasting agonist selective for the nociceptin/orphanin FQ receptor. *Peptides, 28*(6), 1240–1251.

Rizzi, A., Sukhtankar, D. D., Ding, H., Hayashida, K., Ruzza, C., Guerrini, R., et al. (2015). Spinal antinociceptive effects of the novel NOP receptor agonist PWT2-nociceptin/orphanin FQ in mice and monkeys. *British Journal of Pharmacology, 172*(14), 3661–3670.

Rosen, A., Lundeberg, T., Bytner, B., & Nylander, I. (2000). Central changes in nociceptin dynorphin B and Met-enkephalin-Arg-Phe in different models of nociception. *Brain Research, 857*(1-2), 212–218.

Sakurada, T., Katsuyama, S., Sakurada, S., Inoue, M., Tan-No, K., Kisara, K., et al. (1999). Nociceptin-induced scratching, biting and licking in mice: Involvement of spinal NK1 receptors. *British Journal of Pharmacology, 127*(7), 1712–1718.

Salat, K., Jakubowska, A., & Kulig, K. (2015). Cebranopadol: A first-in-class potent analgesic agent with agonistic activity at nociceptin/orphanin FQ and opioid receptors. *Expert Opinion on Investigational Drugs, 24*(6), 837–844.

Schiene, K., Christoph, T., Kogel, B., & Tzschentke, T. M. (2013). Antinociceptive, antihyperalgesic and antiallodynic activity of the NOP receptor agonist Ro65-6570 in rodent models of pain. In *EFIC—8th "Pain in Europe" congress 2013, Florence, Italy*. Abstract 606.

Schlicker, E., & Morari, M. (2000). Nociceptin/orphanin FQ and neurotransmitter release in the central nervous system. *Peptides, 21*(7), 1023–1029.

Schröder, W., Lambert, D. G., Ko, M. C., & Koch, T. (2014). Functional plasticity of the N/OFQ-NOP receptor system determines analgesic properties of NOP receptor agonists. *British Journal of Pharmacology, 171*(16), 3777–3800.

Schunk, S., Linz, K., Hinze, C., Frormann, S., Oberborsch, S., Sundermann, B., et al. (2014). Discovery of a potent analgesic NOP and opioid receptor agonist: Cebranopadol. *ACS Medicinal Chemistry Letters, 5*(8), 857–862.

Scoto, G. M., Arico, G., Iemolo, A., Ronsisvalle, S., & Parenti, C. (2009). Involvement of the nociceptin/orphanin FQ-NOP receptor system in the ventrolateral periaqueductal gray following mechanical allodynia in chronic pain. *Life Sciences, 85*(5-6), 206–210.

Sobczak, M., Mokrowiecka, A., Cygankiewicz, A. I., Zakrzewski, P. K., Salaga, M., Storr, M., et al. (2014). Anti-inflammatory and antinociceptive action of an orally available nociceptin receptor agonist SCH 221510 in a mouse model of inflammatory bowel diseases. *The Journal of Pharmacology and Experimental Therapeutics, 348*(3), 401–409.

Sobczak, M., Salaga, M., Storr, M., & Fichna, J. (2013). Nociceptin/orphanin FQ (NOP) receptors as novel potential target in the treatment of gastrointestinal diseases. *Current Drug Targets, 14*(10), 1203–1209.

Sotgiu, M. L., Bellomi, P., & Biella, G. E. (2004). Efficacy of nociceptin inhibition on WDR neuron activity is enhanced in mononeuropathic rats. *Brain Research, 998*(2), 251–254.

Spagnolo, B., Calo, G., Polgar, W. E., Jiang, F., Olsen, C. M., Berzetei-Gurske, I., et al. (2008). Activities of mixed NOP and mu-opioid receptor ligands. *British Journal of Pharmacology, 153*(3), 609–619.

Stanfa, L. C., Chapman, V., Kerr, N., & Dickenson, A. H. (1996). Inhibitory action of nociceptin on spinal dorsal horn neurones of the rat, in vivo. *British Journal of Pharmacology, 118*(8), 1875–1877.

Sukhtankar, D. D., Lee, H., Rice, K. C., & Ko, M. C. (2014). Differential effects of opioid-related ligands and NSAIDs in nonhuman primate models of acute and inflammatory pain. *Psychopharmacology, 231*(7), 1377–1387.

Sukhtankar, D. D., Zaveri, N. T., Husbands, S. M., & Ko, M. C. (2013). Effects of spinally administered bifunctional nociceptin/orphanin FQ peptide receptor/mu-opioid receptor ligands in mouse models of neuropathic and inflammatory pain. *The Journal of Pharmacology and Experimental Therapeutics, 346*(1), 11–22.

Sun, R. Q., Wang, Y., Zhao, C. S., Chang, J. K., & Han, J. S. (2001). Changes in brain content of nociceptin/orphanin FQ and endomorphin 2 in a rat model of neuropathic pain. *Neuroscience Letters, 311*(1), 13–16.

Sundstrom, G., Dreborg, S., & Larhammar, D. (2010). Concomitant duplications of opioid peptide and receptor genes before the origin of jawed vertebrates. *PLoS One, 5*(5), e10512.

Szolcsanyi, J., & Sandor, Z. (2012). Multisteric TRPV1 nocisensor: A target for analgesics. *Trends in Pharmacological Sciences, 33*(12), 646–655.

Thompson, A. A., Liu, W., Chun, E., Katritch, V., Wu, H., Vardy, E., et al. (2012). Structure of the nociceptin/orphanin FQ receptor in complex with a peptide mimetic. *Nature, 485*(7398), 395–399.

Tian, J. H., Xu, W., Fang, Y., Mogil, J. S., Grisel, J. E., Grandy, D. K., et al. (1997). Bidirectional modulatory effect of orphanin FQ on morphine-induced analgesia: Antagonism in brain and potentiation in spinal cord of the rat. *British Journal of Pharmacology, 120*(4), 676–680.

Toll, L. (2013). The use of bifunctional NOP/mu and NOP receptor selective compounds for the treatment of pain, drug abuse, and psychiatric disorders. *Current Pharmaceutical Design, 19*(42), 7451–7460.

Toll, L., Khroyan, T. V., Polgar, W. E., Jiang, F., Olsen, C., & Zaveri, N. T. (2009). Comparison of the antinociceptive and antirewarding profiles of novel bifunctional

nociceptin receptor/mu-opioid receptor ligands: Implications for therapeutic applications. *The Journal of Pharmacology and Experimental Therapeutics*, *331*(3), 954–964.
Varty, G. B., Lu, S. X., Morgan, C. A., Cohen-Williams, M. E., Hodgson, R. A., Smith-Torhan, A., et al. (2008). The anxiolytic-like effects of the novel, orally active nociceptin opioid receptor agonist 8-[bis(2-methylphenyl)methyl]-3-phenyl-8-azabicyclo[3.2.1] octan-3-ol (SCH 221510). *The Journal of Pharmacology and Experimental Therapeutics*, *326*(2), 672–682.
Wang, J. B., Johnson, P. S., Imai, Y., Persico, A. M., Ozenberger, B. A., Eppler, C. M., et al. (1994). cDNA cloning of an orphan opiate receptor gene family member and its splice variant. *FEBS Letters*, *348*(1), 75–79.
Wang, J. L., Zhu, C. B., Cao, X. D., & Wu, G. C. (1999a). Distinct effect of intracerebroventricular and intrathecal injections of nociceptin/orphanin FQ in the rat formalin test. *Regulatory Peptides*, *79*(2–3), 159–163.
Wang, Y. Q., Zhu, C. B., Cao, X. D., & Wu, G. C. (1999b). Supraspinal hyperalgesia and spinal analgesia by [Phe1psi(CH2-NH)Gly2]nociceptin-(1-13)-NH2 in rat. *European Journal of Pharmacology*, *376*(3), R1–R3.
Witta, J., Palkovits, M., Rosenberger, J., & Cox, B. M. (2004). Distribution of nociceptin/orphanin FQ in adult human brain. *Brain Research*, *997*(1), 24–29.
Wladischkin, K. A., Dysko, R. C., Collins, G. T., Ko, Y. A., Winger, G., & Ko, M. C. (2012). Pharmacological characterization of NOP receptor agonists as abuse-free and constipation-free analgesics in monkeys. *The FASEB Journal*, *26*(Suppl.), 1123.3.
Wu, H., Wacker, D., Mileni, M., Katritch, V., Han, G. W., Vardy, E., et al. (2012). Structure of the human kappa-opioid receptor in complex with JDTic. *Nature*, *485*(7398), 327–332.
Xu, X. J., Hao, J. X., & Wiesenfeld-Hallin, Z. (1996). Nociceptin or antinociceptin: Potent spinal antinociceptive effect of orphanin FQ/nociceptin in the rat. *Neuroreport*, 7(13), 2092–2094.
Yamamoto, T., & Nozaki-Taguchi, N. (1997). Effects of intrathecally administered nociceptin, an opioid receptor-like1 receptor agonist, and N-methyl-D-aspartate receptor antagonists on the thermal hyperalgesia induced by partial sciatic nerve injury in the rat. *Anesthesiology*, *87*(5), 1145–1152.
Yamamoto, T., Nozaki-Taguchi, N., & Kimura, S. (1997a). Analgesic effect of intrathecally administered nociceptin, an opioid receptor-like1 receptor agonist, in the rat formalin test. *Neuroscience*, *81*(1), 249–254.
Yamamoto, T., Nozaki-Taguchi, N., & Kimura, S. (1997b). Effects of intrathecally administered nociceptin, an opioid receptor-like1 (ORL1) receptor agonist, on the thermal hyperalgesia induced by carageenan injection into the rat paw. *Brain Research*, *754*(1-2), 329–332.
Yamamoto, T., Ohtori, S., & Chiba, T. (2000). Effects of pre-emptively administered nociceptin on the development of thermal hyperalgesia induced by two models of experimental mononeuropathy in the rat. *Brain Research*, *871*(2), 192–200.
Yasuda, K., Raynor, K., Kong, H., Breder, C. D., Takeda, J., Reisine, T., et al. (1993). Cloning and functional comparison of kappa and delta opioid receptors from mouse brain. *Proceedings of the National Academy of Sciences of the United States of America*, *90*(14), 6736–6740.
Zaveri, N. T., Jiang, F., Olsen, C., Polgar, W. E., & Toll, L. (2013). Designing bifunctional NOP receptor-mu opioid receptor ligands from NOP receptor-selective scaffolds. Part I. *Bioorganic & Medicinal Chemistry Letters*, *23*(11), 3308–3313.
Zhu, C. B., Cao, X. D., Xu, S. F., & Wu, G. C. (1997). Orphanin FQ potentiates formalin-induced pain behavior and antagonizes morphine analgesia in rats. *Neuroscience Letters*, *235*(1–2), 37–40.

CHAPTER NINE

The Role of Regulatory Transporters in Neuropathic Pain

Muhammad Saad Yousuf*, Bradley J. Kerr*,†,‡,1
*Neuroscience and Mental Health Institute, University of Alberta, Edmonton, Alberta, Canada
†Department of Pharmacology, University of Alberta, Edmonton, Alberta, Canada
‡Department of Anesthesiology and Pain Medicine, University of Alberta, Edmonton, Alberta, Canada
[1]Corresponding author: e-mail address: bradley.kerr@ualberta.ca

Contents

Abstract

Neuropathic pain arises from an injury or disease of the somatosensory nervous system rather than stimulation of pain receptors. As a result, the fine balance between excitation and inhibition is perturbed leading to hyperalgesia and allodynia. Various neuropathic pain models provide considerable evidence that changes in the glutamatergic, GABAergic, and monoaminergic systems. Neurotransmitter reuptake transporter proteins have the potential to change the temporal and spatial profile of various neurotransmitters throughout the nervous system. This, in turn, can affect the downstream effects of these neurotransmitters and hence modulate pain. This chapter explores various reuptake transporter systems and implicates their role in pain processing. Understanding the transporter systems will enhance drug discovery targeting different facets of neuropathic pain.

Advances in Pharmacology, Volume 75
ISSN 1054-3589
http://dx.doi.org/10.1016/bs.apha.2015.12.003

1. INTRODUCTION

The most common symptom across various medical conditions and a major reason for seeking physician consultation is pain (Debono, Hoeksema, & Hobbs, 2013). Pain is defined as "an unpleasant feeling or emotional experience associated with actual or potential tissue damage" (Loeser & Treede, 2008). When pain loses its adaptive value and becomes persistent even after the initial cause has healed, it becomes a disease in itself. As such, neuropathic pain arises from an injury or disease of the somatosensory nervous system. It further has the capacity to severely affect one's quality of life and general activities of daily living (Van Hecke, Austin, Khan, Smith, & Torrance, 2014). While the prevalence of pain is hard to assess, a recent meta-analysis concluded that 6.9–10% of the general population experiences neuropathic pain (Van Hecke et al., 2014).

The molecular basis of the hypersensitivity seen in neuropathic pain is not well understood. It is known, however, that the spinal cord is implicated in modulating pain perception. The Gate Control Theory proposes that local inhibitory interneurons of the spinal cord act as "gates" to dampen or allow nociceptive inputs reaching the brain (Melzack & Wall, 1965). Recent evidence suggests that spinal architecture is more complicated than initially proposed in the Gate Control Theory (Sandkuhler, 2009). Within the spinal cord, various interneurons may form inhibitory or excitatory synapses with projection neurons and other interneurons creating a sophisticated network. This network of local interneurons receives input from primary afferents and descending inputs from the brain. Any form of plasticity in the network may modify pain sensation.

Neuroplasticity may be classified into synaptic plasticity and nonsynaptic plasticity. Synaptic plasticity refers to changes in the strength of a synapse as a result of fluctuations in neural activity (Gerrow & Triller, 2010). Such activity is largely regulated by neurotransmitter secretion, diffusion, and removal from the synapse. However, the effects of a neurotransmitter may vary from cell to cell according to its inherent excitability. Modification of neuronal excitability via changes in cellular mechanisms is known as nonsynaptic plasticity (Kemenes et al., 2006). Modulation of intracellular ion concentrations and changes in action potential propagation are examples of nonsynaptic plasticity. Complex phenomena such as pain are a consequence of synaptic and nonsynaptic mechanisms affecting individual neurons as well as their integration into a larger network (Sandkuhler, 2009).

Transporter proteins are important in moving molecules across a membrane with or against their electrochemical gradient. They can transport ions, neurotransmitters, and large macromolecules such as other proteins. As a result, they can regulate the function of those substances and the cells involved. The Alternating Access Model provides a theoretical guideline that all secondary active transporters should meet (Slotboom, 2014). According to this model, all transporters should (1) have a cavity large enough to fit protein of interest, (2) adopt two different conformations (each opening alternatively into the extracellular or the intracellular matrix), and (3) be able to adjust affinities for protein of interest through conformational change. This chapter aims to implicate transporter proteins in regulating pain processing throughout the nervous system. It will also discuss pharmacological regulation of these transporter proteins in neuropathic pain models.

2. GLUTAMATERGIC SYSTEM

Glutamate (Glu), a nonessential amino acid, is the most prevalent excitatory neurotransmitter in the nervous system. Glu activates downstream neurons by acting on various ionotropic and metabotropic receptors. These receptors are found widely throughout the nervous system and are implicated in a host of functions ranging from cognition (Caddy et al., 2015) to synaptogenesis (Duman & Li, 2012). Under neuropathic pain conditions, changes in Glu levels have also been observed across varying levels of the nervous system. Nociceptive primary afferents mostly relay their activation by releasing Glu onto postsynaptic spinal cord neurons (Gegelashvili & Bjerrum, 2014). Pain perception can be amplified by enhancing the effects of Glu on spinal dorsal horn neurons—a process known as central sensitization (Sandkuhler, 2009). One way that could be achieved is through phosphorylation of receptors which increase membrane trafficking and channel efficacy. Furthermore, modulation of Glu reuptake transporters can affect Glu levels at the synapse and thereby the downstream excitatory consequences of Glu.

2.1 Glutamate Transporters

Majority of the Glu uptake is performed by the Na^+-dependent SLC1A family of Glu transporters (Gegelashvili, Robinson, Trotti, & Rauen, 2001). The SLC1A genes encode for seven high-affinity Glu transporters: EAAT1-5 (excitatory amino acid transporters; Arriza, Eliasof, Kavanaugh, & Amara, 1997;

Fairman, Vandenberg, Arriza, Kavanaugh, & Amara, 1995; Kanai & Hediger, 1992; Pines et al., 1992; Storck, Schulte, Hofmann, & Stoffel, 1992) and ASCT1-2 (alanine/serine/cysteine transporters; Arriza et al., 1993; Utsunomiya-Tate, Endou, & Kanai, 1996). Although the latter group of transporters favors the transport of neutral amino acids, they can transport protonated Glu molecules under acidic conditions. The main driving force for the transport of Glu molecules is the Na^+/K^+ gradient established primarily by the Na^+/K^+ ATPase pump (Danbolt, 2001; Grewer, Gameiro, & Rauen, 2014). Glu is cotransported along with sodium ions across the membrane via facilitated diffusion across the electrochemical gradient of sodium. Moreover, kinetic parameters (K_m and V_{max}) of these transporters are influenced largely by pH, posttranslational modifications, accessibility on the plasma membrane, and scaffold proteins (Beart & O'Shea, 2007; Gegelashvili & Schousboe, 1998; Grewer et al., 2014).

In the brain, EAAT1 and EAAT2 are responsible for majority (>95%) of the Glu reuptake (Danbolt, 2001). Both of these proteins are mainly found on astrocyte soma and processes with minimal expression in oligodendrocytes and activated microglia (Domercq & Matute, 1999; Xin, Weng, & Dougherty, 2009). Neurons only express a small portion (~6–10%) of EAAT2 at the synapse even though significant reuptake by neurons has previously been shown to occur (Furness et al., 2008; Suchak et al., 2003). EAAT3 and EAAT4 are predominantly neuronal with EAAT4 being more prevalent in the cerebellar purkinje neurons (Fairman et al., 1995). EAAT5 is expressed explicitly on retinal cells (Arriza et al., 1997).

Similar cell-type expression profile is seen in the spinal cord as the brain. EAAT1, EAAT2, and EAAT3 are more prevalent in the dorsal horn than in the ventral horn (Queen, Kesslak, & Bridges, 2007). Furthermore, regional specificity is also observed across the spinal cord. The most abundant Glu transporter in the lumbar dorsal horn is EAAT2, whereas EAAT3 expression is more prominent in the thoracic and cervical dorsal horns (Queen et al., 2007).

Glu transporter levels in the periphery are slightly different from the central nervous system. Dorsal root ganglion (DRG) neurons primarily express EAAT1 and EAAT3 on axons and central terminals (Carozzi et al., 2008; Tao et al., 2004). These transporters have also been observed in myelinating Schwann cells of the sciatic nerve (Carozzi et al., 2008). In contrast to the central nervous system, EAAT2 expression is mainly limited to satellite glial cells and axons of the sciatic nerve (Carozzi et al., 2008). In the trigeminal ganglia, reverse action of these transporters has been linked to craniofacial pain (Laursen et al., 2014).

The main purpose of these Glu transporters, under physiological conditions, is to reduce Glu at the synapse, even in short bursts of activation. Under high-throughput conditions, Glu builds up rapidly at the synapse and cannot entirely be cleared only through Glu transporters on the presynaptic membrane (Piet, Vargová, Syková, Poulain, & Oliet, 2004). Instead, dense expression of Glu transporters on astrocytes covering the synapse allows for an efficient diffusion and reuptake of Glu in these conditions. In astrocytes, Glu is converted to glutamine or is used in metabolism primarily as α-ketoglutarate (Nissen, Pajęcka, Stridh, Skytt, & Waagepetersen, 2015). Any Glu that may escape synaptic and astrocytic Glu transporters is rapidly taken up by Glu transporters located extrasynaptically (Tzingounis & Wadiche, 2007). High expression of Glu transporters across the nervous system ensures that Glu only affects intended targets. Excessive extracellular Glu can lead to serious consequences such as excitotoxicity (Kanai et al., 2013).

2.2 Glutamate Transporters: Implications for Pain

Glu is an important neurotransmitter in sensory processing at the level of the spinal cord. Majority of the primary afferents, including those carrying nociceptive information, are glutamatergic (Gegelashvili & Bjerrum, 2014). Modulation of Glu via reuptake processes, thus, has the potential to modify pain perception. Neuropathic pain conditions lead to increased potency of glutamatergic transmission in the dorsal horn via central sensitization (Sandkuhler, 2009). Glu transporters have been reported to mediate this mechanism by being actively suppressed in the spinal cord (Sung, Lim, & Mao, 2003). This leads to an accumulation of extracellular Glu to excitotoxic levels, causing further neuronal cell death (Kanai et al., 2013). Lack of Glu uptake in the spinal cord after partial and complete nerve injury has been known for over a couple of decades (Potashner & Tran, 1984). In these models, changes in Glu transporters correlate with allodynia and hyperalgesia (Cavaliere et al., 2007; Sung et al., 2003). Downregulation of EAAT2 seems to be the most common phenomenon across various models of neuropathic pain (Cavaliere et al., 2007; Olechowski, Tenorio, Sauve, & Kerr, 2013; Putatunda, Hala, Chin, & Lepore, 2014; Sung et al., 2003). In addition to changes in EAAT2, few spinal cord injury studies have also noted a downregulation of EAAT1 and EAAT3

(Cavaliere et al., 2007; Sung et al., 2003). Total change in EAAT2 levels in the spinal dorsal horn is, at best, modest (Ramos et al., 2010). However, nerve injury induces selective internalization of EAAT2 from plasma membranes after nerve injury (Maeda et al., 2008). In the partial sciatic nerve ligation model, a substantial downregulation of total EAAT2 levels was observed, attributable to profound suppression of EAAT2 in astrocytes (Xin et al., 2009). In a large-scale T-cell-mediated disease model of experimental autoimmune encephalomyelitis, EAAT2 levels in the spinal cord decrease, correlating with various pain behaviors in these mice (Olechowski et al., 2013). Furthermore, treatment with β-lactam antibiotic, ceftriaxone, alleviates hyperalgesia associated with the disease by increasing Glu transporter levels (Olechowski et al., 2013). Significant alterations of Glu transporter levels in functional "hot spots" have also been proposed (Napier, Mohammadi, & Christie, 2012). This primarily occurs in and around synapses on neurons, astrocytes, and microglia. The functional consequence of these changes in Glu transporters is accumulation of Glu extrasynaptically where it can act on Glu receptors away from the synapse. Astrocytes have been known to magnify excess Glu response from primary afferents by releasing even more Glu via intracellular calcium signaling (Bezzi et al., 2004; Rojas et al., 2007; Yoshizumi, Eisenach, & Hayashida, 2012). Pharmacological inhibition of Glu transporters results in a similar phenotype for the most part. Administration of DL-TBOA, dihydrokainate, and L-*trans*-pyrrolidine-2,4-dicarboxylic acid inhibits Glu uptake, increases extracellular Glu, and triggers pain behaviors (Liaw et al., 2005; Weng, Chen, & Cata, 2006). Pharmacologically, blocking Glu receptors (both NMDA and non-NMDA receptors) afterward ameliorates hyperalgesia (Liaw et al., 2005). Moreover, upregulation of EAAT2 by viral gene transfer in a mouse model of visceral pain (colon distention) and partial sciatic nerve ligation leads to a significant dampening of pain behaviors (Lin, Roman, et al., 2011; Maeda et al., 2008). These studies implicate Glu transporters in modulating neuropathic pain. Yet, the exact mechanism through which neuropathy leads to an impairment in Glu uptake is still not well understood.

3. GABAergic SYSTEM

γ-Aminobutyric acid (GABA) is another prevalent neurotransmitter in the nervous system. It is responsible for mainly inhibiting neurons in the CNS by acting on ionotropic and metabotropic receptors. As a result, GABA is crucial in maintaining subthreshold membrane potential oscillations and summation of synaptic excitatory inputs (Akam & Kullmann, 2010; Hájos et al., 2004; Mann & Mody, 2010; Pouille & Scanziani, 2001; Stark et al., 2013). This requires a fine balance of GABA release and removal from the synapse. Since GABA cannot be disintegrated enzymatically, clearance of GABA from the synapse requires diffusion and reuptake by GABA transporters. These transporters are widespread throughout the nervous system on different cell types including neurons and astrocytes (Scimemi, 2014). Changes in the expression of GABA transporters are a key mechanism in controlling the effects of GABA in the nervous system.

3.1 GABA Transporters

There are 20 different sodium transporters in the solute carrier 6 (SLC6) family of transporters, grouped into GABA transporters, monoamine transporters, nutrient amino acid/orphan transporters, and neurotransmitter amino acid transporters (Scimemi, 2014). Among them, GABA transporters are classified into vesicular transporters (VGAT), Na^+-dependent high-affinity transporters (GAT1, GAT2, GAT3), and low-affinity transporters (BGT1; Gwak & Hulsebosch, 2011). TauT and CT1, as members of the SLC6 family, also transport GABA across the plasma membrane but much less is known about them (Scimemi, 2014). The nomenclature of the GABA transporters varies from species to species. This chapter uses nomenclature based on rat studies since majority of basic research comes from these animals.

GATs are the most characterized transporters responsible for GABA reuptake. Transport via these proteins is a secondary active mechanism relying on the electrochemical gradient established by Na^+/K^+ ATPase pump (Kanner & Sharon, 1978). Kinetic and thermodynamic studies have revealed that the Na^+ and Cl^- ions are required for GABA transport in a $1GABA:2Na^+:1Cl^-$ ratio (Lu & Hilgemann, 1999a, 1999b). Since GABA is a zwitterion and does not carry an overall charge under physiological conditions, GATs increase influx of a positive charge with every molecule of GABA transported (Kavanaughs, Arriza, North, & Amara, 1992; Mager et al., 1993; Radian & Kanner, 1983). It has been proposed that Cl^- extrusion mechanisms are linked to GATs in order to prevent Cl^- from accumulating in the cells and reversing its physiologically relevant electrochemical gradient (Loo, Eskandari, Boorer, Sarkar, & Wright, 2000). Furthermore, studies using valinomycin, a K^+-selective ionophore, have deduced that GATs are voltage dependent (Kanner & Sharon, 1978). Under the right electrochemical conditions of Na^+/Cl^- ions and high intracellular GABA concentrations, GATs can reverse their action and transport GABA to the extracellular environment (Bicho & Grewer, 2005).

GABA transporters are widely expressed throughout the central nervous system. In particular, the most prevalent GABA transporters are GAT1 and GAT3 (Borden, 1996; Durkin et al., 1995; Scimemi, 2014). High levels of GAT1 are found in the cerebellum, basal ganglia (globus pallidus and ventral pallidum), olfactory bulb, retina, and the interpeduncular nucleus. Moderate levels of GAT1 have been noted throughout the neocortex, amygdala, thalamus, subthalamic nuclei, hypothalamus, substantia nigra, and the spinal cord (laminae I, II, IV, X). The ventral horn of the spinal cord and cerebellar Purkinje cells generally show poor staining for GAT1. Contrary to the wide distribution of GAT1, GAT2 is only expressed in the leptomeninges in order to, perhaps, modulate GABA levels in the cerebrospinal fluid (Scimemi, 2014). GAT3 is abundantly found in the olfactory bulb and the retina. Modest levels of GAT3 are seen in the septum, basal ganglia, amygdala, and thalamus. In contrast to GAT1, the entire neocortex and the spinal cord show minimal GAT3 expression (Borden, 1996; Durkin et al., 1995). Levels of GATs also vary across layers of the cortex. GAT1 is most abundant in layers L2–L4, whereas GAT3 is mainly found in L3 and upper L5 (Minelli, Brecha, Karschin, DeBiasi, & Conti, 1995; Minelli, DeBiasi, Brecha, Zuccarello, & Conti, 1996). GAT2 expression is restricted to the meninges (Conti, Minelli, & Melone, 2004). GABA transporters in the peripheral nervous system remain largely uninvestigated.

In rodents, GAT3 is astrocyte specific with high expression among those surrounding synapses, cell bodies, and basal and apical dendrites (Minelli et al., 1996; Scimemi, 2014). However, other mammals, such as monkeys, cats, and humans, express GAT3 on astrocytes along with oligodendrocytes (Pow et al., 2005). Electron microscopy studies of cortical pyramidal neurons reveal that GAT1 is restricted to axon terminals of symmetrical synapses in the neocortex, largely overlapping with GAD67 presenting neurons (Minelli et al., 1995; Ribak, Tong, & Brecha, 1996; Scimemi, 2014). Interestingly, GAT1 has also been identified on dendritic terminals and soma of non-GABAergic neurons (Yan, Cariaga, & Ribak, 1997). The exact function of this postsynaptic expression is not currently known, but it has been proposed that it aids in sequestering GABA from the synapse and prevents GABA from affecting unintended targets (Scimemi, 2014; Scimemi, Tian, & Diamond, 2009).

The main function of GABA transporters is to remove GABA from extracellular space and thereby terminate its effects. However, under the right conditions, these transporters can reverse their action and release GABA back into the extracellular space (Bicho & Grewer, 2005). As a result, these transporters can affect the time course of GABAergic transmission. Blocking GABA uptake leads to prolonged neuronal response of slow and fast train evoked inhibitory presynaptic currents (IPSCs; Dingledine & Korn, 1985; Isaacson, Solis, & Nicoll, 1993). However, brief fast synaptic IPSCs are largely influenced by GABA diffusion and receptor kinetics rather than GABA reuptake from the synapse (Dingledine & Korn, 1985). This suggests that slower GABAergic currents are regulated by GABA transporters (Szabadics, Tamás, & Soltesz, 2007). Furthermore, different roles of GAT1 and GAT3 have been previously proposed. On thalamic astrocytes, GAT1 is concentrated close to synaptic contacts, whereas GAT3 is found further away from the synapses (Beenhakker & Huguenard, 2010). This subcellular distribution establishes distinct roles of GABA transporters where GAT1 regulates synaptic uptake and GAT3 controls extracellular GABA concentration important in mediating tonic inhibition (Beenhakker & Huguenard, 2010). Recent work has also suggested that GAT1 and GAT3 modulate different signaling pathways depending on vesicular and nonvesicular mechanisms of GABA release during slow or sustained neuronal activity (Kersanté et al., 2013; Song et al., 2013). Interestingly, GABA reuptake mechanisms do not remove all ambient GABA despite the vast distribution of GABA transporters throughout the CNS. This maintains tonic GABAergic currents in order to dampen neuronal transmission (Cavelier, Hamann, Rossi, Mobbs, & Attwell, 2005; Farrant & Nusser, 2005). Therefore, GABA transporters regulate both inhibitory and excitatory conductance, albeit not directly.

3.2 GABA Transporters: Implications for Pain

Under neuropathic pain conditions, the GABAergic system operates inadequately causing a loss of GABAergic tone in the spinal circuits called disinhibition (Coull et al., 2003). Pharmacotherapy that enhances GABAergic function has been shown to reduce pain behaviors and neuronal hyperexcitability postspinal cord injury. Genetically enhancing GAT1 expression results in hyperalgesia while blocking GAT1 with inhibitors, NO-711 and tiagabine, leads to hypoalgesia and a reduction in spontaneous and evoked pain responses after spinal cord injury (Hu et al., 2003; Todorov, Kolchev, & Todorov, 2005). In the paclitaxel-induced neuropathic pain model, the spinal dorsal horn shows an increased expression of GAT1 in presynaptic terminals and astrocytes, while a decrease in GAT3 in astrocytes is observed (Yadav, Yan, Maixner, Gao, & Weng, 2015). The overall result of this is increased GABA reuptake from the synapse and disinhibition. Intrathecal administration of NO-711 ameliorates paclitaxel-induced neuropathic pain (Yadav et al., 2015). On the contrary, antagonizing GAT3 with SNAP5114 yields no significant effect (Yadav et al., 2015). Chronic constriction of the sciatic nerve and spared nerve injury show mixed results. Some studies using chronic constriction of the sciatic nerve and spared nerve injury models have reported an increase in GAT1 expression in the dorsal horn (Daemen, Hoogland, Cijntje, & Spincemaille, 2008), while others have observed a decrease (Miletic, Draganic, Pankratz, & Miletic, 2003; Shih, Miletic, Miletic, & Smith, 2008). Majority of GABA transporter studies have associated GAT1 with neuropathic pain models. However, a few studies have shown that GAT3 inhibition improves allodynia caused by chronic constriction injury in rats and it also ameliorates the second phase response of the formalin model of inflammatory pain (Hu et al., 2003).

4. CHLORIDE HOMEOSTASIS

All of the neurotransmitter transporters mentioned in this chapter depend heavily on the cell's electrochemical potential determined by its intracellular ion concentrations. Ion transporters can use ATP to actively pump ions against their gradients or use the electrochemical potential of another ion (often referred to as ion exchangers). Since sodium and potassium are abundant ions in the body, they are commonly used as a driving ion to transport another ion (known as the driven ion) in the same direction (symporters) or in the opposite direction (antiporters). The nervous system has a plethora of different ion transporters. For brevity, this chapter will focus on chloride cotransporters, Na^+–K^+–$2Cl^-$ cotransporter 1 (NKCC1) and K^+–Cl^- cotransporter 2 (KCC2), as they relate to GABAergic transmission and ultimately to neuropathic pain.

4.1 Chloride Cotransporters

NKCC1 and KCC2 are crucial for determining the strength and polarity of GABA (Price, Cervero, & de Koninck, 2005). NKCC1 actively transports sodium, potassium, and chloride ions into the cell, whereas KCC2 pushes potassium and chloride outward. Phosphorylation of these transporters (pNKCC1, pKCC2) is proposed to enhance transporter activity by improving ion transport rate, cell surface stability, and plasma membrane trafficking (Alessi et al., 2014; Kahle et al., 2013; Modol, Cobianchi, & Navarro, 2014). Their activity is predominantly regulated through this process (Kahle et al., 2013; Modol et al., 2014). When $GABA_A$/glycine receptors are activated, chloride ions either leave or enter the cell. The influx or efflux of chloride is determined by its electrochemical gradient established by these chloride cotransporters (Price et al., 2005). When chloride leaves the cell, intracellular electrochemical potential becomes further depolarized. On the contrary, when chloride extrusion mechanisms are prevalent, chloride seeks to enter the cell leading to greater hyperpolarization. Since the DRG neurons express very little to no KCC2, the intracellular chloride levels are maintained predominantly by NKCC1 (Modol et al., 2014; Price et al., 2005). This leads to an excitatory effect of GABA in the periphery as opposed to an inhibitory effect seen in CNS where KCC2 is abundant (Hasbargen et al., 2010).

Under normal conditions, a neuron's membrane potential is at or around −70 mV, although the exact value depends on a whole host of factors. The anion reversal potential (E_{anion}) of chloride ions is also around −70 mV (Price, Cervero, Gold, Hammond, & Prescott, 2009). In these conditions, opening of $GABA_A$ receptors does not lead to chloride influx since the driving force for chloride ions is minimal, if any. Simultaneous application of excitatory input is significantly dampened as chloride ions seek to maintain an E_{anion} of −70 mV through open $GABA_A$ receptors (Price et al., 2009). This phenomenon is termed shunting and is contrasted with hyperpolarization in which a large driving force pushes K^+ ions out of the cell. In the case of a neuron, the extracellular and intracellular E_{anion} is maintained by a balance of NKCC1 and KCC2 which regulate chloride homeostasis. At birth, NKCC1 levels are abundant in neurons leading to a relatively higher concentration of chloride inside the cell than outside. This makes GABA excitatory during this period. Around about the third week after birth, there is an active suppression of NKCC1 expression and an upregulation of KCC2 in the CNS. Thereby, chloride ions are removed from the cell and E_{anion} is reversed (Falcon, Guendelman, & Stolberg, 1996; Fitzgerald & Gibson, 1984; Jiang & Gebhart, 1998; Marsh, Dickenson, Hatch, & Fitzgerald, 1999; Teng & Abbott, 1998). Neurons in the periphery do not experience such a shift and continue to experience GABAergic input as excitatory into adulthood (Price et al., 2005).

In the spinal cord, local GABAergic interneurons form axo-axonic synapses onto primary afferent terminals leading to primary afferent depolarization (PAD; Zeilhofer, Wildner, & Yévenes, 2012). With abundance of NKCC1 on the primary afferent terminals, intracellular chloride concentration is high compared to the extracellular space. This leads to an efflux of chloride ions in response to GABA and a small depolarization current is passed through the terminal (Price et al., 2005; Zeilhofer et al., 2012). In contrast to depolarizations elsewhere in the nervous system, PAD leads to a decrease in neurotransmitter release by inactivating voltage-gated sodium and voltage-gated calcium channels, and by shunting through open $GABA_A$ channels (Price et al., 2009; Price & Prescott, 2015; Zeilhofer et al., 2012). In this regard, PAD is seen as a form of presynaptic inhibition. However, sufficient increase in PAD may lead to propagation of antidromically conducting action potentials (known as dorsal root reflexes (DRRs)) and further the release of neurotransmitters (Chen et al., 2014; Garcia-Nicas, Laird, & Cervero, 2001; Lin, Wu, & Willis, 1999; Price et al., 2009; Price & Prescott, 2015; Rees, Sluka, Westlund, & Willis, 1994). Administration of $GABA_A$ receptor antagonists (Lin, Li, Xu, Zou, & Fang, 2007; Lin et al., 1999) and NKCC1 antagonist, bumetanide (Valencia-de Ita, Lawand, Lin, Castañeda-Hernandez, & Willis, 2006), prevents the development of DRRs. The exact mechanism of DRRs is not yet resolved.

KCC2 expression in dorsal horn neurons is important in maintaining the inhibitory tone of GABA. It helps maintain a relatively low intracellular chloride concentration such that GABAergic/glycinergic input leads to a chloride influx, hyperpolarization, and ultimately inhibition (Gagnon et al., 2013; Price & Prescott, 2015). Local GABAergic interneurons synapse onto lamina I projection neurons and modulate its activity based on incoming sensory input from primary afferents, descending input from the brain, and complex local circuitry. Reduction of KCC2 expression forms the basis of disinhibition seen in various models of neuropathic pain (Gagnon et al., 2013; Hasbargen et al., 2010; Miletic & Miletic, 2008; Modol et al., 2014; Nomura, Sakai, Nagano, Umino, & Suzuki, 2006; Price & Prescott, 2015; Zhang, Liu, & Xu, 2008). Microglial activation has been shown to cause disinhibition in lamina I neurons (Beggs & Salter, 2013). After peripheral nerve injury, microglia release brain-derived neurotrophic factor (BDNF) as a result of $P2X_4$ receptor activation. BDNF then binds to TrkB receptors on lamina I neurons leading to a downregulation of KCC2. Through disinhibition, projection neurons become less hyperpolarized in response to GABAergic transmission and more sensory and nociceptive information travels to the brain.

4.2 Chloride Cotransporters: Implications for Pain

Chloride cotransporters have the potential to alter the effects of GABA on primary afferent terminals and higher-order neurons of the spinal cord. In various neuropathic pain models, NKCC1 and KCC2 expression and post-translational modifications significantly change across injury and/or disease. In a contusion model of spinal cord injury in rats, NKCC1 levels were shown to increase while KCC2 levels decreased by day 7 postinjury, coinciding with observed hyperalgesia (Hasbargen et al., 2010). In a recent study, peripheral nerve injury lead to an upregulation of NKCC1 in the DRG, a downregulation of KCC2 in the spinal cord, and a temporally later decrease in KCC2 expression in the thalamus and the somatosensory cortex (Modol et al., 2014). Similarly, chronic constriction injury resulted in increased NKCC1 levels in the DRG and decreased KCC2 expression in the dorsal horn 2 days postinjury (Chen et al., 2014). These changes are largely transient and disappear with time even though pain behaviors persist. This indicates that initial response to a neuropathic insult may be due to transient nonsynaptic plasticity while pain at later, chronic stages may be a result of long-lasting synaptic plasticity.

Earlier studies using NKCC1 knockout mice discovered that these mice had impaired noxious heat processing (Sung, Kirby, McDonald, Lovinger, & Delpire, 2000). Although NKCC1 is crucial for development but not necessary, NKCC1 knockout mice have a mortality rate of 30% before weaning (Sung et al., 2000). Those mice that do survive face various comorbidities ranging from poor motor coordination to severe cognitive impairments (Sung et al., 2000). Due to potential confounds in this methodology, later studies have focused on using pharmacological agents, such as bumetanide, to inhibit NKCC1 in neurons. Although bumetanide has been shown to be effective in dampening pain across various models of neuropathic pain (Modol et al., 2014; Pitcher, Price, Entrena, & Cervero, 2007; Sung et al., 2000; Valencia-de Ita et al., 2006), it is a poor agent to study the role of NKCC1 in neurons due to its lack of specificity for NKCC1 and the widespread expression of NKCC1 throughout the body (Price et al., 2009). Intraperitoneal administration of bumetanide affects NKCCs not only in the PNS but also in the kidneys and exocrine glands (Hannaert, Alvarez-Guerra, Pirot, Nazaret, & Garay, 2002). Any effects observed after a systemic injection of bumetanide must be subjected to these confounding factors.

Efforts to identify a pharmacological agent for enhancing KCC2 in the spinal cord have mainly been hindered by lack of specificity. Recent research has, however, identified CLP257 and CLP290 as a selective KCC2 activators (Gagnon et al., 2013). As a prodrug of CLP257, CLP290 was designed to protect its hydroxyl group from glucuronidation. CLP257 generated from the body's metabolism of CLP290 is more potent and longer lasting than CLP257 given intraperitoneally. Regardless, administration of both these compounds has been reported to enhance Cl^- transport and increase recruitment of KCC2 to the plasma membrane (Gagnon et al., 2013). Behaviorally, this alleviates pain hypersensitivity in rats with peripheral nerve injury (Gagnon et al., 2013). Since KCC2 is only found in neurons of the central nervous system, administration of CLP257 and CLP290 is not subjected to the same confounding factors as bumetanide for inhibiting NKCC1. The effects of these compounds have not been widely studied in pain models due to their novelty.

5. MONOAMINERGIC SYSTEM

Monoamine neurotransmitters are a class of neurotransmitters containing one amino group connected to an aromatic ring by a carbon–carbon chain. The most prevalent monoamine neurotransmitters are dopamine (DA), norepinephrine (NE), and serotonin (5-hydroxytryptamine) (Lin, Canales, et al., 2011). These neurotransmitters regulate various cognitive processes from emotions to arousal and even certain forms of memory (Howell & Kimmel, 2008; Seamans & Yang, 2004; Volkow et al., 2000). DA and NE are derived from L-tyrosine (Snyder, 2011), whereas serotonin is synthesized from L-tryptophan (Leu-Semenescu et al., 2010). Although these monoamines are derived from different amino acids, their structure is quite similar. As a result, many monoamine transporters translocate multiple types of monoamines with varying degrees of specificity (Lin, Canales, et al., 2011). Alterations in specificity and expression of monoamine transporters can modify monoamine functioning in the nervous system. Treatment for neuropathic pain has targeted these transport mechanisms via drugs such as selective serotonin reuptake inhibitors (SSRIs), selective NE/DA reuptake inhibitors (SNDRIs), and tricyclic antidepressants (TCAs).

5.1 Monoamine Transporters

Along with GATs, monoamine transporters are part of the solute carrier 6 (SLC6) family of transporters (Scimemi, 2014). They are transmembrane proteins located specifically on monoaminergic neurons. Their expression is highly selective to their respective neurons such that they are often used as markers for their neuron subtype (Lin, Canales, et al., 2011). DA, NE, and serotonin are transported across the plasma membrane by DA transporters (DATs), NE transporters (NETs), and serotonin transporters (SERTs; 5-HTT). Although their nomenclature suggests high specificity, each transporter is capable of carrying another monoamine neurotransmitter, albeit to a lesser extent. Like other transporters discussed, Na^+/Cl^- electrochemical gradients are used to facilitate transport across the membrane (Amara & Kuhar, 1993; Langer & Galzin, 1988). Vesicular monoamine transporters (VMAT1 and VMAT2), however, use a proton motive force to transport monoamines into synaptic vesicles (Henry et al., 1994). VMAT1 and VMAT2 are present in all monoaminergic cell types with VMAT1 transiently expressed only during early development (Hansson, Mezey, & Hoffman, 1998). Each of these transporters is crucial to modulating temporal and spatial aspects of monoaminergic conductance.

Dopaminergic neurons of the ventral tegmental area project to nucleus accumbens (Ikemoto & Panksepp, 1999; Pennartz, Groenewegen, & Lopes Da Silva, 1994) and the prefrontal cortex (Seamans & Yang, 2004), while those originating from the substantia nigra synapse largely onto the striatum (Groenewegen, 2003). All of these dopaminergic neurons selectively express DAT (Lin, Canales, et al., 2011). On the contrary, serotonergic and norepinephrinergic neurons, along with SERT and NET, are more widespread throughout the brain. Serotonergic neurons are largely found in the raphe nuclei of the brain stem from which they spread their axons throughout the telencephalon, diencephalon, and mesencephalon (Moore, Halaris, & Jones, 1978). Similarly, NET is expressed on NE neurons of the locus coeruleus and the lateral tegmental nuclei which project to various areas of the brain (Moore & Bloom, 1978). Furthermore, monoaminergic neurons of the brain provide descending inputs to various levels of the spinal cord, where sensory modulation can occur (Hoshino, Obata, Nakajima, Mieda, & Saito, 2015). The wide expression of these neurotransmitters and their transporters makes them important in modulating various functions of the nervous system.

Subcellular localization of each monoamine transporter varies according to the region being innervated. NET is mainly restricted to the intracellular environment in the prefrontal cortex (Miner et al., 2006). This expression is also highly correlated with the absence of tyrosine hydroxylase which is the enzyme responsible for converting L-tyrosine to L-DOPA, a precursor to DA and NE (Miner et al., 2006). This indicates that most NE neurons in the prefrontal cortex do not synthesize or reuptake NE. As a result, under physiological conditions, NE neurons in the prefrontal cortex conduct action potentials in a low-activity state (Lin, Canales, et al., 2011). With disease, NET plasmalemmal recruitment increases in this area along with the expression of tyrosine hydroxylase to induce a high-activity state of transmission (Miner et al., 2006). On the contrary, SERT and DAT are abundantly expressed on the presynaptic terminals as well as on the surrounding plasma membrane (Nirenberg, Vaughan, Uhl, Kuhar, & Pickel, 1996; Zhou, Tao-Cheng, Segu, Patel, & Wang, 1998). This supports the notion that DA and serotonin are released abundantly under physiological neurotransmission. Recent studies have also shown that DA and serotonin could be released from postsynaptic dendrites (Chen & Rice, 2001; Colgan, Cavolo, Commons, & Levitan, 2012; Roseberry, 2015). DA and serotonin released in this manner are also sequestered by synaptic DATs and SERTs; however, the exact regulatory function of these transporters in this mechanism is not well understood.

Although the primary ligand for DATs is DA, various drugs, both therapeutic and recreational, bind to DATs as either inhibitors or substrates. DAT inhibitors, such as cocaine, bind to the symporter and prevent transport of DA across the membrane (Schmitt, Rothman, & Reith, 2013). On the contrary, DAT substrates, like DA itself, get transported across the membrane and processed intracellularly (Schmitt et al., 2013). As such, amphetaminergic substrates compete for DA binding site on DAT, get translocated across the membrane, and increase the intracellular Na^+ concentration (Sitte et al., 1998). This, in turn, leads to a reversal of DAT activity and DA efflux due to a switch in Na^+ gradient (Khoshbouei, Wang, Lechleiter, Javitch, & Galli, 2003). Both of these mechanisms cause an accumulation of DA extracellularly and thereby enhance its effects, particularly, on reward and addiction systems. Recent research has largely challenged the previous notion of cocaine-like dependence for compounds that affect DAT functioning (Carroll et al., 2010; Schmitt et al., 2013; Vosburg, Hart, Haney, Rubin, & Foltin, 2010). The chemical structure of a DAT ligand can induce a specific conformational change to the protein that elicits a particular downstream process similar to pleiotropic characteristics of G-protein-coupled receptors (Urban et al., 2007). This suggests that each DAT ligand is functionally unique in its behavioral and psychological effects (Li et al., 2011).

5.2 Monoamine Transporters: Implications for Pain

Monoamines in the nervous system are involved in regulating complex behaviors and emotions. Impairment in the monoaminergic system can lead to disease and disorders such as depression, obsessive–compulsive disorder, and attention-deficit hyperactivity disorder (Lin, Canales, et al., 2011). Pain has also been associated with a deterioration of monoaminergic transporters. In this respect, antidepressants, including TCAs, SSRIs, and selective NE reuptake inhibitors (SNRIs), are recommended as first-line treatment for neuropathic pain (Dworkin et al., 2007). These drugs effectively increase NE and DA levels in the spinal cord and mimic or enhance descending antinociceptive inputs from the brain (Nakajima, Obata, Iriuchijima, & Saito, 2012). Intrathecal administration of bupropion inhibits DA–NE reuptake in the spinal cord of rats with a ligated spinal nerve (Hoshino et al., 2015). The accumulation of extracellular DA and NE combined with an upregulation of α2-adrenoceptors and D2 receptors in the substantia gelatinosa dampens pain behaviors in these animals. Other animal studies have reported that α2-adrenoceptor activation leads to downstream activation of inhibitory cholinergic interneurons restoring disinhibition (Bantel, Eisenach, Duflo, Tobin, & Childers, 2005; Eisenach, Zhang, & Duflo, 2005; Obata, Li, & Eisenach, 2005). DA's antinociceptive effects are mediated only as descending inputs since cell bodies in the spinal cord do not produce DA (Holstege et al., 1996). Focal electrical stimulation of dopaminergic neurons of area A11 in the periventricular nucleus attenuates activity of nociceptive fibers in the spinal dorsal horn (Fleetwood-Walker, Hope, & Mitchell, 1988). However, changes in the monoaminergic system in the spinal cord seem to be transient (Hoshino et al., 2015). Tibial and sciatic nerve ligations, both, lead to an initial increase in monoaminergic descending inputs, followed by normalization to control levels around 3 weeks postinjury (Hayashida, Clayton, Johnson, & Eisenach, 2008; Hughes, Hickey, Hulse, Lumb, & Pickering, 2013). Moreover, clinical studies show that TCAs, SNDRIs, and SSRIs yield promising results in treating fibromyalgia pain (Staud, 2010). In this model, SNRIs are more efficacious in treating neuropathic pain compared to TCAs (Evren, Evren, & Guler, 2006; Lin, Canales, et al., 2011). The key in treating pain seems to be a combination of drugs affecting multiple monoamine transporters.

Neuropathic pain is a debilitating disorder that can severely impact an individual's quality of life (Van Hecke et al., 2014). It has long been associated with clinical depression and anxiety (Debono et al., 2013). Since monoamines are important in various cognitive functions, this makes them a worthwhile target for treating pain along with pain-related depression and anxiety. Depression is a complex condition likely to be a result of various impairments, but recent work has implicated the hypofunction of dopaminergic system in the brain to play a role in mediating depression. DAT, NET, and SERT inhibiting compounds, such as cocaine, are associated with euphoria (Cavelier et al., 2005; Lin, Canales, et al., 2011). The wide influence of monoamines can also detrimental because therapeutic agents targeting these systems can cause severe unintended side effects (Schmitt et al., 2013). TCAs, venlafaxine and duloxetine, inhibit serotonin and NE reuptake in the central nervous system but also lead to adverse side effects such as nausea, somnolence, dizziness, and fatigue (Basbaum & Fields, 1984; Jann & Slade, 2007; McQuay et al., 1996). These effects have been associated with increased serotonin in the system rather than increased NE (Angus et al., 2011). Furthermore, classical compounds targeting DATs have cocaine-like abuse liabilities despite analgesic properties. Thus, ideal compounds should have lower affinity to DATs and a higher selectivity for SERT/NET than individual selective inhibitors. Amitifadine, an SNDRI, has recently been identified as such an agent with antinociceptive effects similar to morphine and ketoprofen without the associated abuse potential (Angus et al., 2011). Research on compounds with ideal affinities for each of the three monoamines is still in its infancy.

6. CONCLUSION

Neuropathic pain is a complex disease of the nervous system characterized by injury or disease of the somatosensory nervous system. Various neurotransmitter systems throughout the nervous system are consistently involved in mediating neuropathic pain hypersensitivity. From the release of Glu by primary afferent to the top-down processing in the spinal cord by monoaminergic fibers, neurotransmitter transporters are crucial in modulating pain perception. In essence, increased excitatory and decreased inhibitory tones in the spinal circuitry lead to behavioral manifestation of hyperalgesia and allodynia. Although there have been tremendous advances in this regard, further research is needed to identify ideal pharmacological compounds that would reverse changes across various neurotransmitter systems and resolve pain while minimizing adverse side effects.

CONFLICT OF INTEREST

The authors declare no competing financial interests.

ACKNOWLEDGMENTS

Funding for this project was provided by operating grants from the Canadian Institutes of Health Research (CIHR) MOP-119338 and MOP-86712, the University of Alberta, Alberta Innovates Health Solutions (CRIO), Natural Sciences and Engineering Research Council of Canada (NSERC), and the MS Society of Canada (MSSC). M.S.Y. was supported by a studentship from NSERC and B.J.K. by a Donald Paty Career Development Award from the MSSC.

REFERENCES

Akam, T., & Kullmann, D. M. (2010). Oscillations and filtering networks support flexible routing of information. *Neuron*, *67*, 308–320.

Alessi, D. R., Zhang, J., Khanna, A., Hochdorfer, T., Shang, Y., & Kahle, K. T. (2014). The WNK-SPAK/OSR1 pathway: Master regulator of cation-chloride cotransporters. *Science Signaling*, 7, re3.

Amara, S. G., & Kuhar, M. J. (1993). Neurotransmitter transporters: Recent progress. *Annual Review of Neuroscience*, *16*, 73–93.

Angus, D., Bingham, M., Buchanan, D., Dunbar, N., Gibson, L., Goodwin, R., … Walker, G. (2011). The identification, and optimisation of hERG selectivity, of a mixed NET/SERT re-uptake inhibitor for the treatment of pain. *Bioorganic & Medicinal Chemistry Letters*, *21*, 271–275.

Arriza, J. L., Eliasof, S., Kavanaugh, M. P., & Amara, S. G. (1997). Excitatory amino acid transporter 5, a retinal glutamate transporter coupled to a chloride conductance. *Proceedings of the National Academy of Sciences of the United States of America*, *94*, 4155–4160.

Arriza, J. L., Kavanaugh, M. P., Fairman, W. A., Wu, Y. N., Murdoch, G. H., North, R. A., & Amara, S. G. (1993). Cloning and expression of a human neutral amino acid transporter with structural similarity to the glutamate transporter gene family. *The Journal of Biological Chemistry*, *268*, 15329–15332.

Bantel, C., Eisenach, J. C., Duflo, F., Tobin, J. R., & Childers, S. R. (2005). Spinal nerve ligation increases alpha2-adrenergic receptor G-protein coupling in the spinal cord. *Brain Research*, *1038*, 76–82.

Basbaum, A. I., & Fields, H. L. (1984). Endogenous pain control systems: Brainstem spinal pathways and endorphin circuitry. *Annual Review of Neuroscience*, 7, 309–338.

Beart, P. M., & O'Shea, R. D. (2007). Transporters for L-glutamate: An update on their molecular pharmacology and pathological involvement. *British Journal of Pharmacology*, *150*, 5–17.

Beenhakker, M. P., & Huguenard, J. R. (2010). Astrocytes as gatekeepers of GABAB receptor function. *The Journal of Neuroscience: The Official Journal of the Society for Neuroscience*, *30*, 15262–15276.

Beggs, S., & Salter, M. W. (2013). The known knowns of microglia-neuronal signalling in neuropathic pain. *Neuroscience Letters*, *557*(Pt A), 37–42.

Bezzi, P., Gundersen, V., Galbete, J. L., Seifert, G., Steinhäuser, C., Pilati, E., & Volterra, A. (2004). Astrocytes contain a vesicular compartment that is competent for regulated exocytosis of glutamate. *Nature Neuroscience*, 7, 613–620.

Bicho, A., & Grewer, C. (2005). Rapid substrate-induced charge movements of the GABA transporter GAT1. *Biophysical Journal*, *89*, 211–231.

Borden, L. A. (1996). GABA transporter heterogeneity: Pharmacology and cellular localization. *Neurochemistry International*, *29*, 335–356.

Caddy, C., Amit, B. H., McCloud, T. L., Rendell, J. M., Furukawa, T. A., McShane, R., … Cipriani, A. (2015). Ketamine and other glutamate receptor modulators for depression in adults. *The Cochrane Database of Systematic Reviews*, *9*, CD011612.

Carozzi, V. A., Canta, A., Oggioni, N., Ceresa, C., Marmiroli, P., Konvalinka, J., ... Cavaletti, G. (2008). Expression and distribution of "high affinity" glutamate transporters GLT1, GLAST, EAAC1 and of GCPII in the rat peripheral nervous system. *Journal of Anatomy*, *213*, 539–546.

Carroll, F. I., Blough, B. E., Mascarella, S. W., Navarro, H. A., Eaton, J. B., Lukas, R. J., & Damaj, M. I. (2010). Synthesis and biological evaluation of bupropion analogues as potential pharmacotherapies for smoking cessation. *Journal of Medicinal Chemistry*, *53*, 2204–2214.

Cavaliere, C., Cirillo, G., Rosaria Bianco, M., Rossi, F., De Novellis, V., Maione, S., & Papa, M. (2007). Gliosis alters expression and uptake of spinal glial amino acid transporters in a mouse neuropathic pain model. *Neuron Glia Biology*, *3*, 141–153.

Cavelier, P., Hamann, M., Rossi, D., Mobbs, P., & Attwell, D. (2005). Tonic excitation and inhibition of neurons: Ambient transmitter sources and computational consequences. *Progress in Biophysics and Molecular Biology*, *87*, 3–16.

Chen, J. T., Guo, D., Campanelli, D., Frattini, F., Mayer, F., Zhou, L., ... Hu, J. (2014). Presynaptic GABAergic inhibition regulated by BDNF contributes to neuropathic pain induction. *Nature Communications*, *5*, 5331.

Chen, B. T., & Rice, M. E. (2001). Novel Ca2+ dependence and time course of somatodendritic dopamine release: Substantia nigra versus striatum. *The Journal of Neuroscience: The Official Journal of the Society for Neuroscience*, *21*, 7841–7847.

Colgan, L. A., Cavolo, S. L., Commons, K. G., & Levitan, E. S. (2012). Action potential-independent and pharmacologically unique vesicular serotonin release from dendrites. *The Journal of Neuroscience: The Official Journal of the Society for Neuroscience*, *32*, 15737–15746.

Conti, F., Minelli, A., & Melone, M. (2004). GABA transporters in the mammalian cerebral cortex: Localization, development and pathological implications. *Brain Research Reviews*, *45*, 196–212.

Coull, J. A. M., Boudreau, D., Bachand, K., Prescott, S. A., Nault, F., Sík, A., ... De Koninck, Y. (2003). Trans-synaptic shift in anion gradient in spinal lamina I neurons as a mechanism of neuropathic pain. *Nature*, *424*, 938–942.

Daemen, M. A. R. C., Hoogland, G., Cijntje, J.-M., & Spincemaille, G. H. (2008). Upregulation of the GABA-transporter GAT-1 in the spinal cord contributes to pain behaviour in experimental neuropathy. *Neuroscience Letters*, *444*, 112–115.

Danbolt, N. C. (2001). Glutamate uptake. *Progress in Neurobiology*, *65*, 1–105.

Debono, D. J., Hoeksema, L. J., & Hobbs, R. D. (2013). Caring for patients with chronic pain: Pearls and pitfalls. *The Journal of the American Osteopathic Association*, *113*, 620–627.

Dingledine, R., & Korn, S. J. (1985). Gamma-aminobutyric acid uptake and the termination of inhibitory synaptic potentials in the rat hippocampal slice. *The Journal of Physiology*, *366*, 387–409.

Domercq, M., & Matute, C. (1999). Expression of glutamate transporters in the adult bovine corpus callosum. *Molecular Brain Research*, *67*, 296–302.

Duman, R. S., & Li, N. (2012). A neurotrophic hypothesis of depression: Role of synaptogenesis in the actions of NMDA receptor antagonists. *Philosophical Transactions of the Royal Society, B: Biological Sciences*, *367*, 2475–2484.

Durkin, M. M., Smith, K. E., Borden, L. A., Weinshank, R. L., Branchek, T. A., & Gustafson, E. L. (1995). Localization of messenger RNAs encoding three GABA transporters in rat brain: An in situ hybridization study. *Brain Research. Molecular Brain Research*, *33*, 7–21.

Dworkin, R. H., O'Connor, A. B., Backonja, M., Farrar, J. T., Finnerup, N. B., Jensen, T. S., ... Wallace, M. S. (2007). Pharmacologic management of neuropathic pain: Evidence-based recommendations. *Pain*, *132*, 237–251.

Eisenach, J. C., Zhang, Y., & Duflo, F. (2005). alpha2-Adrenoceptors inhibit the intracellular Ca^{2+} response to electrical stimulation in normal and injured sensory neurons, with increased inhibition of calcitonin gene-related peptide expressing neurons after injury. *Neuroscience, 131*, 189–197.

Evren, B., Evren, C., & Guler, M. H. (2006). An open clinical trial of venlafaxine in the treatment of pain, depressive and anxiety symptoms in fibromyalgia. *The Pain Clinic, 18*, 167–173.

Fairman, W. A., Vandenberg, R. J., Arriza, J. L., Kavanaugh, M. P., & Amara, S. G. (1995). An excitatory amino-acid transporter with properties of a ligand-gated chloride channel. *Nature, 375*, 599–603.

Falcon, M., Guendelman, D., & Stolberg, A. (1996). Development of thermal nociception in rats. *Pain, 67*, 203–208.

Farrant, M., & Nusser, Z. (2005). Variations on an inhibitory theme: Phasic and tonic activation of GABA(A) receptors. *Nature Reviews. Neuroscience, 6*, 215–229.

Fitzgerald, M., & Gibson, S. (1984). The postnatal physiological and neurochemical development of peripheral sensory C fibres. *Neuroscience, 13*, 933–944.

Fleetwood-Walker, S. M., Hope, P. J., & Mitchell, R. (1988). Antinociceptive actions of descending dopaminergic tracts on cat and rat dorsal horn somatosensory neurones. *The Journal of Physiology, 399*, 335–348.

Furness, D. N., Dehnes, Y., Akhtar, A. Q., Rossi, D. J., Hamann, M., Grutle, N. J., … Danbolt, N. C. (2008). A quantitative assessment of glutamate uptake into hippocampal synaptic terminals and astrocytes: New insights into a neuronal role for excitatory amino acid transporter 2 (EAAT2). *Neuroscience, 157*, 80–94.

Gagnon, M., Bergeron, M. J., Lavertu, G., Castonguay, A., Tripathy, S., Bonin, R. P., … De Koninck, Y. (2013). Chloride extrusion enhancers as novel therapeutics for neurological diseases. *Nature Medicine, 19*, 1524–1528.

Garcia-Nicas, E., Laird, J. M., & Cervero, F. (2001). Vasodilatation in hyperalgesic rat skin evoked by stimulation of afferent A beta-fibers: Further evidence for a role of dorsal root reflexes in allodynia. *Pain, 94*, 283–291.

Gegelashvili, G., & Bjerrum, O. J. (2014). High-affinity glutamate transporters in chronic pain: An emerging therapeutic target. *Journal of Neurochemistry, 131*, 712–730.

Gegelashvili, G., Robinson, M. B., Trotti, D., & Rauen, T. (2001). Regulation of glutamate transporters in health and disease. *Progress in Brain Research, 132*, 267–286.

Gegelashvili, G., & Schousboe, A. (1998). Cellular distribution and kinetic properties of high-affinity glutamate transporters. *Brain Research Bulletin, 45*, 233–238.

Gerrow, K., & Triller, A. (2010). Synaptic stability and plasticity in a floating world. *Current Opinion in Neurobiology, 20*, 631–639.

Grewer, C., Gameiro, A., & Rauen, T. (2014). SLC1 glutamate transporters. *Pflügers Archiv/ European Journal of Physiology, 466*, 3–24.

Groenewegen, H. J. (2003). The basal ganglia and motor control. *Neural Plasticity, 10*, 107–120.

Gwak, Y. S., & Hulsebosch, C. E. (2011). GABA and central neuropathic pain following spinal cord injury. *Neuropharmacology, 60*, 799–808.

Hájos, N., Pálhalmi, J., Mann, E. O., Németh, B., Paulsen, O., & Freund, T. F. (2004). Spike timing of distinct types of GABAergic interneuron during hippocampal gamma oscillations in vitro. *The Journal of Neuroscience: The Official Journal of the Society for Neuroscience, 24*, 9127–9137.

Hannaert, P., Alvarez-Guerra, M., Pirot, D., Nazaret, C., & Garay, R. (2002). Rat NKCC2/ NKCC1 cotransporter selectivity for loop diuretic drugs. *Naunyn-Schmiedeberg's Archives of Pharmacology, 365*, 193–199.

Hansson, S. R., Mezey, E., & Hoffman, B. J. (1998). Ontogeny of vesicular monoamine transporter mRNAs VMAT1 and VMAT2. II. Expression in neural crest derivatives and their target sites in the rat. *Brain Research. Developmental Brain Research, 110*, 159–174.

Hasbargen, T., Ahmed, M. M., Miranpuri, G., Li, L., Kahle, K. T., Resnick, D., & Sun, D. (2010). Role of NKCC1 and KCC2 in the development of chronic neuropathic pain following spinal cord injury. *Annals of the New York Academy of Sciences, 1198*, 168–172.

Hayashida, K.-I., Clayton, B. A., Johnson, J. E., & Eisenach, J. C. (2008). Brain derived nerve growth factor induces spinal noradrenergic fiber sprouting and enhances clonidine analgesia following nerve injury in rats. *Pain, 136*, 348–355.

Henry, J. P., Botton, D., Sagne, C., Isambert, M. F., Desnos, C., Blanchard, V., … Gasnier, B. (1994). Biochemistry and molecular biology of the vesicular monoamine transporter from chromaffin granules. *The Journal of Experimental Biology, 196*, 251–262.

Holstege, J. C., Van Dijken, H., Buijs, R. M., Goedknegt, H., Gosens, T., & Bongers, C. M. H. (1996). Distribution of dopamine immunoreactivity in the rat, cat, and monkey spinal cord. *Journal of Comparative Neurology, 376*, 631–652.

Hoshino, H., Obata, H., Nakajima, K., Mieda, R., & Saito, S. (2015). The antihyperalgesic effects of intrathecal bupropion, a dopamine and noradrenaline reuptake inhibitor, in a rat model of neuropathic pain. *Anesthesia and Analgesia, 120*, 460–466.

Howell, L. L., & Kimmel, H. L. (2008). Monoamine transporters and psychostimulant addiction. *Biochemical Pharmacology, 75*, 196–217.

Hu, J.-H., Yang, N., Ma, Y.-H., Zhou, X.-G., Jiang, J., Duan, S.-H., … Guo, L.-H. (2003). Hyperalgesic effects of gamma-aminobutyric acid transporter I in mice. *Journal of Neuroscience Research, 73*, 565–572.

Hughes, S. W., Hickey, L., Hulse, R. P., Lumb, B. M., & Pickering, A. E. (2013). Endogenous analgesic action of the pontospinal noradrenergic system spatially restricts and temporally delays the progression of neuropathic pain following tibial nerve injury. *Pain, 154*, 1680–1690.

Ikemoto, S., & Panksepp, J. (1999). The role of nucleus accumbens dopamine in motivated behavior: A unifying interpretation with special reference to reward-seeking. *Brain Research. Brain Research Reviews, 31*, 6–41.

Isaacson, J. S., Solis, J. M., & Nicoll, R. A. (1993). Local and diffuse synaptic actions of GABA in the hippocampus. *Neuron, 10*, 165–175.

Jann, M. W., & Slade, J. H. (2007). Antidepressant agents for the treatment of chronic pain and depression. *Pharmacotherapy, 27*, 1571–1587.

Jiang, M. C., & Gebhart, G. F. (1998). Development of mustard oil-induced hyperalgesia in rats. *Pain, 77*, 305–313.

Kahle, K. T., Deeb, T. Z., Puskarjov, M., Silayeva, L., Liang, B., Kaila, K., & Moss, S. J. (2013). Modulation of neuronal activity by phosphorylation of the K-Cl cotransporter KCC2. *Trends in Neurosciences, 36*, 726–737.

Kanai, Y., Clémençon, B., Simonin, A., Leuenberger, M., Lochner, M., Weisstanner, M., & Hediger, M. A. (2013). The SLC1 high-affinity glutamate and neutral amino acid transporter family. *Molecular Aspects of Medicine, 34*, 108–120.

Kanai, Y., & Hediger, M. A. (1992). Primary structure and functional characterization of a high-affinity glutamate transporter. *Nature, 360*, 467–471.

Kanner, B. I., & Sharon, I. (1978). Active transport of L-glutamate by membrane vesicles isolated from rat brain. *Biochemistry, 17*, 3949–3953.

Kavanaughs, M. P., Arriza, J. L., North, R. A., & Amara, S. G. (1992). Electrogenic uptake of GABA by a cloned transporter expressed in Xenopus oocytes. *Journal of Biological Chemistry, 267*, 22007–22009.

Kemenes, I., Straub, V. A., Nikitin, E. S., Staras, K., O'Shea, M., Kemenes, G., & Benjamin, P. R. (2006). Role of delayed nonsynaptic neuronal plasticity in long-term associative memory. *Current Biology, 16*, 1269–1279.

Kersanté, F., Rowley, S. C. S., Pavlov, I., Gutièrrez-Mecinas, M., Semyanov, A., Reul, J. M. H. M., … Gutierrez-Mecinas, M. (2013). A functional role for both GABA transporter-1 and GABA transporter-3 in the modulation of extracellular GABA and

GABAergic tonic conductances in the rat hippocampus. *The Journal of Physiology, 591*, 2429–2441.

Khoshbouei, H., Wang, H., Lechleiter, J. D., Javitch, J. A., & Galli, A. (2003). Amphetamine-induced dopamine efflux: A voltage-sensitive and intracellular Na^+-dependent mechanism. *Journal of Biological Chemistry, 278*, 12070–12077.

Langer, S. Z., & Galzin, A. M. (1988). Studies on the serotonin transporter in platelets. *Experientia, 44*, 127–130.

Laursen, J. C., Cairns, B. E., Dong, X. D., Kumar, U., Somvanshi, R. K., Arendt-Nielsen, L., & Gazerani, P. (2014). Glutamate dysregulation in the trigeminal ganglion: A novel mechanism for peripheral sensitization of the craniofacial region. *Neuroscience, 256*, 23–35.

Leu-Semenescu, S., Arnulf, I., Decaix, C., Moussa, F., Clot, F., Boniol, C., ... Roze, E. (2010). Sleep and rhythm consequences of a genetically induced loss of serotonin. *Sleep, 33*, 307–314.

Li, S.-M., Kopajtic, T. A., O'Callaghan, M. J., Agoston, G. E., Cao, J., Newman, A. H., & Katz, J. L. (2011). N-substituted benztropine analogs: Selective dopamine transporter ligands with a fast onset of action and minimal cocaine-like behavioral effects. *The Journal of Pharmacology and Experimental Therapeutics, 336*, 575–585.

Liaw, W. J., Stephens, R. L., Binns, B. C., Chu, Y., Sepkuty, J. P., Johns, R. A., ... Tao, Y. X. (2005). Spinal glutamate uptake is critical for maintaining normal sensory transmission in rat spinal cord. *Pain, 115*, 60–70.

Lin, Z., Canales, J. J., Björgvinsson, T., Thomsen, M., Qu, H., Liu, Q. R., ... Caine, S. B. (2011). Monoamine transporters: Vulnerable and vital doorkeepers. *Progress in Molecular Biology and Translational Science, 98*, 1–46. http://dx.doi.org/10.1016/B978-0-12-385506-0.00001-6.

Lin, Q., Li, D., Xu, X., Zou, X., & Fang, L. (2007). Roles of TRPV1 and neuropeptidergic receptors in dorsal root reflex-mediated neurogenic inflammation induced by intradermal injection of capsaicin. *Molecular Pain, 3*, 30.

Lin, Y., Roman, K., Foust, K. D., Kaspar, B. K., Bailey, M. T., & Stephens, R. L. (2011). Glutamate transporter GLT-1 upregulation attenuates visceral nociception and hyperalgesia via spinal mechanisms not related to anti-inflammatory or probiotic effects. *Pain Research and Treatment, 2011*, 507029.

Lin, Q., Wu, J., & Willis, W. D. (1999). Dorsal root reflexes and cutaneous neurogenic inflammation after intradermal injection of capsaicin in rats. *Journal of Neurophysiology, 82*, 2602–2611.

Loeser, J. D., & Treede, R. D. (2008). The Kyoto protocol of IASP Basic Pain Terminology. *Pain, 137*, 473–477.

Loo, D. D., Eskandari, S., Boorer, K. J., Sarkar, H. K., & Wright, E. M. (2000). Role of Cl^- in electrogenic Na^+-coupled cotransporters GAT1 and SGLT1. *The Journal of Biological Chemistry, 275*, 37414–37422.

Lu, C. C., & Hilgemann, D. W. (1999a). GAT1 (GABA:Na^+:Cl^-) cotransport function. Kinetic studies in giant Xenopus oocyte membrane patches. *The Journal of General Physiology, 114*, 445–457.

Lu, C. C., & Hilgemann, D. W. (1999b). GAT1 (GABA:Na^+:Cl^-) cotransport function. Steady state studies in giant Xenopus oocyte membrane patches. *The Journal of General Physiology, 114*, 429–444.

Maeda, S., Kawamoto, A., Yatani, Y., Shirakawa, H., Nakagawa, T., & Kaneko, S. (2008). Gene transfer of GLT-1, a glial glutamate transporter, into the spinal cord by recombinant adenovirus attenuates inflammatory and neuropathic pain in rats. *Molecular Pain, 4*, 65.

Mager, S., Naeve, J., Quick, M., Labarca, C., Davidson, N., & Lester, H. A. (1993). Steady states, charge movements, and rates for a cloned GABA transporter expressed in Xenopus oocytes. *Neuron, 10*, 177–188.

Mann, E. O., & Mody, I. (2010). Control of hippocampal gamma oscillation frequency by tonic inhibition and excitation of interneurons. *Nature Neuroscience, 13*, 205–212.

Marsh, D., Dickenson, A., Hatch, D., & Fitzgerald, M. (1999). Epidural opioid analgesia in infant rats I: Mechanical and heat responses. *Pain*, *82*, 23–32.
McQuay, H. J., Tramèr, M., Nye, B. A., Carroll, D., Wiffen, P. J., & Moore, R. A. (1996). A systematic review of antidepressants in neuropathic pain. *Pain*, *68*, 217–227.
Melzack, R., & Wall, P. D. (1965). Pain mechanisms: A new theory. *Science*, *150*, 971–979.
Miletic, G., Draganic, P., Pankratz, M. T., & Miletic, V. (2003). Muscimol prevents long-lasting potentiation of dorsal horn field potentials in rats with chronic constriction injury exhibiting decreased levels of the GABA transporter GAT-1. *Pain*, *105*, 347–353.
Miletic, G., & Miletic, V. (2008). Loose ligation of the sciatic nerve is associated with TrkB receptor-dependent decreases in KCC2 protein levels in the ipsilateral spinal dorsal horn. *Pain*, *137*, 532–539.
Minelli, A., Brecha, N. C., Karschin, C., DeBiasi, S., & Conti, F. (1995). GAT-1, a high-affinity GABA plasma membrane transporter, is localized to neurons and astroglia in the cerebral cortex. *The Journal of Neuroscience: The Official Journal of the Society for Neuroscience*, *15*, 7734–7746.
Minelli, A., DeBiasi, S., Brecha, N. C., Zuccarello, L. V., & Conti, F. (1996). GAT-3, a high-affinity GABA plasma membrane transporter, is localized to astrocytic processes, and it is not confined to the vicinity of GABAergic synapses in the cerebral cortex. *The Journal of Neuroscience : The Official Journal of the Society for Neuroscience*, *16*, 6255–6264.
Miner, L. H., Jedema, H. P., Moore, F. W., Blakely, R. D., Grace, A. A., & Sesack, S. R. (2006). Chronic stress increases the plasmalemmal distribution of the norepinephrine transporter and the coexpression of tyrosine hydroxylase in norepinephrine axons in the prefrontal cortex. *The Journal of Neuroscience: The Official Journal of the Society for Neuroscience*, *26*, 1571–1578.
Modol, L., Cobianchi, S., & Navarro, X. (2014). Prevention of NKCC1 phosphorylation avoids downregulation of KCC2 in central sensory pathways and reduces neuropathic pain after peripheral nerve injury. *Pain*, *155*, 1577–1590.
Moore, R. Y., & Bloom, F. E. (1978). Central catecholamine neuron systems: Anatomy and physiology of the dopamine systems. *Annual Review of Neuroscience*, *1*, 129–169.
Moore, R. Y., Halaris, A. E., & Jones, B. E. (1978). Serotonin neurons of the midbrain raphe: Ascending projections. *The Journal of Comparative Neurology*, *180*, 417–438.
Nakajima, K., Obata, H., Iriuchijima, N., & Saito, S. (2012). An increase in spinal cord noradrenaline is a major contributor to the antihyperalgesic effect of antidepressants after peripheral nerve injury in the rat. *Pain*, *153*, 990–997.
Napier, I. A., Mohammadi, S. A., & Christie, M. J. (2012). Glutamate transporter dysfunction associated with nerve injury-induced pain in mice. *Journal of Neurophysiology*, *107*, 649–657.
Nirenberg, M. J., Vaughan, R. A., Uhl, G. R., Kuhar, M. J., & Pickel, V. M. (1996). The dopamine transporter is localized to dendritic and axonal plasma membranes of nigrostriatal dopaminergic neurons. *The Journal of Neuroscience: The Official Journal of the Society for Neuroscience*, *16*, 436–447.
Nissen, J. D., Pajęcka, K., Stridh, M. H., Skytt, D. M., & Waagepetersen, H. S. (2015). Dysfunctional TCA-cycle metabolism in glutamate dehydrogenase deficient astrocytes. *Glia*, *63*, 2313–2326. http://dx.doi.org/10.1002/glia.22895.
Nomura, H., Sakai, A., Nagano, M., Umino, M., & Suzuki, H. (2006). Expression changes of cation chloride cotransporters in the rat spinal cord following intraplantar formalin. *Neuroscience Research*, *56*, 435–440.
Obata, H., Li, X., & Eisenach, J. C. (2005). alpha2-Adrenoceptor activation by clonidine enhances stimulation-evoked acetylcholine release from spinal cord tissue after nerve ligation in rats. *Anesthesiology*, *102*, 657–662.
Olechowski, C. J., Tenorio, G., Sauve, Y., & Kerr, B. J. (2013). Changes in nociceptive sensitivity and object recognition in experimental autoimmune encephalomyelitis (EAE). *Experimental Neurology*, *241*, 113–121.

Pennartz, C. M. A., Groenewegen, H. J., & Lopes Da Silva, F. H. (1994). The nucleus accumbens as a complex of functionally distinct neuronal ensembles: An integration of behavioural, electrophysiological and anatomical data. *Progress in Neurobiology*, *42*, 719–761.

Piet, R., Vargová, L., Syková, E., Poulain, D. A., & Oliet, S. H. R. (2004). Physiological contribution of the astrocytic environment of neurons to intersynaptic crosstalk. *Proceedings of the National Academy of Sciences of the United States of America*, *101*, 2151–2155.

Pines, G., Danbolt, N. C., Bjørås, M., Zhang, Y., Bendahan, A., Eide, L., … Kanner, B. I. (1992). Cloning and expression of a rat brain L-glutamate transporter. *Nature*, *360*, 464–467.

Pitcher, M. H., Price, T. J., Entrena, J. M., & Cervero, F. (2007). Spinal NKCC1 blockade inhibits TRPV1-dependent referred allodynia. *Molecular Pain*, *3*, 17.

Potashner, S. J., & Tran, P. L. (1984). Decreased uptake and release of D-aspartate in the guinea pig spinal cord after dorsal root section. *Journal of Neurochemistry*, *42*, 1135–1144.

Pouille, F., & Scanziani, M. (2001). Enforcement of temporal fidelity in pyramidal cells by somatic feed-forward inhibition. *Science (New York, NY)*, *293*, 1159–1163.

Pow, D. V., Sullivan, R. K. P., Williams, S. M., Scott, H. L., Dodd, P. R., & Finkelstein, D. (2005). Differential expression of the GABA transporters GAT-1 and GAT-3 in brains of rats, cats, monkeys and humans. *Cell and Tissue Research*, *320*, 379–392.

Price, T. J., Cervero, F., & de Koninck, Y. (2005). Role of cation-chloride-cotransporters (CCC) in pain and hyperalgesia. *Current Topics in Medicinal Chemistry*, *5*, 547–555.

Price, T. J., Cervero, F., Gold, M. S., Hammond, D. L., & Prescott, S. A. (2009). Chloride regulation in the pain pathway. *Brain Research Reviews*, *60*, 149–170.

Price, T. J., & Prescott, S. A. (2015). Inhibitory regulation of the pain gate and how its failure causes pathological pain. *Pain*, *156*, 789–792.

Putatunda, R., Hala, T. J., Chin, J., & Lepore, A. C. (2014). Chronic at-level thermal hyperalgesia following rat cervical contusion spinal cord injury is accompanied by neuronal and astrocyte activation and loss of the astrocyte glutamate transporter, GLT1, in superficial dorsal horn. *Brain Research*, *1581*, 64–79.

Queen, S. A., Kesslak, J. P., & Bridges, R. J. (2007). Regional distribution of sodium-dependent excitatory amino acid transporters in rat spinal cord. *The Journal of Spinal Cord Medicine*, *30*, 263–271.

Radian, R., & Kanner, B. I. (1983). Stoichiometry of sodium- and chloride-coupled gamma-aminobutyric acid transport by synaptic plasma membrane vesicles isolated from rat brain. *Biochemistry*, *22*, 1236–1241.

Ramos, K. M., Lewis, M. T., Morgan, K. N., Crysdale, N. Y., Kroll, J. L., Taylor, F. R., … Watkins, L. R. (2010). Spinal upregulation of glutamate transporter GLT-1 by ceftriaxone: Therapeutic efficacy in a range of experimental nervous system disorders. *Neuroscience*, *169*, 1888–1900.

Rees, H., Sluka, K. A., Westlund, K. N., & Willis, W. D. (1994). Do dorsal root reflexes augment peripheral inflammation? *Neuroreport*, *5*, 821–824.

Ribak, C. E., Tong, W. M., & Brecha, N. C. (1996). Astrocytic processes compensate for the apparent lack of GABA transporters in the axon terminals of cerebellar Purkinje cells. *Anatomy and Embryology*, *194*, 379–390.

Rojas, H., Colina, C., Ramos, M., Benaim, G., Jaffe, E. H., Caputo, C., & DiPolo, R. (2007). Na+ entry via glutamate transporter activates the reverse Na+/Ca2+ exchange and triggers Ca(i)2+-induced Ca2+ release in rat cerebellar type-1 astrocytes. *Journal of Neurochemistry*, *100*, 1188–1202.

Roseberry, A. G. (2015). Acute fasting increases somatodendritic dopamine release in the ventral tegmental area. *Journal of Neurophysiology*, *114*, 1072–1082. http://dx.doi.org/10.1152/jn.01008.2014.

Sandkuhler, J. (2009). Models and mechanisms of hyperalgesia and allodynia. *Physiological Reviews*, *89*, 707–758.

Schmitt, K. C., Rothman, R. B., & Reith, M. E. (2013). Nonclassical pharmacology of the dopamine transporter: Atypical inhibitors, allosteric modulators, and partial substrates. *The Journal of Pharmacology and Experimental Therapeutics*, *346*, 2–10.

Scimemi, A. (2014). Structure, function, and plasticity of GABA transporters. *Frontiers in Cellular Neuroscience*, *8*, 1–14.

Scimemi, A., Tian, H., & Diamond, J. S. (2009). Neuronal transporters regulate glutamate clearance, NMDA receptor activation, and synaptic plasticity in the hippocampus. *The Journal of Neuroscience: The Official Journal of the Society for Neuroscience*, *29*, 14581–14595.

Seamans, J. K., & Yang, C. R. (2004). The principal features and mechanisms of dopamine modulation in the prefrontal cortex. *Progress in Neurobiology*, *74*, 1–57.

Shih, A., Miletic, V., Miletic, G., & Smith, L. J. (2008). Midazolam administration reverses thermal hyperalgesia and prevents gamma-aminobutyric acid transporter loss in a rodent model of neuropathic pain. *Anesthesia and Analgesia*, *106*, 1296–1302.

Sitte, H. H., Huck, S., Reither, H., Boehm, S., Singer, E. A., & Pifl, C. (1998). Carrier-mediated release, transport rates, and charge transfer induced by amphetamine, tyramine, and dopamine in mammalian cells transfected with the human dopamine transporter. *Journal of Neurochemistry*, *71*, 1289–1297.

Slotboom, D. J. (2014). Structural and mechanistic insights into prokaryotic energy-coupling factor transporters. *Nature Reviews. Microbiology*, *12*, 79–87.

Snyder, S. H. (2011). What dopamine does in the brain. *Proceedings of the National Academy of Sciences of the United States of America*, *108*, 18869–18871.

Song, I., Volynski, K., Brenner, T., Ushkaryov, Y., Walker, M., & Semyanov, A. (2013). Different transporter systems regulate extracellular GABA from vesicular and non-vesicular sources. *Frontiers in Cellular Neuroscience*, *7*, 23.

Stark, E., Eichler, R., Roux, L., Fujisawa, S., Rotstein, H. G., & Buzsáki, G. (2013). Inhibition-induced theta resonance in cortical circuits. *Neuron*, *80*, 1263–1276.

Staud, R. (2010). Pharmacological treatment of fibromyalgia syndrome: New developments. *Drugs*, *70*, 1–14.

Storck, T., Schulte, S., Hofmann, K., & Stoffel, W. (1992). Structure, expression, and functional analysis of a Na(+)-dependent glutamate/aspartate transporter from rat brain. *Proceedings of the National Academy of Sciences of the United States of America*, *89*, 10955–10959.

Suchak, S. K., Baloyianni, N. V., Perkinton, M. S., Williams, R. J., Meldrum, B. S., & Rattray, M. (2003). The "glial" glutamate transporter, EAAT2 (G1t-1) accounts for high affinity glutamate uptake into adult rodent nerve endings. *Journal of Neurochemistry*, *84*, 522–532.

Sung, K. W., Kirby, M., McDonald, M. P., Lovinger, D. M., & Delpire, E. (2000). Abnormal GABAA receptor-mediated currents in dorsal root ganglion neurons isolated from Na-K-2Cl cotransporter null mice. *The Journal of Neuroscience: The Official Journal of the Society for Neuroscience*, *20*, 7531–7538.

Sung, B., Lim, G., & Mao, J. (2003). Altered expression and uptake activity of spinal glutamate transporters after nerve injury contribute to the pathogenesis of neuropathic pain in rats. *The Journal of Neuroscience: The Official Journal of the Society for Neuroscience*, *23*, 2899–2910.

Szabadics, J., Tamás, G., & Soltesz, I. (2007). Different transmitter transients underlie presynaptic cell type specificity of GABAA,slow and GABAA,fast. *Proceedings of the National Academy of Sciences of the United States of America*, *104*, 14831–14836.

Tao, F., Liaw, W.-J., Zhang, B., Yaster, M., Rothstein, J. D., Johns, R. A., & Tao, Y.-X. (2004). Evidence of neuronal excitatory amino acid carrier 1 expression in rat dorsal root ganglion neurons and their central terminals. *Neuroscience*, *123*, 1045–1051.

Teng, C. J., & Abbott, F. V. (1998). The formalin test: A dose-response analysis at three developmental stages. *Pain*, *76*, 337–347.

Todorov, A. A., Kolchev, C. B., & Todorov, A. B. (2005). Tiagabine and gabapentin for the management of chronic pain. *The Clinical Journal of Pain*, *21*, 358–361.

Tzingounis, A. V., & Wadiche, J. I. (2007). Glutamate transporters: Confining runaway excitation by shaping synaptic transmission. *Nature Reviews. Neuroscience*, *8*, 935–947.

Urban, J. D., Clarke, W. P., von Zastrow, M., Nichols, D. E., Kobilka, B., Weinstein, H., ... Mailman, R. B. (2007). Functional selectivity and classical concepts of quantitative pharmacology. *The Journal of Pharmacology and Experimental Therapeutics*, *320*, 1–13.

Utsunomiya-Tate, N., Endou, H., & Kanai, Y. (1996). Cloning and functional characterization of a system ASC-like Na^+-dependent neutral amino acid transporter. *The Journal of Biological Chemistry*, *271*, 14883–14890.

Valencia-de Ita, S., Lawand, N. B., Lin, Q., Castañeda-Hernandez, G., & Willis, W. D. (2006). Role of the Na^+-K^+-$2Cl^-$ cotransporter in the development of capsaicin-induced neurogenic inflammation. *Journal of Neurophysiology*, *95*, 3553–3561.

Van Hecke, O., Austin, S. K., Khan, R. A., Smith, B. H., & Torrance, N. (2014). Neuropathic pain in the general population: A systematic review of epidemiological studies. *Pain*, *155*, 654–662.

Volkow, N. D., Wang, G. J., Fischman, M. W., Foltin, R., Fowler, J. S., Franceschi, D., ... Pappas, N. (2000). Effects of route of administration on cocaine induced dopamine transporter blockade in the human brain. *Life Sciences*, *67*, 1507–1515.

Vosburg, S. K., Hart, C. L., Haney, M., Rubin, E., & Foltin, R. W. (2010). Modafinil does not serve as a reinforcer in cocaine abusers. *Drug and Alcohol Dependence*, *106*, 233–236.

Weng, H.-R., Chen, J. H., & Cata, J. P. (2006). Inhibition of glutamate uptake in the spinal cord induces hyperalgesia and increased responses of spinal dorsal horn neurons to peripheral afferent stimulation. *Neuroscience*, *138*, 1351–1360.

Xin, W.-J., Weng, H.-R., & Dougherty, P. M. (2009). Plasticity in expression of the glutamate transporters GLT-1 and GLAST in spinal dorsal horn glial cells following partial sciatic nerve ligation. *Molecular Pain*, *5*, 15.

Yadav, R., Yan, X., Maixner, D. W., Gao, M., & Weng, H.-R. (2015). Blocking the GABA transporter GAT-1 ameliorates spinal GABAergic disinhibition and neuropathic pain induced by paclitaxel. *Journal of Neurochemistry*, *133*, 857–869.

Yan, X. X., Cariaga, W. A., & Ribak, C. E. (1997). Immunoreactivity for GABA plasma membrane transporter, GAT-1, in the developing rat cerebral cortex: Transient presence in the somata of neocortical and hippocampal neurons. *Developmental Brain Research*, *99*, 1–19.

Yoshizumi, M., Eisenach, J. C., & Hayashida, K. (2012). Riluzole and gabapentinoids activate glutamate transporters to facilitate glutamate-induced glutamate release from cultured astrocytes. *European Journal of Pharmacology*, *677*, 87–92.

Zeilhofer, H. U., Wildner, H., & Yévenes, G. E. (2012). Fast synaptic inhibition in spinal sensory processing and pain control. *Physiological Reviews*, *92*, 193–235.

Zhang, W., Liu, L.-Y., & Xu, T.-L. (2008). Reduced potassium-chloride co-transporter expression in spinal cord dorsal horn neurons contributes to inflammatory pain hypersensitivity in rats. *Neuroscience*, *152*, 502–510.

Zhou, F. C., Tao-Cheng, J. H., Segu, L., Patel, T., & Wang, Y. (1998). Serotonin transporters are located on the axons beyond the synaptic junctions: Anatomical and functional evidence. *Brain Research*, *805*, 241–254.

CHAPTER TEN

The Pharmacology of Visceral Pain

Anthony C. Johnson*, Beverley Greenwood-Van Meerveld*,†,‡,1
*Oklahoma Center for Neuroscience, University of Oklahoma Health Sciences Center, Oklahoma City, Oklahoma, USA
†Veterans Affairs Medical Center, Oklahoma City, Oklahoma, USA
‡Department of Physiology, University of Oklahoma Health Sciences Center, Oklahoma City, Oklahoma, USA
[1]Corresponding author: e-mail address: beverley-greenwood@ouhsc.edu

Contents

Abstract

Visceral pain describes pain emanating from the internal thoracic, pelvic, or abdominal organs. Unlike somatic pain, visceral pain is generally vague, poorly localized, and characterized by hypersensitivity to a stimulus such as organ distension. While current therapeutics provides some relief from somatic pain, drugs used for treatment of chronic visceral pain are typically less efficacious and limited by multiple adverse side effects. Thus, the treatment of visceral pain represents a major unmet medical need. Further, more basic research into the physiology and pathophysiology of visceral pain is needed to provide novel targets for future drug development. In concert with chronic visceral pain, there is a high comorbidity with stress-related psychiatric disorders including anxiety and depression. The mechanisms linking visceral pain with these overlapping comorbidities remain to be elucidated. However, persistent stress facilitates pain perception and sensitizes pain pathways, leading to a feed-forward cycle promoting chronic visceral pain disorders. We will focus on stress-induced exacerbation of chronic visceral pain and provide supporting evidence that centrally acting drugs targeting the pain and stress-responsive brain regions may represent a valid target for the development of novel and effective therapeutics.

Advances in Pharmacology, Volume 75
ISSN 1054-3589
http://dx.doi.org/10.1016/bs.apha.2015.11.002

ABBREVIATIONS

2-AG 2-arachidonoylglycerol
$5HT_3$ serotonin type-3 receptor
$5HT_4$ serotonin type-4 receptor
ACC anterior cingulate cortex
ACTH adrenocorticotropic hormone
AEA anandamide
AMPA alpha-amino-3-hydroxy-5-methyl-4-isoxazolepropionic acid
ASO antisense oligodeoxynucleotides
BDNF brain-derived neurotropic factor
CB_1 cannabinoid receptor type 1
CB_2 cannabinoid receptor type 2
CeA central nucleus of the amygdala
cGMP cyclic guanosine monophosphate
ClC-2 chloride channel type 2
CORT cortisol/corticosterone
CRH corticotropin-releasing hormone
CRH_1 CRH type-1 receptor
CRH_2 CRH type-2 receptor
DRG dorsal root ganglia
FD functional dyspepsia
GABA gamma-aminobutyric acid
$GABA_A$ GABA receptor type A
$GABA_B$ GABA receptor type B
GC-C guanylate cyclase-C
GERD gastroesophageal reflux disease
GI gastrointestinal
GR glucocorticoid receptor
HPA hypothalamic–pituitary–adrenal
IBD inflammatory bowel disease
IBS irritable bowel syndrome
IBS-C IBS with constipation
IBS-D IBS with diarrhea
IC interstitial cystitis
LC locus coeruleus
MCC midcingulate cortex
mGluRs metabotropic glutamate receptors
miR microRNA
MR mineralocorticoid receptor
N/OFQ nociceptin/orphanin FQ
NMDA *N*-methyl-D-aspartate
NOP N/OFQ peptide receptor
NSAID nonsteroidal anti-inflammatory drug
NTS nucleus tractus solitarius
PACAP pituitary adenylate cyclase-activating polypeptide
PAG periaqueductal gray
PBS painful bladder syndrome

PFC prefrontal cortex
PVN paraventricular nucleus of the hypothalamus
RVM rostroventral medulla
trkB tyrosine receptor kinase B receptor
TRPV1 transient receptor potential cation channel, subfamily V, type 1
WAS water avoidance stress

1. INTRODUCTION

Visceral pain describes pain from internal organs and is generally described as dull, diffuse, poorly localized and characterized by hypersensitivity to a provocative stimulus such as organ distension. An interesting feature of visceral pain is that it is commonly "referred" to somatic sites or organs distant from the source of the pain itself. Chronic visceral pain is the hallmark feature of many disorders, some with distinct organ pathology, including inflammatory bowel disease (IBD), pancreatitis, interstitial cystitis (IC)/painful bladder syndrome (PBS), and gynecological pain, whereas in other visceral pain disorders such as irritable bowel syndrome (IBS) and functional dyspepsia (FD), there is no evidence of any structural or histological abnormalities to explain the pain. However, abdominal pain represents one of the main reasons patients seek medical attention. Currently, despite large numbers of patients with chronic, and often debilitating visceral pain, the clinical management of these patients is largely inadequate. There are few effective therapies to treat patients with chronic visceral pain due in part to a lack of knowledge related to the underlying mechanisms. In this chapter, we will briefly discuss visceral pain pathways and the potential mechanisms leading to chronic visceral pain. This will be followed by a description of the current therapies for treating chronic visceral pain with an emphasis on abdominal pain associated with IBS. The remaining section of the chapter will summarize the latest research linking nociception to the stress axis and will highlight future targets for visceral pain therapeutics that lie within this visceral pain–stress axis.

2. VISCERAL PAIN PATHWAYS

Pain pathways innervating the gastrointestinal (GI) tract arise from extrinsic splanchnic primary afferents from the spinal cord with cell bodies in the dorsal root ganglia (DRG). Visceral afferents innervating the GI tract playing a pivotal role in visceral sensation arise from parasympathetic primary afferents within the vagus and pelvic nerves. Cell bodies of these vagal primary afferents are localized to the nodose ganglia, which terminate in the nucleus tractus solitarius (NTS) within the medulla. Upon stimulation within the peripheral organ, the extrinsic nociceptors (Aδ- and C-fibers) synapse in the dorsal horn of the spinal cord. Second-order neurons then ascend to the brain through anterolateral pathways such as the spinothalamic and the spinoreticular tracts. A parallel pain pathway ascends through the dorsal columns to the medial lemniscus. Within the brain tertiary neurons in the thalamus distribute the pain signal to cortical areas, such as primary and secondary somatosensory cortex to provide localization of the signal. Other regions, such as the insula and the anterior and midcingulate cortex (ACC/MCC), are activated to provide the "feel" of the stimulus (sharp, dull, aching, burning) and the perception of unpleasantness. Collateral brainstem connections activate the amygdala to integrate the pain signal with outflow to the autonomic nervous system and the hypothalamic–pituitary–adrenal (HPA) axis. A pivotal characteristic of visceral pain is that it is often referred to remote sites. There are two potential pathways to explain this referred pain, which include viscerosomatic and viscerovisceral convergence at the level of the spinal cord. Both pathways involve convergence at the same second-order neuron within the dorsal horn of the spinal cord, whereas dichotomizing afferents may also play a role in viscerovisceral convergence.

2.1 Mechanisms of Visceral Pain: Visceral afferent Sensitization

The pathophysiology of visceral is mediated by multiple mechanisms at peripheral, spinal, and supraspinal sites. Sensitization of peripheral and/or central pathways is responsible for increase perception of luminal stimuli and leads to visceral hypersensitivity, which can be affected by multiple mechanisms, including stress, mood, and chronic inflammation. Additionally, some individuals have vulnerabilities or resilience to chronic pain due to receptor polymorphisms neurotransmitter receptors or reuptake mechanisms.

2.1.1 Peripheral Sensitization

Increases in epithelial permeability allow luminal antigens, toxins, and microbial fermentation products to translocate the epithelial barrier to activate afferent nerve endings leading to visceral afferent sensitization. Additionally, inflammation produces long-term alterations in the physiology of the afferent terminals due to immune mediators released at the site of injury. Inflammatory mediators can directly sensitize afferent terminals leading to visceral hypersensitivity. Mediators such as cytokines, prostaglandins, histamine, proteases, and low pH at the site of an acute injury (Arroyo-Novoa et al., 2009; Widgerow & Kalaria, 2012) activate receptors on the afferent terminals to increase intracellular second messengers causing the release of neurotransmitters, such as substance P, calcitonin gene-related peptide, and nitric oxide, which can further sensitize visceral afferents. The second messenger systems (protein kinase A, protein kinase C) also lead to changes in gene expression that induces neuronal plasticity to alter the expression of receptors (neurokinin receptor 1, tyrosine receptor kinase A, prostaglandin receptor, protease-activated receptors, etc.) that leads to persistent changes in the excitability of the neuron (Woolf & Salter, 2000), through modifying the expression or function of ion channels (sodium, calcium, and potassium) that produce the action potentials that transmit the pain signal to the spinal cord (Schaible, Ebersberger, & Natura, 2011; Stemkowski & Smith, 2012).

2.1.2 Central Sensitization

Pain sensitization also involves neuronal remodeling within the dorsal horn of the spinal cord. At the level of the superficial lamina of the spinal cord, the primary visceral afferent releases glutamate to activate a second-order neuron, causing activation of sodium-permeable alpha-amino-3-hydroxy-5-methyl-4-isoxazolepropionic acid (AMPA) receptors followed by the subsequent activation of sodium and calcium-permeable *N*-methyl-D-aspartate (NMDA) receptors. Primary afferents also release algesic mediators, such as substance P, which activates second messenger signaling that initiates neuronal remodeling leading to changes in the properties of the receptors present in the dendritic structure of the second-order neuron (Woolf & Salter, 2000). With the persistent activation of the second-order neuron by the primary nociceptor, a phenotypic switch occurs in the dendrites causing an increase in the expression of a calcium-permeable variant of the AMPA receptor resulting in an increased excitability of the second-order neuron (Tao, 2012). At the level of the spinal interneurons, a parallel mechanism leads to hypersensitivity within the dorsal horn of the spinal cord via the release of neurotransmitters from the primary nociceptive afferent activating presynaptic receptors on the inhibitory interneuron, causing hyperpolarization of the inhibitory interneuron and a decreased release of gamma-aminobutyric acid (GABA) and/or glycine onto the second-order neuron (Braz, Solorzano, Wang, & Basbaum, 2014;

Zeilhofer, Wildner, & Yevenes, 2012). Thus, a combination of increased excitation and disinhibition can produce a persistent hyperexcitable state in the second-order neuron and chronic nociceptive signaling.

A similar mechanism to produce chronic visceral pain can be invoked within the central pain matrix in the brain (Jaggi & Singh, 2011). Ascending afferent information from the second-order spinal neurons promotes hyperexcitability within the central pain matrix by increasing the sensory signals reaching the tertiary neurons within the thalamus, raphe, or parabrachial nucleus, which then enhances signaling to secondary cortical and limbic structures. Remodeling of integration nuclei (amygdala, ACC/MCC, insula) can make the perception of the noxious stimulus more unpleasant, producing an enhanced negative emotional response (Staud, 2012). Imaging studies have demonstrated that in patients with chronic visceral pain, there is increased activation of brain regions that integrate pain signals and produce negative affect, such as the amygdala and insula, along with a decreased activity in pain inhibitory/positive affect nuclei, such as the prefrontal cortex (PFC) and cingulate (Labus et al., 2013; Wilder-Smith, 2011). Additionally, the altered signaling within the central pain matrix disrupts the descending dorsal column inhibitory pathway by modulating of activity in the periaqueductal gray (PAG) and rostroventral medulla (RVM) (Heinricher, Tavares, Leith, & Lumb, 2009; Ossipov, Lai, Malan, & Porreca, 2000).

2.2 Mechanisms of Visceral Pain: Stress Modulation

There is a high degree of comorbidity between visceral pain disorders, such as IBS and IBD, and psychological disorders, such as anxiety and depression; a potential common link between visceral pain and the comorbid psychological disorders is that periods of stress worsen the patient's symptoms (Grover & Drossman, 2010; Ringel & Drossman, 2002; Whitehead, Palsson, & Jones, 2002). Acute stress invokes two parallel physiological responses. The first response in the classical "flight or fight" response mediated by the sympathomedullary axis, which actives the sympathetic nervous system resulting in the release of adrenaline (epinephrine) into the blood circulation from the adrenal medulla. The adrenaline activates adrenergic receptors to increase heart rate, decrease blood flow to the skin, while increasing blood to the muscles, decrease most GI functions, and dilate the pupil. The second response, occurring simultaneously, is the activation of the neuroendocrine HPA axis. The HPA axis is initiated when the paraventricular nucleus of the hypothalamus (PVN) releases corticotropin-releasing hormone (CRH) into the hypophyseal portal circulation so that CRH will bind to its type-1 receptor (CRH_1) in the anterior pituitary. Following synthesis of precursors, the anterior pituitary will secrete adrenocorticotropic hormone (ACTH) into the blood circulation, where it binds to ACTH receptors in the adrenal cortex. Cortisol (corticosterone in rat and mice; CORT) is then rapidly synthesized, released into circulation, binds to cortisol binding globulin, and is distributed throughout the body to adjust glucose metabolism (to restore energy used by the sympathomedullary axis) and to bind within the brain and pituitary for feedback-inhibition of the HPA axis (Herman & Cullinan, 1997) via binding to the high-affinity mineralocorticoid receptor (MR) and the low-affinity glucocorticoid receptor (GR) (Reul & de Kloet, 1985; Sapolsky, McEwen, & Rainbow, 1983). In opposition to the feedback-inhibition, CORT binding in the amygdala will facilitate the HPA axis through increased CRH expression (Schulkin, Gold, & McEwen, 1998; Shepard, Barron, & Myers, 2000), leading to an increase in visceral hypersensitivity (Myers & Greenwood-Van Meerveld, 2010, 2012). Chronic stress can also remodel limbic brain regions that participate in the central pain matrix, such as increasing dendritic arborization in the amygdala and decreasing dendritic arborization in the hippocampus and PFC (Mitra & Sapolsky, 2008; Radley, Anderson, Hamilton, Alcock, & Romig-Martin, 2013; Vyas, Mitra, Shankaranarayana Rao, & Chattarji, 2002; Woolley, Gould, & McEwen, 1990), resulting in a chronic facilitation of both the HPA axis and visceral pain. The descending pain inhibitory systems (PAG, RVM, locus coeruleus (LC)) (Giesler & Liebeskind, 1976; Ness & Gebhart, 1987; Traub, Silva, Gebhart, & Solodkin, 1996) within the brainstem are also stress sensitive. Activation of the PAG, which also modulates the raphe and RVM, is partially controlled by opposing regulation from the PFC and amygdala, which is disrupted in periods of chronic stress (da Costa Gomez & Behbehani, 1995; Price, 1999). In addition to signals from the spinoreticular pathway, the RVM also integrates signaling from the PAG and amygdala and can directly modulate visceral nociception (Zhuo & Gebhart, 2002), while there are reciprocal connections between the amygdala, hypothalamus, and LC to link activity between the HPA and sympathomedullary axis (Reyes, Carvalho, Vakharia, & Van Bockstaele, 2011; Sawchenko & Swanson, 1981). Dysfunction of these pain facilitatory and inhibitory circuits can lead to persistent visceral pain following repeated and/or chronic stressors, with each region presenting different receptors that could be targeted with novel therapeutics to treat visceral pain.

2.3 Therapeutic Approaches for Treating Chronic Visceral Pain

Visceral pain is a complex condition that is poorly managed. Patients worry that their abdominal pain may underlie a more sinister condition and frequently visit their physician for reassurance and an effective analgesic. Unfortunately, there are no approved pharmacological treatments specifically for visceral pain and patients are usually exposed to a trial-and-error approach to treat their pain. Opioidergic drugs are a primary choice for the management of patients experiencing severe visceral pain (Inturrisi & Lipman, 2010; Trescot, 2013). Examples of drugs in this class include morphine, oxycodone, and fentanyl. These compounds can produce significant pain relief through a direct effect on visceral pain pathways; however, the use of these drugs is limited by side effects including nausea, constipation, and respiratory depression as well as the potential for analgesic tolerance and dependence with chronic use. Evidence also suggests that nociceptive sensitization and opioid-induced hyperalgesia can develop with prolonged use of opioids. Another approach for visceral pain management is to use over the counter nonsteroidal anti-inflammatory agents (NSAIDs) (Buvanendran, 2013; Buvanendran & Lipman, 2010). This class of compounds includes drugs such as ibuprofen, naproxen sodium, celecoxib, and meloxicam. NSAIDs relieve pain by indirectly suppressing cyclooxygenase activity and thus preventing prostaglandin formation in response to injury. With this class of compound, careful dosage compliance is essential to avoid gastric ulcer formation and harmful effects on renal function. Acetaminophen (alone or in combination with an opiate) can be administered as an alternative therapy, but has the potential to damage the liver especially if taken with alcohol. In patients with chronic abdominal pain associated with IBS older treatment approaches have included the use of anticholinergics/antispasmodics such as dicyclomine and hyoscyamine as smooth muscle relaxants as well as antidepressants neither of which has proven efficacy against visceral pain. However, serotonergic compounds such as alosetron ($5HT_3$ antagonist) (Camilleri et al., 2001) and tegaserod ($5HT_4$ agonist) (Novick et al., 2002) have demonstrated proven efficacy over placebo to treat symptoms of IBS including visceral pain. However, both alosetron and tegaserod were withdrawn from the market, for life-threatening GI effects and adverse cardiovascular effects, respectively. However, alosetron has been reintroduced with restricted availability for IBS with constipation. Recently, newer approaches have been approved for treating symptoms in patients with IBS. A minimally absorbed guanylate cyclase-C (GC-C) agonist, linaclotide, has proven efficacy over placebo in reducing abdominal pain in patients with IBS-C (Quigley et al., 2013). Although the mechanism by which linaclotide relieves abdominal pain is poorly understood, preclinical experiments suggest a reduction in visceral hypersensitivity through an analgesic mechanism involving activation of GC-C expressed on mucosal epithelial cells, resulting in the production and release of cGMP to inhibit visceral nociceptors (Castro et al., 2013). In contrast, lubiprostone, a chloride channel type 2 (ClC-2) agonist, which also has been approved for IBS-C, provides improvement in overall quality of life for patients, but only modest improvement in pain scores that were not significantly better than placebo (Wilson & Schey, 2015). In addition, two recently FDA approved IBS therapies eluxadoline (Dove et al., 2013), a mixed opioid agonist/antagonist, and rifaximin (Pimentel et al., 2011) a nonabsorbable broad spectrum antimicrobial both improve symptoms associated with IBS including abdominal pain. However, further basic research is required to determine whether these newer therapies approved to treat IBS attenuate visceral pain via an effect on visceral pain pathways or provide relief by normalizing stool production.

2.4 Receptors That Modulate Visceral Nociception

Due to the limited therapeutic options for treating chronic visceral pain, there is a need for further basic research to investigate targets for new pharmaceuticals. To address the myriad of possible targets, there have been multiple excellent reviews focusing on different potential mechanisms for chronic visceral pain (Camilleri, 2013; Dekel, Drossman, & Sperber, 2013; Elsenbruch, 2014; Greenwood-Van Meerveld, Prusator, & Johnson, 2015; Lee & Lee, 2014; Moloney, O'Mahony, Dinan, & Cryan, 2015; Srinath, Young, & Szigethy, 2014). The next section will focus on the overlap between the visceral pain and stress neurocircuitry that could provide novel pharmaceutical targets for treating chronic visceral pain. For information on the overlap between chronic somatic and neuropathic pain with stress, we refer the reader to our recent review (Johnson & Greenwood-Van Meerveld, 2014).

2.4.1 Brain-Derived Neurotropic Factor Receptor

Brain-derived neurotropic factor (BDNF) signals through the tyrosine receptor kinase B (trkB) receptor and participates in a variety of functions throughout the central nervous system including neurogenesis, neuronal survival, and synaptic remodeling and is implicated as a potential mediator of pain because it has been shown to participate in central sensitization (Binder & Scharfman, 2004). With regard to visceral pain disorders, BDNF expression in pancreatic tissue correlated with pain ratings in patients with chronic pancreatitis (Zhu, Friess, Wang, Zimmermann, & Buchler, 2001), and increased esophageal sensitivity in normal volunteers was associated with a BDNF polymorphism (Vasant, Payton, Mistry, Thompson, & Hamdy, 2013). In IBS patients, particularly the IBS-D subtype, there was more BDNF expression in mucosal biopsies, the level of expression correlated with pain severity in the patients (Yu et al., 2012), and fecal supernatants induced increased BDNF expression in Caco-2 cell culture (Wang et al., 2015). Preclinical studies supporting a role of BDNF in visceral hypersensitivity have demonstrated reduced colonic sensitivity to distension in BDNF heterozygous mice (Yang et al., 2010; Yu et al., 2012) and increased colonic sensitivity following exogenous BDNF administration (Wang et al., 2015; Yu et al., 2012). Similarly, rat models involving adverse neonatal manipulation induced gastric or colonic hypersensitivity in adulthood that was mediated by increased BDNF expression in the spinal cord (Winston, Li, & Sarna, 2014; Winston & Sarna, 2013). In contrast, BDNF has also been shown to be antinociceptive in models visceral pain involving an acute inflammation (Li, Zhang, Liu, Gong, et al., 2012; Li et al., 2010), emphasizing that the duration and underlying causes of the visceral pain are important variables when trying to test the efficacy of novel therapeutics.

2.4.2 Corticotropin-Releasing Hormone Receptors

Wylie Vale's laboratory at the Salk Institute first sequenced the 41-amino acid peptide, now called CRH, from sheep hypothalamus (Vale, Spiess, Rivier, & Rivier, 1981), and subsequently from rat hypothalamus (Rivier, Spiess, & Vale, 1983), that induced secretion of ACTH from rat pituitary cell cultures. CRH has one high-affinity receptor, CRH_1, and a lower affinity receptor, CRH_2, which are both G-protein-coupled receptors (Alexander et al., 2013; Alexander, Mathie, & Peters, 2011). There is preclinical evidence for opposing roles for central CRH_1 and CRH_2 in the regulation of visceral and somatic nociceptive behaviors (Fukudo, 2007; Ji & Neugebauer, 2007, 2008; Tran, Schulkin, & Greenwood-Van Meerveld, 2014; Yarushkina, Bagaeva, & Filaretova, 2009). Subsequent research has identified CRH and its receptors throughout the brain's stress and pain circuitry, including the CeA (Gallagher, Orozco-Cabal, Liu, & Shinnick-Gallagher, 2008), as well as within the GI tract (Larauche, Kiank, & Tache, 2009), where peripheral CRH_1 may provide an additional level of regulation of visceral nociception (Larauche et al., 2009). In IBS patients, clinical studies have demonstrated abnormal ACTH secretion in response to a stressor (Chang et al., 2009) or exogenous CRH (Dinan et al., 2006) along with changes in cytokine expression in the colon, and increases in colonic motility (Fukudo, Nomura, & Hongo, 1998). Additional studies found that a nonselective CRH antagonist decreased both colonic motility and patient's pain ratings (Sagami et al., 2004), while a CRH_1 antagonist produced changes in functional connectivity within the central pain matrix in response to anticipation of visceral pain, particularly between the amygdala, insula, and the orbitofrontal cortex (Hubbard et al., 2011). Preclinical studies have evaluated the effects of systemically, centrally, and/or peripherally restricted CRH antagonists in multiple models of visceral nociception. In particular, colonic hypersensitivity induced by intracerebroventricular administration of CRH was inhibited by peripheral administration of a CRH_1 antagonist, antalarmin, that crosses the blood–brain barrier (Greenwood-Van Meerveld, Johnson, Cochrane, Schulkin, & Myers, 2005), and CRH_1 knockout mice demonstrate colonic hyposensitivity to balloon distension (Trimble, Johnson, Foster, & Greenwood-van Meerveld, 2007). Additional evidence supporting the central role for CRH in maintenance of visceral pain was recently demonstrated with the mechanism for colonic hypersensitivity induced by prolonged CRH upregulation within the CeA involving epigenetically induced down-regulation of GR (Tran, Schulkin, Ligon, & Greenwood-Van Meerveld, 2015), which could then be inhibited through CRF ASO (Johnson, Tran, & Greenwood-Van Meerveld, 2015) or through infusion of a CRH_1 antagonist directly into the CeA (Johnson, Tran, Schulkin, & Greenwood-Van Meerveld, 2012). Despite clear preclinical experimental results in multiple animal models, clinical evidence of pain relief for CRH antagonists has been equivocal (Sagami et al., 2004; Sweetser et al., 2009). The reason for this disparity between the preclinical efficacy of CRH_1 antagonism and the lack of clinical efficacy in patients with visceral pain associated with IBS remains to be resolved but likely reflects the complexity of patients with IBS, the high placebo response rate in these patients as well as the pharmacokinetic characteristics of the lead compounds that were moved into clinical trials (Tache & Million, 2015). Thus, based upon the neuroanatomical distribution of CRH and its receptors, as well as more recent preclinical data, there continues to be strong experimental evidence suggesting the potential therapeutic value of CRH antagonists for visceral pain.

2.4.3 Endocannabinoid Receptors

Anandamide (AEA) and 2-arachidonoylglycerol (2-AG) are the endogenous ligands for the two G-protein-coupled endocannabinoid receptors, CB_1 and CB_2 (Pertwee et al., 2010). Beyond central expression of CB_1 and CB_2 within the central pain matrix and limbic areas (Butler & Finn, 2009; Gorzalka, Hill, & Hillard, 2008; Hill & McEwen, 2010; Luongo, Maione, & Di Marzo, 2014), both receptors are also expressed within the enteric nervous system where they modulate sensation, motility, and inflammation (Duncan, Davison, & Sharkey, 2005). A positron emission tomography imagining study demonstrated an increase in CB_1 receptor availability throughout the brain of FD patients, suggesting that a deficit in central endocannabinoid signaling may be contributing to the pain experienced in this disorder (Ly et al., 2015). However, a recent review summarizing the findings of clinical studies in IBS or gastroesophageal reflux disease (GERD) patients on the effects of endocannabinoid agonists found a decrease in pain perception only in GERD patients and no change in pain perception for most IBS patients (Malik, Baik, & Schey, 2015). In contrast to the clinical findings, there are multiple preclinical models of visceral hypersensitivity that have demonstrated that both CB_1 and CB_2 receptors can reduce hypersensitivity, in a model-dependent fashion (reviewed by Izzo & Sharkey, 2010). The disconnect between the preclinical and clinical results for these compounds may be in part due to central psychotropic side effects that are difficult to detect in animal models. New pharmaceuticals that are designed to minimize the central side effects of these receptors should provide better efficacy for chronic visceral pain.

2.4.4 GABA Receptors

The major inhibitory transmitter, GABA, which is expressed throughout the brain and spinal cord, has two receptor subtypes: type A are ionotropic chloride channels (Barnard et al., 1998; Olsen & Sieghart, 2008), and type B are metabotropic G-protein-coupled receptors (Bowery et al., 2002). GABA and its receptors are also expressed throughout the enteric nervous system (Krantis, 2000). The potential roles of $GABA_A$ and $GABA_B$ as analgesic targets have been recently reviewed (Goudet et al., 2009; Munro, Hansen, & Mirza, 2013). For visceral pain behaviors, preclinical studies have demonstrated that the baclofen, a $GABA_B$ agonist, reduces hypersensitivity to gastric or colonic distension (Brusberg et al., 2009; Lindstrom et al., 2011; Liu, Shenoy, & Pasricha, 2011). Similarly, a role for $GABA_A$ regulation of neonatal cystitis-induced colonic hypersensitivity, mediated by miR-181a, has also been demonstrated (Sengupta et al., 2013), providing additional evidence for dysregulation of GABA receptors underlying some chronic visceral pain disorders. Thus, development of novel subtype-selective GABA agonists that are devoid of central side effects may represent a useful therapy for chronic visceral pain.

2.4.5 Glucocorticoid and Mineralocorticoid Receptors

The central nucleus of the amygdala (CeA) is a key regulatory nucleus that integrates visceral, neuroendocrine, and autonomic signals to modulate nociception and behavior (Myers & Greenwood-Van Meerveld, 2009). A direct, nonredundant role for GR and MR signaling in the CeA to modulate colonic nociception has been demonstrated by using a model of targeted CeA exposure to corticosteroids (CORT, dexamethasone, aldosterone) and/or GR (mifepristone) or MR (spironolactone) antagonists (Myers & Greenwood-Van Meerveld, 2007, 2010). A recent study also demonstrated that directly targeting the CeA with CORT induces bladder hypersensitivity to distension (DeBerry, Robbins, & Ness, 2015), suggesting a possible central site regulating the comorbid visceral pain experienced by patients with PBS and IBS. Additionally, in both the CeA-targeted model and a model of psychological stress, repeated water avoidance stress (WAS), visceral hypersensitivity was associated with persistent decreases in expression of GR and increases in expression of CRH (Tran, Chaloner, Sawalha, & Greenwood Van-Meerveld, 2013; Tran & Greenwood-Van Meerveld, 2012). The role of GR expression in the CeA to modulate visceral pain has been investigated through two approaches: first, the decrease in GR expression can be induced by CORT through decreases in histone 3-lysine 9, mediated by increased expression of the histone deacetylase sirtuin 6, which leads to a persistent disinhibition of CRH expression (Tran et al., 2015); second, using antisense oligodeoxynucleotides (ASO) targeting GR mRNA to transiently knockdown expression of GR within the CeA-induced visceral hypersensitivity in normal, stress-naïve rats (Johnson & Greenwood-Van Meerveld, 2015). Knockdown of MR in the CeA using ASO was also able to increase visceral sensitivity in normal rats, confirming the nonredundant role for GR and MR in the CeA for the regulation of noxious visceral sensation (Johnson & Greenwood-Van Meerveld, 2015). Further, there is evidence from preclinical studies that systemic CORT can directly modulate visceral sensation. Elevating plasma CORT to a physiologically relevant stress-exposed level through either a single session of WAS repeated for 10 days or a single bolus CORT injection induced visceral hypersensitivity that could be inhibited through systemic mifepristone administration (Hong et al., 2011). Additional studies demonstrated that mechanism for the WAS- or CORT-induced visceral hypersensitivity involved reciprocal changes in the cannabinoid receptor type 1 (CB_1) and the transient receptor potential cation channel, subfamily V, type 1 (TRPV1) within the L6-S2 DRG, which were mediated by epigenetically induced changes in the expression of those receptors (Hong, Zheng, & Wiley, 2015). An alternative mechanism for bladder hypersensitivity induced by WAS combined with colonic irritation demonstrated changes in NMDA subunit phosphorylation within the L6-S1 dorsal horn that was inhibited following adrenalectomy or mifepristone administration (Peng et al., 2012). In contrast, a 4-day dosing regimen of dexamethasone, that reduced levels of immune activation, failed to modify colonic hypersensitivity in two different mouse models (La & Gebhart, 2014), indicating that the role of corticosteroids in the modulation of visceral pain may vary based on the cause of the hypersensitivity.

2.4.6 Glutamate Receptors

As the primary excitatory neurotransmitter, glutamate and its receptors—AMPA, NMDA, and metabotropic glutamatergic receptors (mGluRs)—are expressed throughout the central nervous system, participate central sensitization, and also modulate visceral pain (Kannampalli & Sengupta, 2015). Several preclinical studies have demonstrated roles for both AMPA and NMDA receptors in the ACC in the modulation of visceral hypersensitivity (Cao et al., 2008; Li, Zhang, Liu, Cao, et al., 2012; Wu et al., 2008; Zhou, Huang, Gao, Zhang, & Jiang, 2014). There is also preclinical evidence for NMDA receptors in the spinal cord modulating postinflammatory colonic hypersensitivity (Zhou, Price, Caudle, & Verne, 2009) and pancreatitis-induced hypersensitivity (Zhang, Zhang, & Westlund, 2004). The mGluRs, divided into three functional groups with group 1 (mGluR1 and mGluR5) producing excitation, group 2 (mGluR2 and mGluR3), and group 3 (mGluR4, mGluR6, mGluR7, and mGluR8) producing inhibition, are also potential therapeutic targets for chronic visceral pain (Blackshaw, Page, & Young, 2011). Models of colonic hypersensitivity have demonstrated a general role for mGluR5 antagonists to inhibit colonic nociception (Lindstrom et al., 2008), and a specific role for mGluR5 receptors in the CeA to modulate both colonic (Ji & Neugebauer, 2010) and bladder hypersensitivity (Crock et al., 2012). Further, group 2 mGluRs were demonstrated to participate in estradiol-induced colonic hypersensitivity

(Cao, Bai, Ji, & Traub, 2015), and an acute dose of a nonselective group 2 mGluR antagonist produced a transient inhibition of pancreatitis-induced hypersensitivity (McIlwrath & Westlund, 2015). While there is one report of subtype-selective group 3 mGluR agonists and antagonists producing opposing effects on cardiac nociceptive responses (Liu et al., 2012), and there is expression of group 3 mGluRs in the GI tract that should modulate motility and secretion (Julio-Pieper, O'Connor, Dinan, & Cryan, 2013), further studies of the role of group 3 mGluRs in visceral pain have not been reported in the literature. Overall, selective pharmacological tools targeting glutamatergic receptors should provide new therapies for chronic visceral pain.

2.4.7 Pituitary Adenylate Cyclase-Activating Polypeptide Receptors

Pituitary adenylate cyclase-activating polypeptide (PACAP) is a short polypeptide that occurs as two splice variants, PACAP27 (27 amino acids) or PACAP38 (38 amino acids), which is expressed within the limbic brain and serves to modify stress responsiveness through its high-affinity receptor, PAC_1 (Hammack & May, 2015). Preclinical evidence supports a role for PACAP in the modulation of not only visceral but also neuropathic and inflammatory pain (Bon, Lanteri-Minet, Michiels, & Menetrey, 1998; Ohsawa et al., 2002; Shimizu, Katahira, Sugawara, Inoue, & Miyata, 2004). While there are currently no nonpeptide antagonists for PACAP, studies of responses to visceral pain in PACAP or PAC_1 knockout mice have shown a decrease in writhing behaviors in those animals (Martin et al., 2003; Sandor et al., 2010), along with a modest decrease in writhing following peripheral administration of PACAP38 and mixed effects in somatic and neuropathic pain models (Sandor et al., 2009). Since PACAP modulates stress and pain behaviors, once additional pharmacological tools are available, the PAC_1 receptor may be a useful target for the treatment of chronic, functional visceral pain.

2.4.8 Other Receptor Targets

2.4.8.1 Mast Cell Stabilizers

While not targeting a single specific receptor, drugs that prevent mast cell degranulation are potential therapeutic targets for functional visceral pain as experienced in IBS. Mast cells have been found in close proximity to sensory afferents with the GI tract; activated mast cells release a variety of mediators that can activate nociceptors, and mast cells express receptors for neuropeptides released by the afferents that can cause further mast cell degranulation (van Diest, Stanisor, Boeckxstaens, de Jonge, & van den Wijngaard, 2012). Additionally, multiple clinical studies have demonstrated increased overall numbers of mast cells in IBS patients (Ford & Talley, 2011), which were further associated with defects in tight junctions that could lead to additional afferent sensitization and/or mast cell activation due to exposure to luminal contents (Piche, 2014; Walker, Warwick, Ung, & Talley, 2011). However, to date, there have been no formal clinical trials of mast cell stabilizers for the treatment of chronic visceral pain.

2.4.8.2 Nociceptin/Orphanin FQ (N/OFQ) Peptide (NOP) Receptor

N/OFQ and the NOP receptor have been implicated in playing a role in modulation of pain, inflammation, stress, and anxiety disorders due to expression in a variety of cell types throughout the body (Donica, Awwad, Thakker, & Standifer, 2013; Witkin et al., 2014). There have been limited investigations of the role of the NOP receptor in visceral pain disorders, mainly focusing on inflammatory models, along a few clinical observations of decreased NOP receptor expression in some IBS and IBD patient biopsies (Agostini & Petrella, 2014). Thus, while there is some rational for using NOP agonists in select patient populations, a drawback of this receptor is the potential for biphasic responses that will require careful dose titration to avoid unwanted side effects.

2.4.8.3 Sigma-1 Receptors

Recent reviews have highlighted the potential for sigma-1 receptors to be a target for novel pain therapeutics due to their expression within the central pain matrix and colocalization with glutamatergic and opioidergic neurons (Maurice & Su, 2009; Zamanillo, Romero, Merlos, & Vela, 2013). In a model of colonic pain induced by an enema of 1% capsaicin, sigma-1 receptor knockout mice displayed less pain behaviors than wild-type mice, and three sigma-1 receptor antagonists dose-dependently decrease pain behaviors in wild-type mice without effect in knockout mice (Gonzalez-Cano, Merlos, Baeyens, & Cendan, 2013).

2.4.8.4 Transient Receptor Potential Cation Channel, Subtype V, Type 1 (TRPV1) Receptor

TRPV1 receptors are respond to polymodal stimuli including capsaicin, low pH, and heat and is expressed on most nociceptive afferent fibers throughout the body (Bevan, Quallo, & Andersson, 2014; Scholz & Woolf, 2002). There have been two studies demonstrating increased TRPV1-positive nerve fibers in mucosal biopsies from IBS patients and IBD patients in remission with IBS-like pain, which also showed that the TRPV1 content correlated with overall pain ratings (Akbar et al., 2010, 2008). A recent study of IBS-D patients provided evidence for a mechanism by which a decrease in miR-199 expression, which was inversely correlated with pain ratings, induces an increase in TRPV1 expression in the colon (Zhou et al., 2015), indicating that colonic TRPV1 activation may regulate pain in some IBS subtypes. Preclinical studies of TRPV1 antagonists have also demonstrated efficacy in models of acute irritant-induced, active-, and postinflammatory-induced colonic hypersensitivity (Miranda et al., 2007; Wiskur et al., 2010). However, some clinical studies have not demonstrated a role for TRPV1 in mediating pain in IBS patients (Cenac et al., 2015; van Wanrooij et al., 2014), and an issue with the pharmacology of the TRPV1 antagonists is that the TRPV1 receptor also plays a role in basal thermoregulation (Gavva, 2008).

3. EVALUATION OF PAIN BEHAVIORS IN EXPERIMENTAL MODELS

Multiple rodent models are available to evaluate the efficacy of novel therapeutics to treat visceral pain. To assess visceral pain behaviors, contractile response to hollow organ distension (stomach, colon, uterus, bladder) is typically monitored. The reader is referred to one of our recent reviews that highlights in detail the experimental models currently used to assess visceral pain (Greenwood-Van Meerveld et al., 2015). In general, rodent models attempt to recapitulate visceral pain in patients in response to peripheral insults such as inflammation or following exposure to chronic stress. In these behavioral assays, the ability of the novel therapeutic to produce analgesia is measured as a decrease in the evoked nociceptive response. Although these are widely used and validated assays for investigating the analgesic efficacy of novel therapeutics, there have been important lessons learned from these experimental models. Additionally, there are challenges and limitations that must be considered in the interpretation of the data from experimental models and their translatability to humans. Specific challenges are that visceral pain is a global term for complex clinical phenotypes that are highly multifactorial and involve complex interactions with biological, psychological, and sociological variables. As such, visceral pain is comorbid with many other clinical disorders making it virtually impossible to recapitulate all the symptoms of visceral pain in a single experimental model. Another important consideration is that until recently most research was performed using male animals to investigate the efficacy of novel compounds. However, visceral pain is a more frequent complaint in females, and we believe that future research must provide information taken from both male and female animals to increase translatability of the findings.

4. CONCLUSION

Chronic visceral pain, despite its high prevalence, represents a significant unmet therapeutic need. The complex pathophysiology and lack of biomarkers are likely culprits surrounding the paucity of therapeutics to treat visceral pain disorders. In this review, we have provided evidence to highlight for the reader the future potential of CNS-directed therapies to target common neural mechanisms that facilitate both stress and nociception. However, this does not rule out future opportunities for selective targeting of treatments directed at the periphery to treat visceral pain. An important message is the need for more research focusing on potential synergistic mechanisms between the overlapping central and peripheral components of the pain neurocircuits, which may produce therapeutic targets with increased efficacy and fewer unwanted side effects.

CONFLICT OF INTEREST

Dr. B.G.-V.M. has preclinical animal pharmacology based grant support from Ironwood Pharmaceutics, Glaxo-Smith Kline Pharmaceuticals, and White Sands Pharmaceuticals, who are developing treatments for gastrointestinal disorders.

Dr. A.C. Johnson has no conflict of interest to declare.

ACKNOWLEDGMENT

Dr. B.G.-V.M. would like to acknowledge the support she receives from the Department of Veterans Affairs, USA.

REFERENCES

Agostini, S., & Petrella, C. (2014). The endogenous nociceptin/orphanin FQ-NOP receptor system as a potential therapeutic target for intestinal disorders. *Neurogastroenterology and Motility*, *26*(11), 1519–1526. http://dx.doi.org/10.1111/nmo.12460.

Akbar, A., Yiangou, Y., Facer, P., Brydon, W. G., Walters, J. R., Anand, P., et al. (2010). Expression of the TRPV1 receptor differs in quiescent inflammatory bowel disease with or without abdominal pain. *Gut*, *59*(6), 767–774. http://dx.doi.org/10.1136/gut.2009.194449.

Akbar, A., Yiangou, Y., Facer, P., Walters, J. R., Anand, P., & Ghosh, S. (2008). Increased capsaicin receptor TRPV1-expressing sensory fibres in irritable bowel syndrome and their correlation with abdominal pain. *Gut*, *57*(7), 923–929. http://dx.doi.org/10.1136/gut.2007.138982.

Alexander, S. P., Benson, H. E., Faccenda, E., Pawson, A. J., Sharman, J. L., Spedding, M., et al. (2013). The Concise Guide to PHARMACOLOGY 2013/14: G protein-coupled receptors. *British Journal of Pharmacology*, *170*(8), 1459–1581. http://dx.doi.org/10.1111/bph.12445.

Alexander, S. P., Mathie, A., & Peters, J. A. (2011). Guide to receptors and channels (GRAC), 5th edition. *British Journal of Pharmacology*, *164*(Suppl. 1), S1–S324. http://dx.doi.org/10.1111/j.1476-5381.2011.01649_1.x.

Arroyo-Novoa, C. M., Figueroa-Ramos, M. I., Miaskowski, C., Padilla, G., Stotts, N., & Puntillo, K. A. (2009). Acute wound pain: Gaining a better understanding. *Advances in Skin & Wound Care*, *22*(8), 373–380. http://dx.doi.org/10.1097/01.ASW.0000358637.38161.8f. quiz 381–382.

Barnard, E. A., Skolnick, P., Olsen, R. W., Mohler, H., Sieghart, W., Biggio, G., et al. (1998). International Union of Pharmacology. XV. Subtypes of gamma-aminobutyric acid A receptors: Classification on the basis of subunit structure and receptor function. *Pharmacological Reviews*, *50*(2), 291–313.

Bevan, S., Quallo, T., & Andersson, D. A. (2014). Trpv1. *Handbook of Experimental Pharmacology*, *222*, 207–245. http://dx.doi.org/10.1007/978-3-642-54215-2_9.

Binder, D. K., & Scharfman, H. E. (2004). Brain-derived neurotrophic factor. *Growth Factors*, *22*(3), 123–131.

Blackshaw, L. A., Page, A. J., & Young, R. L. (2011). Metabotropic glutamate receptors as novel therapeutic targets on visceral sensory pathways. *Frontiers in Neuroscience*, *5*, 40. http://dx.doi.org/10.3389/fnins.2011.00040.

Bon, K., Lanteri-Minet, M., Michiels, J. F., & Menetrey, D. (1998). Cyclophosphamide cystitis as a model of visceral pain in rats: A c-fos and Krox-24 study at telencephalic levels, with a note on pituitary adenylate cyclase activating polypeptide (PACAP). *Experimental Brain Research*, *122*(2), 165–174.

Bowery, N. G., Bettler, B., Froestl, W., Gallagher, J. P., Marshall, F., Raiteri, M., et al. (2002). International Union of Pharmacology. XXXIII. Mammalian gamma-aminobutyric acid(B) receptors: Structure and function. *Pharmacological Reviews*, *54*(2), 247–264.

Braz, J., Solorzano, C., Wang, X., & Basbaum, A. I. (2014). Transmitting pain and itch messages: A contemporary view of the spinal cord circuits that generate gate control. *Neuron*, *82*(3), 522–536. http://dx.doi.org/10.1016/j.neuron.2014.01.018.

Brusberg, M., Ravnefjord, A., Martinsson, R., Larsson, H., Martinez, V., & Lindstrom, E. (2009). The GABA(B) receptor agonist, baclofen, and the positive allosteric modulator, CGP7930, inhibit visceral pain-related responses to colorectal distension in rats. *Neuropharmacology*, *56*(2), 362–367. http://dx.doi.org/10.1016/j.neuropharm.2008.09.006.

Butler, R. K., & Finn, D. P. (2009). Stress-induced analgesia. *Progress in Neurobiology*, *88*(3), 184–202. http://dx.doi.org/10.1016/j.pneurobio.2009.04.003.

Buvanendran, A. (2013). Nonsteroidal anti-inflammatory drugs. In A. Buvanendran, T. R. Deer, V. Gordin, P. S. Kim, M. S. Leong, S. J. Panchal, & A. L. Ray (Eds.), *Comprehensive treatment of chronic pain by medical, interventional, and integrative approaches: The AMERICAN ACADEMY Of PAIN MEDICINE textbook on patient management* (pp. 35–44). New York: Springer. http://dx.doi.org/10.1007/978-1-4614-1560-2.

Buvanendran, A., & Lipman, A. G. (2010). Nonsteroidal anti-inflammatory drugs and acetaminophen. In J. C. Ballantyne, S. M. Fishman, & J. P. Rathmell (Eds.), *Bonica's management of pain* (4th ed., pp. 1157–1171). Philadelphia: Lippincott Williams & Wilkins.

Camilleri, M. (2013). Pharmacological agents currently in clinical trials for disorders in neurogastroenterology. *Journal of Clinical Investigation*, *123*(10), 4111–4120. http://dx.doi.org/10.1172/JCI70837.

Camilleri, M., Chey, W. Y., Mayer, E. A., Northcutt, A. R., Heath, A., Dukes, G. E., et al. (2001). A randomized controlled clinical trial of the serotonin type 3 receptor antagonist alosetron in women with diarrhea-predominant irritable bowel syndrome. *Archives of Internal Medicine*, *161*(14), 1733–1740.

Cao, D. Y., Bai, G., Ji, Y., & Traub, R. J. (2015). Epigenetic upregulation of metabotropic glutamate receptor 2 in the spinal cord attenuates oestrogen-induced visceral hypersensitivity. *Gut*, *64*(12), 1913–1920. http://dx.doi.org/10.1136/gutjnl-2014-307748.

Cao, Z., Wu, X., Chen, S., Fan, J., Zhang, R., Owyang, C., et al. (2008). Anterior cingulate cortex modulates visceral pain as measured by visceromotor responses in viscerally hypersensitive rats. *Gastroenterology*, *134*(2), 535–543. http://dx.doi.org/10.1053/j.gastro.2007.11.057.

Castro, J., Harrington, A. M., Hughes, P. A., Martin, C. M., Ge, P., Shea, C. M., et al. (2013). Linaclotide inhibits colonic nociceptors and relieves abdominal pain via guanylate cyclase-C and extracellular cyclic guanosine 3',5'-monophosphate. *Gastroenterology*, *145*(6), 1334–1346.e1-11. http://dx.doi.org/10.1053/j.gastro.2013.08.017.

Cenac, N., Bautzova, T., Le Faouder, P., Veldhuis, N. A., Poole, D. P., Rolland, C., et al. (2015). Quantification and potential functions of endogenous agonists of transient receptor potential channels in patients with irritable bowel syndrome. *Gastroenterology*. *149*(2), 433.e7-444.e7. http://dx.doi.org/10.1053/j.gastro.2015.04.011.

Chang, L., Sundaresh, S., Elliott, J., Anton, P. A., Baldi, P., Licudine, A., et al. (2009). Dysregulation of the hypothalamic-pituitary-adrenal (HPA) axis in irritable bowel syndrome. *Neurogastroenterology and Motility*, *21*(2), 149–159. http://dx.doi.org/10.1111/j.1365-2982.2008.01171.x.

Crock, L. W., Kolber, B. J., Morgan, C. D., Sadler, K. E., Vogt, S. K., Bruchas, M. R., et al. (2012). Central amygdala metabotropic glutamate receptor 5 in the modulation of visceral pain. *Journal of Neuroscience*, *32*(41), 14217–14226. http://dx.doi.org/10.1523/JNEUROSCI.1473-12.2012.

da Costa Gomez, T. M., & Behbehani, M. M. (1995). An electrophysiological characterization of the projection from the central nucleus of the amygdala to the periaqueductal gray of the rat: The role of opioid receptors. *Brain Research*, *689*(1), 21–31.

DeBerry, J. J., Robbins, M. T., & Ness, T. J. (2015). The amygdala central nucleus is required for acute stress-induced bladder hyperalgesia in a rat visceral pain model. *Brain Research*, *1606*, 77–85. http://dx.doi.org/10.1016/j.brainres.2015.01.008.

Dekel, R., Drossman, D. A., & Sperber, A. D. (2013). The use of psychotropic drugs in irritable bowel syndrome. *Expert Opinion on Investigational Drugs*, *22*(3), 329–339. http://dx.doi.org/10.1517/13543784.2013.761205.

Dinan, T. G., Quigley, E. M., Ahmed, S. M., Scully, P., O'Brien, S., O'Mahony, L., et al. (2006). Hypothalamic-pituitary-gut axis dysregulation in irritable bowel syndrome: Plasma cytokines as a potential biomarker? *Gastroenterology*, *130*(2), 304–311. http://dx.doi.org/10.1053/j.gastro.2005.11.033.

Donica, C. L., Awwad, H. O., Thakker, D. R., & Standifer, K. M. (2013). Cellular mechanisms of nociceptin/orphanin FQ (N/OFQ) peptide (NOP) receptor regulation and heterologous regulation by N/OFQ. *Molecular Pharmacology*, *83*(5), 907–918. http://dx.doi.org/10.1124/mol.112.084632.

Dove, L. S., Lembo, A., Randall, C. W., Fogel, R., Andrae, D., Davenport, J. M., et al. (2013). Eluxadoline benefits patients with irritable bowel syndrome with diarrhea in a phase 2 study. *Gastroenterology*. *145*(2), 329.e1-338.e1. http://dx.doi.org/10.1053/j.gastro.2013.04.006.

Duncan, M., Davison, J. S., & Sharkey, K. A. (2005). Review article: Endocannabinoids and their receptors in the enteric nervous system. *Alimentary Pharmacology & Therapeutics*, *22*(8), 667–683. http://dx.doi.org/10.1111/j.1365-2036.2005.02648.x.

Elsenbruch, S. (2014). How positive and negative expectations shape the experience of visceral pain. *Handbook of Experimental Pharmacology*, *225*, 97–119. http://dx.doi.org/10.1007/978-3-662-44519-8_6.

Ford, A. C., & Talley, N. J. (2011). Mucosal inflammation as a potential etiological factor in irritable bowel syndrome: A systematic review. *Journal of Gastroenterology*, *46*(4), 421–431. http://dx.doi.org/10.1007/s00535-011-0379-9.

Fukudo, S. (2007). Role of corticotropin-releasing hormone in irritable bowel syndrome and intestinal inflammation. *Journal of Gastroenterology*, *42*(Suppl. 17), 48–51. http://dx.doi.org/10.1007/s00535-006-1942-7.

Fukudo, S., Nomura, T., & Hongo, M. (1998). Impact of corticotropin-releasing hormone on gastrointestinal motility and adrenocorticotropic hormone in normal controls and patients with irritable bowel syndrome. *Gut*, *42*(6), 845–849.

Gallagher, J. P., Orozco-Cabal, L. F., Liu, J., & Shinnick-Gallagher, P. (2008). Synaptic physiology of central CRH system. *European Journal of Pharmacology*, *583*(2–3), 215–225. http://dx.doi.org/10.1016/j.ejphar.2007.11.075.

Gavva, N. R. (2008). Body-temperature maintenance as the predominant function of the vanilloid receptor TRPV1. *Trends in Pharmacological Sciences*, *29*(11), 550–557. http://dx.doi.org/10.1016/j.tips.2008.08.003.

Giesler, G. J., Jr., & Liebeskind, J. C. (1976). Inhibition of visceral pain by electrical stimulation of the periaqueductal gray matter. *Pain*, *2*(1), 43–48.

Gonzalez-Cano, R., Merlos, M., Baeyens, J. M., & Cendan, C. M. (2013). sigma1 receptors are involved in the visceral pain induced by intracolonic administration of capsaicin in mice. *Anesthesiology*, *118*(3), 691–700. http://dx.doi.org/10.1097/ALN.0b013e318280a60a.

Gorzalka, B. B., Hill, M. N., & Hillard, C. J. (2008). Regulation of endocannabinoid signaling by stress: Implications for stress-related affective disorders. *Neuroscience and Biobehavioral Reviews*, *32*(6), 1152–1160. http://dx.doi.org/10.1016/j.neubiorev.2008.03.004.

Goudet, C., Magnaghi, V., Landry, M., Nagy, F., Gereau, R. W. t., & Pin, J. P. (2009). Metabotropic receptors for glutamate and GABA in pain. *Brain Research Reviews*, *60*(1), 43–56. http://dx.doi.org/10.1016/j.brainresrev.2008.12.007.

Greenwood-Van Meerveld, B., Johnson, A. C., Cochrane, S., Schulkin, J., & Myers, D. A. (2005). Corticotropin-releasing factor 1 receptor-mediated mechanisms inhibit colonic hypersensitivity in rats. *Neurogastroenterology and Motility*, *17*(3), 415–422. http://dx.doi.org/10.1111/j.1365-2982.2005.00648.x.

Greenwood-Van Meerveld, B., Prusator, D. K., & Johnson, A. C. (2015). Animal models of gastrointestinal and liver diseases. Animal models of visceral pain: Pathophysiology, translational relevance, and challenges. *American Journal of Physiology. Gastrointestinal and Liver Physiology*, *308*(11), G885–G903. http://dx.doi.org/10.1152/ajpgi.00463.2014.

Grover, M., & Drossman, D. A. (2010). Functional abdominal pain. *Current Gastroenterology Reports*, *12*(5), 391–398. http://dx.doi.org/10.1007/s11894-010-0125-0.

Hammack, S. E., & May, V. (2015). Pituitary adenylate cyclase activating polypeptide in stress-related disorders: Data convergence from animal and human studies. *Biological Psychiatry*, *78*(3), 167–177. http://dx.doi.org/10.1016/j.biopsych.2014.12.003.

Heinricher, M. M., Tavares, I., Leith, J. L., & Lumb, B. M. (2009). Descending control of nociception: Specificity, recruitment and plasticity. *Brain Research Reviews*, *60*(1), 214–225. http://dx.doi.org/10.1016/j.brainresrev.2008.12.009.

Herman, J. P., & Cullinan, W. E. (1997). Neurocircuitry of stress: Central control of the hypothalamo-pituitary-adrenocortical axis. *Trends in Neurosciences*, *20*(2), 78–84.

Hill, M. N., & McEwen, B. S. (2010). Involvement of the endocannabinoid system in the neurobehavioural effects of stress and glucocorticoids. *Progress in*

Neuropsychopharmacology & Biological Psychiatry, *34*(5), 791–797. http://dx.doi.org/10.1016/j.pnpbp.2009.11.001.

Hong, S., Zheng, G., & Wiley, J. W. (2015). Epigenetic regulation of genes that modulate chronic stress-induced visceral pain in the peripheral nervous system. *Gastroenterology*. *148*(1), 148.e7-157.e7. http://dx.doi.org/10.1053/j.gastro.2014.09.032.

Hong, S., Zheng, G., Wu, X., Snider, N. T., Owyang, C., & Wiley, J. W. (2011). Corticosterone mediates reciprocal changes in CB 1 and TRPV1 receptors in primary sensory neurons in the chronically stressed rat. *Gastroenterology*. *140*(2), 627.e4-637.e4. http://dx.doi.org/10.1053/j.gastro.2010.11.003.

Hubbard, C. S., Labus, J. S., Bueller, J., Stains, J., Suyenobu, B., Dukes, G. E., et al. (2011). Corticotropin-releasing factor receptor 1 antagonist alters regional activation and effective connectivity in an emotional-arousal circuit during expectation of abdominal pain. *Journal of Neuroscience*, *31*(35), 12491–12500. http://dx.doi.org/10.1523/JNEUROSCI.1860-11.2011.

Inturrisi, C. E., & Lipman, A. G. (2010). Opioid analgesics. In J. C. Ballantyne, S. M. Fishman, & J. P. Rathmell (Eds.), *Bonica's management of pain* (4th ed., pp. 1172–1187). Philadelphia: Lippincott Williams & Wilkins.

Izzo, A. A., & Sharkey, K. A. (2010). Cannabinoids and the gut: New developments and emerging concepts. *Pharmacology & Therapeutics*, *126*(1), 21–38. http://dx.doi.org/10.1016/j.pharmthera.2009.12.005.

Jaggi, A. S., & Singh, N. (2011). Role of different brain areas in peripheral nerve injury-induced neuropathic pain. *Brain Research*, *1381*, 187–201. http://dx.doi.org/10.1016/j.brainres.2011.01.002.

Ji, G., & Neugebauer, V. (2007). Differential effects of CRF1 and CRF2 receptor antagonists on pain-related sensitization of neurons in the central nucleus of the amygdala. *Journal of Neurophysiology*, *97*(6), 3893–3904. http://dx.doi.org/10.1152/jn.00135.2007.

Ji, G., & Neugebauer, V. (2008). Pro- and anti-nociceptive effects of corticotropin-releasing factor (CRF) in central amygdala neurons are mediated through different receptors. *Journal of Neurophysiology*, *99*(3), 1201–1212. http://dx.doi.org/10.1152/jn.01148.2007.

Ji, G., & Neugebauer, V. (2010). Reactive oxygen species are involved in group I mGluR-mediated facilitation of nociceptive processing in amygdala neurons. *Journal of Neurophysiology*, *104*(1), 218–229. http://dx.doi.org/10.1152/jn.00223.2010.

Johnson, A. C., & Greenwood-Van Meerveld, B. (2014). Stress-induced pain: A target for the development of novel therapeutics. *Journal of Pharmacology and Experimental Therapeutics*, *351*(2), 327–335. http://dx.doi.org/10.1124/jpet.114.218065.

Johnson, A. C., & Greenwood-Van Meerveld, B. (2015). Knockdown of steroid receptors in the central nucleus of the amygdala induces heightened pain behaviors in the rat. *Neuropharmacology*, *93C*, 116–123. http://dx.doi.org/10.1016/j.neuropharm.2015.01.018.

Johnson, A. C., Tran, L., & Greenwood-Van Meerveld, B. (2015). Knockdown of corticotropin-releasing factor in the central amygdala reverses persistent viscerosomatic hyperalgesia. *Translational Psychiatry*, *5*, e517. http://dx.doi.org/10.1038/tp.2015.16.

Johnson, A. C., Tran, L., Schulkin, J., & Greenwood-Van Meerveld, B. (2012). Importance of stress receptor-mediated mechanisms in the amygdala on visceral pain perception in an intrinsically anxious rat. *Neurogastroenterology and Motility*, *24*(5), 479–486. http://dx.doi.org/10.1111/j.1365-2982.2012.01899.x. e219.

Julio-Pieper, M., O'Connor, R. M., Dinan, T. G., & Cryan, J. F. (2013). Regulation of the brain-gut axis by group III metabotropic glutamate receptors. *European Journal of Pharmacology*, *698*(1–3), 19–30. http://dx.doi.org/10.1016/j.ejphar.2012.10.027.

Kannampalli, P., & Sengupta, J. N. (2015). Role of principal ionotropic and metabotropic receptors in visceral pain. *Journal of Neurogastroenterology and Motility*, *21*(2), 147–158. http://dx.doi.org/10.5056/jnm15026.

Krantis, A. (2000). GABA in the mammalian enteric nervous system. *News in Physiological Sciences*, *15*, 284–290.

La, J. H., & Gebhart, G. F. (2014). Condition-specific role of colonic inflammatory molecules in persistent functional colorectal hypersensitivity in the mouse. *Neurogastroenterology and Motility*, *26*(12), 1730–1742. http://dx.doi.org/10.1111/nmo.12455.

Labus, J. S., Gupta, A., Coveleskie, K., Tillisch, K., Kilpatrick, L., Jarcho, J., et al. (2013). Sex differences in emotion-related cognitive processes in irritable bowel syndrome and healthy control subjects. *Pain*, *154*(10), 2088–2099. http://dx.doi.org/10.1016/j.pain.2013.06.024.

Larauche, M., Gourcerol, G., Wang, L., Pambukchian, K., Brunnhuber, S., Adelson, D. W., et al. (2009). Cortagine, a CRF1 agonist, induces stresslike alterations of colonic function and visceral hypersensitivity in rodents primarily through peripheral pathways. *American Journal of Physiology, Gastrointestinal and Liver Physiology*, *297*(1), G215–G227. http://dx.doi.org/10.1152/ajpgi.00072.2009.

Larauche, M., Kiank, C., & Tache, Y. (2009). Corticotropin releasing factor signaling in colon and ileum: Regulation by stress and pathophysiological implications. *Journal of Physiology and Pharmacology*, *60*(Suppl. 7), 33–46.

Lee, K. N., & Lee, O. Y. (2014). Intestinal microbiota in pathophysiology and management of irritable bowel syndrome. *World Journal of Gastroenterology*, *20*(27), 8886–8897. http://dx.doi.org/10.3748/wjg.v20.i27.8886.

Li, Y., Zhang, X., Liu, H., Cao, Z., Chen, S., Cao, B., et al. (2012). Phosphorylated CaMKII post-synaptic binding to NR2B subunits in the anterior cingulate cortex mediates visceral pain in visceral hypersensitive rats. *Journal of Neurochemistry*, *121*(4), 662–671. http://dx.doi.org/10.1111/j.1471-4159.2012.07717.x.

Li, Q., Zhang, X., Liu, K., Gong, L., Li, J., Yao, W., et al. (2012). Brain-derived neurotrophic factor exerts antinociceptive effects by reducing excitability of colon-projecting dorsal root ganglion neurons in the colorectal distention-evoked visceral pain model. *Journal of Neuroscience Research*, *90*(12), 2328–2334. http://dx.doi.org/10.1002/jnr.23119.

Li, F., Zhang, J. W., Wei, R., Luo, X. G., Zhang, J. Y., Zhou, X. F., et al. (2010). Sex-differential modulation of visceral pain by brain derived neurotrophic factor (BDNF) in rats. *Neuroscience Letters*, *478*(3), 184–187. http://dx.doi.org/10.1016/j.neulet.2010.05.013.

Lindstrom, E., Brusberg, M., Hughes, P. A., Martin, C. M., Brierley, S. M., Phillis, B. D., et al. (2008). Involvement of metabotropic glutamate 5 receptor in visceral pain. *Pain*, *137*(2), 295–305. http://dx.doi.org/10.1016/j.pain.2007.09.008.

Lindstrom, E., Brusberg, M., Ravnefjord, A., Kakol-Palm, D., Pahlman, I., Noven, A., et al. (2011). Oral baclofen reduces visceral pain-related pseudo-affective responses to colorectal distension in rats: Relation between plasma exposure and efficacy. *Scandinavian Journal of Gastroenterology*, *46*(6), 652–662. http://dx.doi.org/10.3109/00365521.2011.560677.

Liu, X. H., Han, M., Zhu, J. X., Sun, N., Tang, J. S., Huo, F. Q., et al. (2012). Metabotropic glutamate subtype 7 and 8 receptors oppositely modulate cardiac nociception in the rat nucleus tractus solitarius. *Neuroscience*, *220*, 322–329. http://dx.doi.org/10.1016/j.neuroscience.2012.05.024.

Liu, L. S., Shenoy, M., & Pasricha, P. J. (2011). The analgesic effects of the GABAB receptor agonist, baclofen, in a rodent model of functional dyspepsia. *Neurogastroenterology and Motility*, *23*(4), 356–361. http://dx.doi.org/10.1111/j.1365-2982.2010.01649.x.e160–351.

Luongo, L., Maione, S., & Di Marzo, V. (2014). Endocannabinoids and neuropathic pain: Focus on neuron-glia and endocannabinoid-neurotrophin interactions. *European Journal of Neuroscience*, *39*(3), 401–408. http://dx.doi.org/10.1111/ejn.12440.

Ly, H. G., Ceccarini, J., Weltens, N., Bormans, G., Van Laere, K., Tack, J., et al. (2015). Increased cerebral cannabinoid-1 receptor availability is a stable feature of functional dyspepsia: A [F]MK-9470 PET study. *Psychotherapy and Psychosomatics*, *84*(3), 149–158. http://dx.doi.org/10.1159/000375454.

Malik, Z., Baik, D., & Schey, R. (2015). The role of cannabinoids in regulation of nausea and vomiting, and visceral pain. *Current Gastroenterology Reports*, *17*(2), 429. http://dx.doi.org/10.1007/s11894-015-0429-1.

Martin, M., Otto, C., Santamarta, M. T., Torrecilla, M., Pineda, J., Schutz, G., et al. (2003). Morphine withdrawal is modified in pituitary adenylate cyclase-activating polypeptide type I-receptor-deficient mice. *Brain Research. Molecular Brain Research*, *110*(1), 109–118.

Maurice, T., & Su, T. P. (2009). The pharmacology of sigma-1 receptors. *Pharmacology & Therapeutics*, *124*(2), 195–206. http://dx.doi.org/10.1016/j.pharmthera.2009.07.001.

McIlwrath, S. L., & Westlund, K. N. (2015). Pharmacological attenuation of chronic alcoholic pancreatitis induced hypersensitivity in rats. *World Journal of Gastroenterology*, *21*(3), 836–853. http://dx.doi.org/10.3748/wjg.v21.i3.836.

Miranda, A., Nordstrom, E., Mannem, A., Smith, C., Banerjee, B., & Sengupta, J. N. (2007). The role of transient receptor potential vanilloid 1 in mechanical and chemical visceral hyperalgesia following experimental colitis. *Neuroscience*, *148*(4), 1021–1032. http://dx.doi.org/10.1016/j.neuroscience.2007.05.034.

Mitra, R., & Sapolsky, R. M. (2008). Acute corticosterone treatment is sufficient to induce anxiety and amygdaloid dendritic hypertrophy. *Proceedings of the National Academy of Sciences of the United States of America*, *105*(14), 5573–5578. http://dx.doi.org/10.1073/pnas.0705615105.

Moloney, R. D., O'Mahony, S. M., Dinan, T. G., & Cryan, J. F. (2015). Stress-induced visceral pain: Toward animal models of irritable-bowel syndrome and associated comorbidities. *Frontiers in Psychiatry*, *6*, 15. http://dx.doi.org/10.3389/fpsyt.2015.00015.

Munro, G., Hansen, R. R., & Mirza, N. R. (2013). GABA(A) receptor modulation: Potential to deliver novel pain medicines? *European Journal of Pharmacology*, *716*(1–3), 17–23. http://dx.doi.org/10.1016/j.ejphar.2013.01.070.

Myers, B., & Greenwood-Van Meerveld, B. (2007). Corticosteroid receptor-mediated mechanisms in the amygdala regulate anxiety and colonic sensitivity. *American Journal of Physiology, Gastrointestinal and Liver Physiology*, *292*(6), G1622–G1629. http://dx.doi.org/10.1152/ajpgi.00080.2007.

Myers, B., & Greenwood-Van Meerveld, B. (2009). Role of anxiety in the pathophysiology of irritable bowel syndrome: Importance of the amygdala. *Frontiers in Neuroscience*, *3*, 47. http://dx.doi.org/10.3389/neuro.21.002.2009.

Myers, B., & Greenwood-Van Meerveld, B. (2010). Divergent effects of amygdala glucocorticoid and mineralocorticoid receptors in the regulation of visceral and somatic pain. *American Journal of Physiology, Gastrointestinal and Liver Physiology*, *298*(2), G295–G303. http://dx.doi.org/10.1152/ajpgi.00298.2009.

Myers, B., & Greenwood-Van Meerveld, B. (2012). Differential involvement of amygdala corticosteroid receptors in visceral hyperalgesia following acute or repeated stress. *American Journal of Physiology, Gastrointestinal and Liver Physiology*, *302*(2), G260–G266. http://dx.doi.org/10.1152/ajpgi.00353.2011.

Ness, T. J., & Gebhart, G. F. (1987). Quantitative comparison of inhibition of visceral and cutaneous spinal nociceptive transmission from the midbrain and medulla in the rat. *Journal of Neurophysiology*, *58*(4), 850–865.

Novick, J., Miner, P., Krause, R., Glebas, K., Bliesath, H., Ligozio, G., et al. (2002). A randomized, double-blind, placebo-controlled trial of tegaserod in female patients suffering from irritable bowel syndrome with constipation. *Alimentary Pharmacology & Therapeutics*, *16*(11), 1877–1888.

Ohsawa, M., Brailoiu, G. C., Shiraki, M., Dun, N. J., Paul, K., & Tseng, L. F. (2002). Modulation of nociceptive transmission by pituitary adenylate cyclase activating polypeptide in the spinal cord of the mouse. *Pain, 100*(1–2), 27–34.

Olsen, R. W., & Sieghart, W. (2008). International Union of Pharmacology. LXX. Subtypes of gamma-aminobutyric acid(A) receptors: Classification on the basis of subunit composition, pharmacology, and function. Update. *Pharmacological Reviews, 60*(3), 243–260. http://dx.doi.org/10.1124/pr.108.00505.

Ossipov, M. H., Lai, J., Malan, T. P., Jr., & Porreca, F. (2000). Spinal and supraspinal mechanisms of neuropathic pain. *Annals of the New York Academy of Sciences, 909*, 12–24.

Peng, H. Y., Hsieh, M. C., Lai, C. Y., Chen, G. D., Huang, Y. P., & Lin, T. B. (2012). Glucocorticoid mediates water avoidance stress-sensitized colon-bladder cross-talk via RSK2/PSD-95/NR2B in rats. *American Journal of Physiology, Endocrinology and Metabolism, 303*(9), E1094–E1106. http://dx.doi.org/10.1152/ajpendo.00235.2012.

Pertwee, R. G., Howlett, A. C., Abood, M. E., Alexander, S. P., Di Marzo, V., Elphick, M. R., et al. (2010). International Union of Basic and Clinical Pharmacology. LXXIX. Cannabinoid receptors and their ligands: Beyond CB(1) and CB(2). *Pharmacological Reviews, 62*(4), 588–631. http://dx.doi.org/10.1124/pr.110.003004.

Piche, T. (2014). Tight junctions and IBS—The link between epithelial permeability, low-grade inflammation, and symptom generation? *Neurogastroenterology and Motility, 26*(3), 296–302. http://dx.doi.org/10.1111/nmo.12315.

Pimentel, M., Lembo, A., Chey, W. D., Zakko, S., Ringel, Y., Yu, J., et al. (2011). Rifaximin therapy for patients with irritable bowel syndrome without constipation. *New England Journal of Medicine, 364*(1), 22–32. http://dx.doi.org/10.1056/NEJMoa1004409.

Price, J. L. (1999). Prefrontal cortical networks related to visceral function and mood. *Annals of the New York Academy of Sciences, 877*, 383–396.

Quigley, E. M., Tack, J., Chey, W. D., Rao, S. S., Fortea, J., Falques, M., et al. (2013). Randomised clinical trials: Linaclotide phase 3 studies in IBS-C—A prespecified further analysis based on European Medicines Agency-specified endpoints. *Alimentary Pharmacology & Therapeutics, 37*(1), 49–61. http://dx.doi.org/10.1111/apt.12123.

Radley, J. J., Anderson, R. M., Hamilton, B. A., Alcock, J. A., & Romig-Martin, S. A. (2013). Chronic stress-induced alterations of dendritic spine subtypes predict functional decrements in an hypothalamo-pituitary-adrenal-inhibitory prefrontal circuit. *Journal of Neuroscience, 33*(36), 14379–14391. http://dx.doi.org/10.1523/JNEUROSCI.0287-13.2013.

Reul, J. M., & de Kloet, E. R. (1985). Two receptor systems for corticosterone in rat brain: Microdistribution and differential occupation. *Endocrinology, 117*(6), 2505–2511. http://dx.doi.org/10.1210/endo-117-6-2505.

Reyes, B. A., Carvalho, A. F., Vakharia, K., & Van Bockstaele, E. J. (2011). Amygdalar peptidergic circuits regulating noradrenergic locus coeruleus neurons: Linking limbic and arousal centers. *Experimental Neurology, 230*(1), 96–105. http://dx.doi.org/10.1016/j.expneurol.2011.04.001.

Ringel, Y., & Drossman, D. A. (2002). Irritable bowel syndrome: Classification and conceptualization. *Journal of Clinical Gastroenterology, 35*(1 Suppl.), S7–S10.

Rivier, J., Spiess, J., & Vale, W. (1983). Characterization of rat hypothalamic corticotropin-releasing factor. *Proceedings of the National Academy of Sciences of the United States of America, 80*(15), 4851–4855.

Sagami, Y., Shimada, Y., Tayama, J., Nomura, T., Satake, M., Endo, Y., et al. (2004). Effect of a corticotropin releasing hormone receptor antagonist on colonic sensory and motor function in patients with irritable bowel syndrome. *Gut, 53*(7), 958–964.

Sandor, K., Bolcskei, K., McDougall, J. J., Schuelert, N., Reglodi, D., Elekes, K., et al. (2009). Divergent peripheral effects of pituitary adenylate cyclase-activating polypeptide-38 on nociception in rats and mice. *Pain, 141*(1–2), 143–150. http://dx.doi.org/10.1016/j.pain.2008.10.028.

Sandor, K., Kormos, V., Botz, B., Imreh, A., Bolcskei, K., Gaszner, B., et al. (2010). Impaired nocifensive behaviours and mechanical hyperalgesia, but enhanced thermal allodynia in pituitary adenylate cyclase-activating polypeptide deficient mice. *Neuropeptides, 44*(5), 363–371. http://dx.doi.org/10.1016/j.npep.2010.06.004.

Sapolsky, R. M., McEwen, B. S., & Rainbow, T. C. (1983). Quantitative autoradiography of [3H]corticosterone receptors in rat brain. *Brain Research, 271*(2), 331–334.

Sawchenko, P. E., & Swanson, L. W. (1981). Central noradrenergic pathways for the integration of hypothalamic neuroendocrine and autonomic responses. *Science, 214*(4521), 685–687.

Schaible, H. G., Ebersberger, A., & Natura, G. (2011). Update on peripheral mechanisms of pain: Beyond prostaglandins and cytokines. *Arthritis Research & Therapy, 13*(2), 210. http://dx.doi.org/10.1186/ar3305.

Scholz, J., & Woolf, C. J. (2002). Can we conquer pain? *Nature Neuroscience, 5*(Suppl.), 1062–1067. http://dx.doi.org/10.1038/nn942.

Schulkin, J., Gold, P. W., & McEwen, B. S. (1998). Induction of corticotropin-releasing hormone gene expression by glucocorticoids: Implication for understanding the states of fear and anxiety and allostatic load. *Psychoneuroendocrinology, 23*(3), 219–243.

Sengupta, J. N., Pochiraju, S., Kannampalli, P., Bruckert, M., Addya, S., Yadav, P., et al. (2013). MicroRNA-mediated GABA Aalpha-1 receptor subunit down-regulation in adult spinal cord following neonatal cystitis-induced chronic visceral pain in rats. *Pain, 154*(1), 59–70. http://dx.doi.org/10.1016/j.pain.2012.09.002.

Shepard, J. D., Barron, K. W., & Myers, D. A. (2000). Corticosterone delivery to the amygdala increases corticotropin-releasing factor mRNA in the central amygdaloid nucleus and anxiety-like behavior. *Brain Research, 861*(2), 288–295.

Shimizu, T., Katahira, M., Sugawara, H., Inoue, K., & Miyata, A. (2004). Diverse effects of intrathecal pituitary adenylate cyclase-activating polypeptide on nociceptive transmission in mice spinal cord. *Regulatory Peptides, 123*(1–3), 117–122. http://dx.doi.org/10.1016/j.regpep.2004.05.019.

Srinath, A., Young, E., & Szigethy, E. (2014). Pain management in patients with inflammatory bowel disease: Translational approaches from bench to bedside. *Inflammatory Bowel Diseases, 20*(12), 2433–2449. http://dx.doi.org/10.1097/MIB.0000000000000170.

Staud, R. (2012). Abnormal endogenous pain modulation is a shared characteristic of many chronic pain conditions. *Expert Review of Neurotherapeutics, 12*(5), 577–585. http://dx.doi.org/10.1586/ern.12.41.

Stemkowski, P. L., & Smith, P. A. (2012). Sensory neurons, ion channels, inflammation and the onset of neuropathic pain. *Canadian Journal of Neurological Sciences, 39*(4), 416–435.

Sweetser, S., Camilleri, M., Linker Nord, S. J., Burton, D. D., Castenada, L., Croop, R., et al. (2009). Do corticotropin releasing factor-1 receptors influence colonic transit and bowel function in women with irritable bowel syndrome? *American Journal of Physiology, Gastrointestinal and Liver Physiology, 296*(6), G1299–G1306. http://dx.doi.org/10.1152/ajpgi.00011.2009.

Tache, Y., & Million, M. (2015). Role of corticotropin-releasing factor signaling in stress-related alterations of colonic motility and hyperalgesia. *Journal of Neurogastroenterology and Motility, 21*(1), 8–24. http://dx.doi.org/10.5056/jnm14162.

Tao, Y. X. (2012). AMPA receptor trafficking in inflammation-induced dorsal horn central sensitization. *Neuroscience Bulletin, 28*(2), 111–120. http://dx.doi.org/10.1007/s12264-012-1204-z.

Tran, L., Chaloner, A., Sawalha, A. H., & Greenwood Van-Meerveld, B. (2013). Importance of epigenetic mechanisms in visceral pain induced by chronic water avoidance stress. *Psychoneuroendocrinology, 38*(6), 898–906. http://dx.doi.org/10.1016/j.psyneuen.2012.09.016.

Tran, L., & Greenwood-Van Meerveld, B. (2012). Altered expression of glucocorticoid receptor and corticotropin-releasing factor in the central amygdala in response to elevated corticosterone. *Behavioural Brain Research, 234*(2), 380–385. http://dx.doi.org/10.1016/j.bbr.2012.07.010.

Tran, L., Schulkin, J., & Greenwood-Van Meerveld, B. (2014). Importance of CRF receptor-mediated mechanisms of the bed nucleus of the stria terminalis in the processing of anxiety and pain. *Neuropsychopharmacology, 39*(11), 2633–2645. http://dx.doi.org/10.1038/npp.2014.117.

Tran, L., Schulkin, J., Ligon, C. O., & Greenwood-Van Meerveld, B. (2015). Epigenetic modulation of chronic anxiety and pain by histone deacetylation. *Molecular Psychiatry, 20*(10), 1219–1231. http://dx.doi.org/10.1038/mp.2014.122.

Traub, R. J., Silva, E., Gebhart, G. F., & Solodkin, A. (1996). Noxious colorectal distention induced-c-Fos protein in limbic brain structures in the rat. *Neuroscience Letters, 215*(3), 165–168.

Trescot, A. (2013). Clinical use of opioids. In A. Buvanendran, T. R. Deer, V. Gordin, P. S. Kim, M. S. Leong, S. J. Panchal, et al. (Eds.), *Comprehensive treatment of chronic pain by medical, interventional, and integrative approaches: THE AMERICAN ACADEMY OF PAIN MEDICINE textbook on patient management* (pp. 99–110). New York: Springer. http://dx.doi.org/10.1007/978-1-4614-1560-2.

Trimble, N., Johnson, A. C., Foster, A., & Greenwood-van Meerveld, B. (2007). Corticotropin-releasing factor receptor 1-deficient mice show decreased anxiety and colonic sensitivity. *Neurogastroenterology and Motility, 19*(9), 754–760. http://dx.doi.org/10.1111/j.1365-2982.2007.00951.x.

Vale, W., Spiess, J., Rivier, C., & Rivier, J. (1981). Characterization of a 41-residue ovine hypothalamic peptide that stimulates secretion of corticotropin and beta-endorphin. *Science, 213*(4514), 1394–1397.

van Diest, S. A., Stanisor, O. I., Boeckxstaens, G. E., de Jonge, W. J., & van den Wijngaard, R. M. (2012). Relevance of mast cell-nerve interactions in intestinal nociception. *Biochimica et Biophysica Acta, 1822*(1), 74–84. http://dx.doi.org/10.1016/j.bbadis.2011.03.019.

van Wanrooij, S. J., Wouters, M. M., Van Oudenhove, L., Vanbrabant, W., Mondelaers, S., Kollmann, P., et al. (2014). Sensitivity testing in irritable bowel syndrome with rectal capsaicin stimulations: Role of TRPV1 upregulation and sensitization in visceral hypersensitivity? *American Journal of Gastroenterology, 109*(1), 99–109. http://dx.doi.org/10.1038/ajg.2013.371.

Vasant, D. H., Payton, A., Mistry, S., Thompson, D. G., & Hamdy, S. (2013). The val66met polymorphism of brain-derived neurotrophic factor is associated with human esophageal hypersensitivity. *Neurogastroenterology and Motility, 25*(2), 162–e185. http://dx.doi.org/10.1111/nmo.12021.

Vyas, A., Mitra, R., Shankaranarayana Rao, B. S., & Chattarji, S. (2002). Chronic stress induces contrasting patterns of dendritic remodeling in hippocampal and amygdaloid neurons. *Journal of Neuroscience, 22*(15), 6810–6818http://dx.doi.org/20026655.

Walker, M. M., Warwick, A., Ung, C., & Talley, N. J. (2011). The role of eosinophils and mast cells in intestinal functional disease. *Current Gastroenterology Reports, 13*(4), 323–330. http://dx.doi.org/10.1007/s11894-011-0197-5.

Wang, P., Chen, F. X., Du, C., Li, C. Q., Yu, Y. B., Zuo, X. L., et al. (2015). Increased production of BDNF in colonic epithelial cells induced by fecal supernatants from diarrheic IBS patients. *Scientific Reports, 5*, 10121. http://dx.doi.org/10.1038/srep10121.

Whitehead, W. E., Palsson, O., & Jones, K. R. (2002). Systematic review of the comorbidity of irritable bowel syndrome with other disorders: What are the causes and implications? *Gastroenterology, 122*(4), 1140–1156.

Widgerow, A. D., & Kalaria, S. (2012). Pain mediators and wound healing—Establishing the connection. *Burns, 38*(7), 951–959. http://dx.doi.org/10.1016/j.burns.2012.05.024.

Wilder-Smith, C. H. (2011). The balancing act: Endogenous modulation of pain in functional gastrointestinal disorders. *Gut*, *60*(11), 1589–1599. http://dx.doi.org/10.1136/gutjnl-2011-300253.

Wilson, N., & Schey, R. (2015). Lubiprostone in constipation: Clinical evidence and place in therapy. *Therapeutic Advances in Chronic Disease*, *6*(2), 40–50. http://dx.doi.org/10.1177/2040622314567678.

Winston, J. H., Li, Q., & Sarna, S. K. (2014). Chronic prenatal stress epigenetically modifies spinal cord BDNF expression to induce sex-specific visceral hypersensitivity in offspring. *Neurogastroenterology & Motility*, *26*(5), 715–730. http://dx.doi.org/10.1111/nmo.12326.

Winston, J. H., & Sarna, S. K. (2013). Developmental origins of functional dyspepsia-like gastric hypersensitivity in rats. *Gastroenterology*, *144*(3), 570–579. http://dx.doi.org/10.1053/j.gastro.2012.11.001. e573.

Wiskur, B. J., Tyler, K., Campbell-Dittmeyer, K., Chaplan, S. R., Wickenden, A. D., & Greenwood-Van Meerveld, B. (2010). A novel TRPV1 receptor antagonist JNJ-17203212 attenuates colonic hypersensitivity in rats. *Methods & Findings in Experimental & Clinical Pharmacology*, *32*(8), 557–564. http://dx.doi.org/10.1358/mf.2010.32.8.1507853.

Witkin, J. M., Statnick, M. A., Rorick-Kehn, L. M., Pintar, J. E., Ansonoff, M., Chen, Y., et al. (2014). The biology of Nociceptin/Orphanin FQ (N/OFQ) related to obesity, stress, anxiety, mood, and drug dependence. *Pharmacology & Therapeutics*, *141*(3), 283–299. http://dx.doi.org/10.1016/j.pharmthera.2013.10.011.

Woolf, C. J., & Salter, M. W. (2000). Neuronal plasticity: Increasing the gain in pain. *Science*, *288*(5472), 1765–1769.

Woolley, C. S., Gould, E., & McEwen, B. S. (1990). Exposure to excess glucocorticoids alters dendritic morphology of adult hippocampal pyramidal neurons. *Brain Research*, *531*(1–2), 225–231.

Wu, X., Gao, J., Yan, J., Fan, J., Owyang, C., & Li, Y. (2008). Role for NMDA receptors in visceral nociceptive transmission in the anterior cingulate cortex of viscerally hypersensitive rats. *American Journal of Physiology-Gastrointestinal and Liver Physiology*, *294*(4), G918–G927. http://dx.doi.org/10.1152/ajpgi.00452.2007.

Yang, J., Yu, Y., Yu, H., Zuo, X., Liu, C., Gao, L., et al. (2010). The role of brain-derived neurotrophic factor in experimental inflammation of mouse gut. *European Journal of Pain*, *14*(6), 574–579. http://dx.doi.org/10.1016/j.ejpain.2009.10.007.

Yarushkina, N. I., Bagaeva, T. R., & Filaretova, L. P. (2009). Analgesic actions of corticotropin-releasing factor (CRF) on somatic pain sensitivity: Involvement of glucocorticoid and CRF-2 receptors. *Neuroscience and Behavioral Physiology*, *39*(9), 819–823. http://dx.doi.org/10.1007/s11055-009-9212-9.

Yu, Y. B., Zuo, X. L., Zhao, Q. J., Chen, F. X., Yang, J., Dong, Y. Y., et al. (2012). Brain-derived neurotrophic factor contributes to abdominal pain in irritable bowel syndrome. *Gut*, *61*(5), 685–694. http://dx.doi.org/10.1136/gutjnl-2011-300265.

Zamanillo, D., Romero, L., Merlos, M., & Vela, J. M. (2013). Sigma 1 receptor: A new therapeutic target for pain. *European Journal of Pharmacology*, *716*(1–3), 78–93. http://dx.doi.org/10.1016/j.ejphar.2013.01.068.

Zeilhofer, H. U., Wildner, H., & Yevenes, G. E. (2012). Fast synaptic inhibition in spinal sensory processing and pain control. *Physiological Reviews*, *92*(1), 193–235. http://dx.doi.org/10.1152/physrev.00043.2010.

Zhang, L., Zhang, X., & Westlund, K. N. (2004). Restoration of spontaneous exploratory behaviors with an intrathecal NMDA receptor antagonist or a PKC inhibitor in rats with acute pancreatitis. *Pharmacology Biochemistry & Behavior*, *77*(1), 145–153.

Zhou, L., Huang, J., Gao, J., Zhang, G., & Jiang, J. (2014). NMDA and AMPA receptors in the anterior cingulate cortex mediates visceral pain in visceral hypersensitivity rats. *Cellular Immunology*, *287*(2), 86–90. http://dx.doi.org/10.1016/j.cellimm.2013.12.001.

Zhou, Q., Price, D. D., Caudle, R. M., & Verne, G. N. (2009). Spinal NMDA NR1 subunit expression following transient TNBS colitis. *Brain Research*, *1279*, 109–120. http://dx.doi.org/10.1016/j.brainres.2009.04.038.
Zhou, Q., Yang, L., Larson, S., Basra, S., Merwat, S., Tan, A., et al. (2015). Decreased miR-199 augments visceral pain in patients with IBS through translational upregulation of TRPV1. *Gut*. http://dx.doi.org/10.1136/gutjnl-2013-306464, pii: gutjnl-2013-306464.
Zhu, Z. W., Friess, H., Wang, L., Zimmermann, A., & Buchler, M. W. (2001). Brain-derived neurotrophic factor (BDNF) is upregulated and associated with pain in chronic pancreatitis. *Digestive Diseases and Sciences*, *46*(8), 1633–1639.
Zhuo, M., & Gebhart, G. F. (2002). Facilitation and attenuation of a visceral nociceptive reflex from the rostroventral medulla in the rat. *Gastroenterology*, *122*(4), 1007–1019.

CHAPTER ELEVEN

Preclinical Pharmacological Approaches in Drug Discovery for Chronic Pain

Garth T. Whiteside*, James D. Pomonis†, Jeffrey D. Kennedy‡,1

*Discovery Research, Purdue Pharma L.P., Cranbury, New Jersey, USA
†American Preclinical Services, LLC, Minneapolis, Minnesota, USA
‡JK Associates BioPharma Consulting, LLC, Carmel, Indiana, USA
1Corresponding author: e-mail address: jdkennedy2@gmail.com

Contents

Abstract

In recent years, animal behavioral models, particularly those used in pain research, have been increasingly scrutinized and criticized for their role in the poor translation of novel pharmacotherapies for chronic pain. This chapter addresses the use of animal models of pain used in drug discovery research. It highlights how, when, and why animal models of pain are used as one of the many experimental tools used to gain better understanding of target mechanisms and rank-order compounds in the iterative process of establishing structure–activity relationship. Together, these models help create an "analgesic signature" for a compound and inform the indications most likely to yield success in clinical trials. In addition, the authors discuss some often underappreciated aspects of currently used (traditional) animal models of pain, including simply applying basic pharmacological principles to study design and data interpretation as well as consideration of efficacy alongside side effect measures as part of the overall conclusion of efficacy. This is provided to add perspective regarding current efforts to develop new models and endpoints both in rodents and in larger animal species as well as assess cognitive and/or affective aspects of pain. Finally, the authors suggest ways in which efficacy evaluation in animal models of pain, whether traditional or new, might better align with clinical standards of analysis,

Advances in Pharmacology, Volume 75
ISSN 1054-3589
http://dx.doi.org/10.1016/bs.apha.2015.12.002

citing examples where applying effect size and number needed to treat estimations to animal model data suggest that the efficacy bar often may be set too low preclinically to allow successful translation to the clinical setting.

1. INTRODUCTION

Discovering and developing novel drugs for use in humans are arduous. Obstacles are present at many levels, including biology, chemistry, intellectual property, and regulatory considerations. When pursuing unprecedented targets, these obstacles are associated with even greater risk. As such, only a fraction of preclinical effort will translate to successful clinical studies, a challenge for drug discovery in any therapeutic arena. Although pharmacokinetic (PK) parameters were once a main reason for clinical development failures, this is no longer the case (Kola & Landis, 2004). In recent years, criticism has been widely levied against the animal models used in pain research and analgesic drug development (Blackshaw, 2012; Mao, 2012; Oertel & Lötsch, 2013; Taneja, Di lorio, Danhof, & Della Pasqua, 2012). The widespread belief that these models have limited or no translational value comes from both academia and industry, with many suggesting that the paucity of new analgesic drugs results from animal model data that are misleading in their conclusion of efficacy and/or poorly reflect clinical pain signs and symptoms (Blackburn-Munro, 2004; Rice et al., 2008; Vierck, Hansson, & Yezierski, 2008). With that said, it is our firm belief that current translational challenges should not in any way lessen the value of, or confidence in, animal models of pain.

Drug development efforts fail for numerous reasons: toxicity, dose-limiting side effects, failure to show improvement or otherwise differentiate versus standard of care (SOC) drugs, or poor selection of indication or patient cohort, among others. While a few examples exist where efficacy demonstrated in animal models of pain has failed to translate to clinical efficacy (Hill, 2000; Huggins, Smart, Langman, Taylor, & Young, 2012; Pande et al., 1996), in general, such failures have been poorly documented with little published data. Thus, a definitive conclusion that animal models yield "false-positive" data is not clearly supported. Likewise, it is all but certain the converse has never been tested, namely identification of a "false-negative" through clinical trial of a mechanism that failed to show efficacy preclinically. In this light, it is worth noting that there have been successes in translating preclinical efficacy to the clinic, including the approval of ziconitide, the still evolving development of antinerve growth factor therapies, and the more recently published successful trial of a TRPV1 antagonist compound, albeit in the context of third molar extraction (Quiding et al., 2013); whether TRPV1 antagonist compounds prove efficacious in more complex, chronic pain conditions await data from further clinical pain studies. In this chapter, the authors put forward a perspective on existing, "traditional" models of pain as well as new models being developed. We offer a rationale for how animal models are used across the drug discovery process, one that may differ in some notable aspects from their use in academic research. While recognizing the limitations of these models, we hope to highlight some of the current misconceptions around animal models of pain and suggest for consideration potential improvements. (Aspects of the work described in this chapter have been published elsewhere: Whiteside, Pomonis, & Kennedy, 2013.)

2. THE NEEDS OF DRUG DISCOVERY

The endgame for pharmaceutical companies is to bring new drugs to market. The steps required to do so are numerous and span, on average, 12 years or longer and involve a number of science and business functions. Drug discovery is often described as beginning with target identification, proceeding to target validation, and culminating in identification and production of a development candidate/potential new therapeutic agent. Each step involves "go/no-go" criteria that must be met in order to move to the next step. As a consequence, the tools employed at each step are likely to change as the process progresses, including the use of animal models.

In the target identification phase, animal models are very important in order to monitor gene expression or protein levels in specific tissues during disease progression. These studies utilize multiple, often complex, models to interrogate the role of a protein in the underlying biology. In the target validation phase, genetically modified animals may be used to "validate" a target mechanism's role in pathobiology by determining the consequence of disrupting its function; additionally at this stage, if any probe molecules are available to assess pharmacology, they are often used to obtain an initial understanding of potential efficacy, although these molecules typically exhibit poor drug-like properties. Upon reaching a decision to initiate a drug discovery program aimed at a particular target, drug discovery groups need suitable animal models of pain amenable to screening tens to hundreds of compounds in a manner that will enable description of efficacy and potency in a dose-responsive fashion, PKs, pharmacodynamics (PDs), and side effects, all within a time frame of months and with a high degree of reproducibility and precision (see Fig. 1). Once a suitable candidate is identified using screening and second tier models, additional compound characterization is frequently conducted, including use of novel models/endpoints that may more specifically model a particular pain syndrome and may help inform the clinical conditions that should be targeted.

As such, the requirements for advancement vary over the course of the drug discovery process. At the target validation stage, the cost, throughput, and feasibility of pharmacological manipulation are of lesser importance than at later time points. Conversely, once a target has been identified and preclinically validated, the animal models used must be chosen primarily based on relevance to the pharmacology under investigation but throughput, sensitivity, ability to determine relative potency, reproducibility, and cost, among others are also critically important. The final stage of characterization is seen as adding to what is known for a particular compound and enriching the preclinical dataset. What might be considered an appropriate model in one part of the process may not be suitable for other parts. Ultimately, successful drug discovery and development is not predicated on developing the "holy grail" of animal models of neuropathic pain (or any other painful condition), but more-so on understanding the benefits and

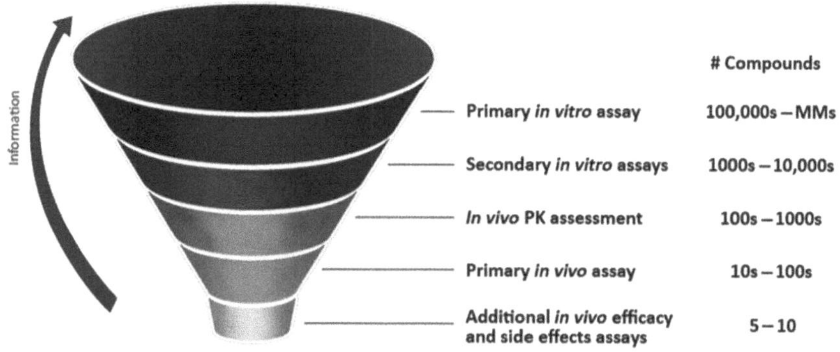

Figure 1 A simplified flowchart representing the use of biological assays, including *in vivo* assays, in industry. The range of compound numbers typically tested at each tier is indicated, although this will vary by company and project. Compounds move down "through the funnel" if prespecified criteria in the biological assays are met, while information is fed back in order to improve the characteristics of newly synthesized compounds and increase the chances of a compound being advanced into development. PK, pharmacokinetics, MMs, millions.

limitations inherent to all the assays and models that together are used to establish confidence in a target and compounds so that data-driven decisions can be made when considering advancement of candidate compounds at each stage of the process.

3. CURRENT STATUS AND NEW PERSPECTIVES ON ANIMAL MODELS OF PAIN

Numerous animal models of pain have been designed as a means to investigate mechanisms underlying nociceptive, inflammatory, and nerve injury pain. It is beyond the scope and intent of this chapter to describe these models, their methodology, variations, and endpoints, but the reader is directed to review by Mogil (2009) as well as Joshi and Honore (2006) for more details. To assess pain in animals as part of drug discovery, most models in use couple a method for inducing a hypersensitive state, such as mechanical trauma or injection of an algogenic substance (the model), to a behavioral assessment (the endpoint). Endpoints traditionally include either direct observation of nonevoked, spontaneous behaviors such as flinching, licking, biting, or altered weight bearing, or evoked responses such as paw withdrawal, vocalization, or struggle following application of a stimulus (heat, blunt pressure, focused tactile probing, etc.). These behaviors are believed to represent pain being experienced by the animal and have been referred to as "pain stimulated" (Stevenson et al., 2009). Advances are being made in establishing disease models to represent osteoarthritis (OA), fibromyalgia, postoperative, visceral, and thermal injury pain, among others. Likewise, the methodology for developing new endpoints is growing and now includes an array of measures such as electroencephalograms (Granmo, Jensen, & Schouenborg, 2013), alterations in sleep (Leys et al., 2013; Silva, Andersen, & Tufik, 2008), movement (thigmotaxis) (Huang et al., 2013), or gait (Piesla et al., 2009), changes in social or "well-being" behaviors such as burrowing (Andrews et al., 2012), and choice (preference, aversion) paradigms (Hummel, Lu, Cummons, & Whiteside, 2008; King et al., 2009; Sufka, 1994; van der Kam, Vry, Schiene, & Tzschentke, 2008), intracranial self-stimulation and other pain-depressed behaviors (Negus et al., 2006; Pereira Do Carmo, Stevenson, Carlezon, & Negus, 2009), even facial expressions (Langford et al., 2010). It is safe to say that hundreds of model/endpoint combinations are now possible and being described in the literature.

Interest has also grown in the development and implementation of large animal and/or naturally developing (naturalistic) models of pain based on the assumption these will show greater face, construct and, ultimately, predictive validity. There is support for the view that new models utilizing novel endpoints are needed in order to overcome the current translational impasse in the development of novel pain drugs (Langford et al., 2010; Mao, 2012). A number of academic and industrial groups are accelerating efforts around, for example, dog models of OA (Brown, Boston, Coyne, & Farrar, 2008), and nonhuman primate models of inflammatory or nerve injury pain (Henze & Urban, 2010). Although these models ultimately may reveal insights into pain behaviors not readily apparent in rodents and provide translational benefits from both PK/PD and toxicology perspectives, they also present a number of challenges, not the least of which relates to greater heterogeneity in the manifestations of "spontaneous" pain relative to that induced in rodents by directed means. While rodent models utilizing homogeneous age, sex, weight, and strain are criticized as not being representative of clinical pain, naturalistic models in larger animals make establishing robust endpoints and reproducibility between experiments much more difficult, even if they may more closely mimic human-like disease heterogeneity. Power calculations for compound assessments in a typical behavioral study over a 3-point dose response, most often covering a 10-fold dose range, typically suggest group sizes of 8–10 animals; including positive and negative control groups, this approaches a total experiment size of 50 animals, a number not feasible when using larger animals. In addition, because injury and, hence, pain severity is not controlled as it is when applying a uniform insult to groups of rodents, intra- and intergroup variability is likely to obscure conclusions of statistical efficacy. Assays using thermal or mechanical stimuli to evoke nocifensive responses in large animal models of pain are the same as those criticized for use in rodent models. Unfortunately, measurement of nonevoked pain endpoints in larger species is still rudimentary and highly variable, although advances are being made (Brown et al., 2008; Walton, Cowderoy, Lascelles, & Innes, 2013). The caution is to maintain perspective regarding the fact that animal models, even those utilizing nonhuman primates, represent, at best, only an approximation of human biology and behavior. In an almost paradoxical way, many, while acknowledging this gap, remain keen to anthropomorphize animal behavior.

Efforts to generate new behavioral data, particularly those revealing insights into cognitive and affective aspects of pain, are certain to enrich our understanding of pain pathobiology and may ultimately increase translational success; however, in our view, there are other gaps in the translational chain more readily accessible and likely to yield positive results in the short term. These include better patient phenotyping and stratification, implementation of trial designs that may help minimize placebo effects, and, in the preclinical realm, setting the bar higher with respect to what is viewed as efficacious enough to merit advancement into development (discussed below).

Gaining confidence in the predictive validity of any behavioral assessment is a lengthy process. Ideally, compounds proven clinically efficacious should have entered into development based, in part, on robust efficacy in an animal model(s). Establishing such a connection for a new model could take many years. While back translation is more rapid and provides some level of confidence in established mechanisms, this is not possible if no clinically efficacious treatments are available or for new mechanisms that have yet to be tested clinically. Only time and significant experience will determine whether new models represent an improvement over those currently in use. It is our opinion that any new model should be used in addition to, and not as a replacement for, established models. All models are "predictive" for some aspect of pain; the key lies in determining which model/endpoint combination, whether traditional or new, best reflects the pharmacology and clinical phenotype of interest. Moreover, as more extensive pharmacologic validation using new models accumulates, we would suggest that a failure to align efficacy across these and the traditional models does not necessarily invalidate either but instead adds greater depth to our overall understanding of pain pathophysiology. Indeed, if endpoints do align, as recently found for spared nerve injury-induced hypersensitivity to von Frey fibers and spared nerve injury-induced reduction in burrowing behavior (Lau et al., 2013), the challenge for the field is to justify and to demonstrate that new models constitute an improvement as predictors of translational success. The true test of this will come only with successful development of an unprecedented mechanism; we already know that the clinically efficacious pain drugs back translate into the traditional models both with respect to exposure and model type (Whiteside, Adedoyin, & Leventhal, 2008).

Because there are numerous combinations of model and endpoint, it is not sensible to group all under a single heading of "animal models of pain" and deem the lot neither valid nor predictive; a more specific analysis is warranted. For example, a simple nociceptive pain model such as tail flick is responsive to several classes of compounds given intrathecally in addition to systemically administered opioids. If developing a new opioid drug, this assay may be highly predictive of clinical efficacy. In addition, such a model, among the simplest in the spectrum of model/endpoint combinations, may even allow for accurate determinations of expected efficacious exposure levels across a dose range, as supported by comparative analysis of other molecules from the same class and route of administration for which both preclinical and clinical data exist. The corollary is also true, in that currently used models must be used appropriately to have the best chance of providing a solid translational bridge to clinical pain. For example, the complete Freund's adjuvant (CFA) model most closely recapitulates the etiology and symptomatology of inflammatory arthritis conditions such as rheumatoid arthritis yet is often used as a bridge to OA. It is unreasonable to expect efficacy achieved in the CFA model to accurately predict clinical efficacy in OA let alone in animal models of OA. Furthermore, because clinically used compounds display efficacy against traditional models/endpoints, the development of new therapies will require they, too, be tested in those assays; decision makers in pharmaceutical and biotech companies and, ultimately, payors demand that any new drug differentiates from SOC drugs by demonstrating some aspect of superiority. And as additional preclinical endpoints are developed, their sensitivities to differing pharmacologies will have to be established. These are unlikely to align perfectly (Huntjens, Spalding, Danhof, & Della Pasqua, 2009), given that sensory, affective, and cognitive manifestations of pain have different, if overlapping, neural substrates and so would be expected to respond differently to treatments. Thus, sorting out the relative importance of one endpoint versus another will further complicate the ability to establish predictive PK/PD relationships. The trend toward increased use of evoked endpoints in the clinic, including quantitative sensory testing (QST), as a means to diagnose and to stratify patient subpopulations (Baron, Förster, & Binder, 2012) may also inform alignment between clinical and preclinical endpoints if these can be shown to have utility for assessing drug efficacy. Our prediction is that aligning preclinical model/endpoint with well-circumscribed disease phenotypes and as well expanding the use of evoked endpoints, in addition to currently used patient-reported outcome measures to assess clinical drug efficacy, will improve the overall translational success.

We view as essential practices that experiments are conducted employing blinding and randomization, that dose response curves are established to determine whether they inform/confirm both mechanism and PK/PD relationships and that motor deficits are ruled out as potential confounds against accurate conclusions of efficacy (Whiteside et al., 2008). In addition, we further advocate the use of multiple models, species, and endpoints (including nonevoked) combined with models of affect, cognition, and other behaviors that together are integrated to create an analgesic signature for a given mechanism. This serves the purpose of not overemphasizing any one model or technique, given clear evidence from both clinical experience and back-translation studies that no drug/mechanism yields equivalent efficacy in all models or on all endpoints; hence, no single model or technique should be used to drive a drug discovery and development effort. In addition, establishing efficacy across a variety of models reduces translational risk associated with the target mechanism, and observed variability in potency or maximal effects can help inform both clinical trial design and patient population selection.

4. THE CRITICAL ROLE OF BEHAVIORAL PHARMACOLOGY IN DRUG DEVELOPMENT

Animal efficacy models constitute but one step in an array of molecular, cell- and tissue-based biological assays that in concert with synthetic chemistry are used to screen many molecules and then to more thoroughly characterize smaller numbers of compounds with the goal of identifying one, or a few, candidates for clinical development. There are many steps in this process (see Fig. 1) including creation and validation of cell lines used to conclude appropriate activity at, and selectivity for, the molecular target, PK assessments both *in vitro* and in animals, electrophysiology assays, side effect profiling, biomarker, target engagement and other "translational" models, as well as toxicity assessments. Together, these assays and models are used to establish converging lines of evidence in support of a target mechanism's role in pain and to build confidence that a candidate molecule, whether protein or small organic compound, by robustly modifying the target's activity, will demonstrate activity against a clinical pain condition(s).

A lack of translatability of any of the aforementioned assays, not just *in vivo* efficacy assessments, may lead to a negative clinical trial. Questions regarding the predictive validity of cell-based assays are rarely discussed in the context of successful clinical translation, as there is an appreciation that such assays are highly contrived, artificial, and serve primarily as a means to allow researchers to rank-order compounds according to a limited set of criteria. In contrast, a similar acknowledgment of assay limitations is rarely, if ever, extended to the interpretation of data from animal models of pain, which are also contrived and artificial; however, the fact that the models are contrived and artificial understates their utility in the drug discovery process. It is sometimes underappreciated that during drug development, these models are used not only to determine efficacy interrogated in the context of some insult/disease but also to play critical roles in generating credible dose–response curves that can be used to establish PK/PD relationships and help rank-order compounds as part of the structure–activity relationship (SAR) paradigm.

In drug discovery, a novel compound is not determined to be efficacious following administration of a single dose in a single model. A typical behavioral experiment might involve a range of doses followed by efficacy measurement at a number of time points following dosing, often centered around the projected T_{max} (time of maximal plasma exposure) based on prior PK evaluation. If a limited number of time points are used, then such an evaluation provides only a snapshot-in-time of a compound's performance. Indeed, the thorough profiling of potential drug candidate compounds requires the application of basic pharmacological principles to determine the extent of a compound's dose–response qualities, its minimum or median effective dose (ED_{50}) as a measure of potency, and its maximal effect as a measure of efficacy (see Fig. 2A). Assuming that the biological effect of a novel drug is driven by on-target mechanisms, robust dose–response relationships must be present so that pharmaceutical techniques (such as dosage formulation) can be used to overcome pharmacological issues (e.g., obtaining desired plasma levels of the drug). As such, efficacy cannot be simplified to a single time point or a single dose but must be inferred from the entirety of a compound's pharmacological profile (and the entire class of compounds). Therefore, the need for the ability to provide meaningful data over a range of doses and multiple time points is critical for drug discovery.

Another important aspect of the SAR paradigm of drug discovery is gaining an understanding of compound efficacy in relationship to undesirable side effects. In the case of pain drugs, many of which require CNS exposure in order to achieve maximal efficacy, researchers typically employ models of motoric impairment, such as the ability of a test animal to walk without falling off a rotating drum (rotarod assay). As shown in Fig. 2A, comparing doses that produce efficacy in a pain model to those leading to motoric impairment allows the researcher to both accurately conclude efficacy (as opposed to an inability to respond to a painful stimulus) and establish a therapeutic index (TI) based on the separation of doses (or ideally, plasma drug concentrations) between an efficacious and an impairing dose. This is

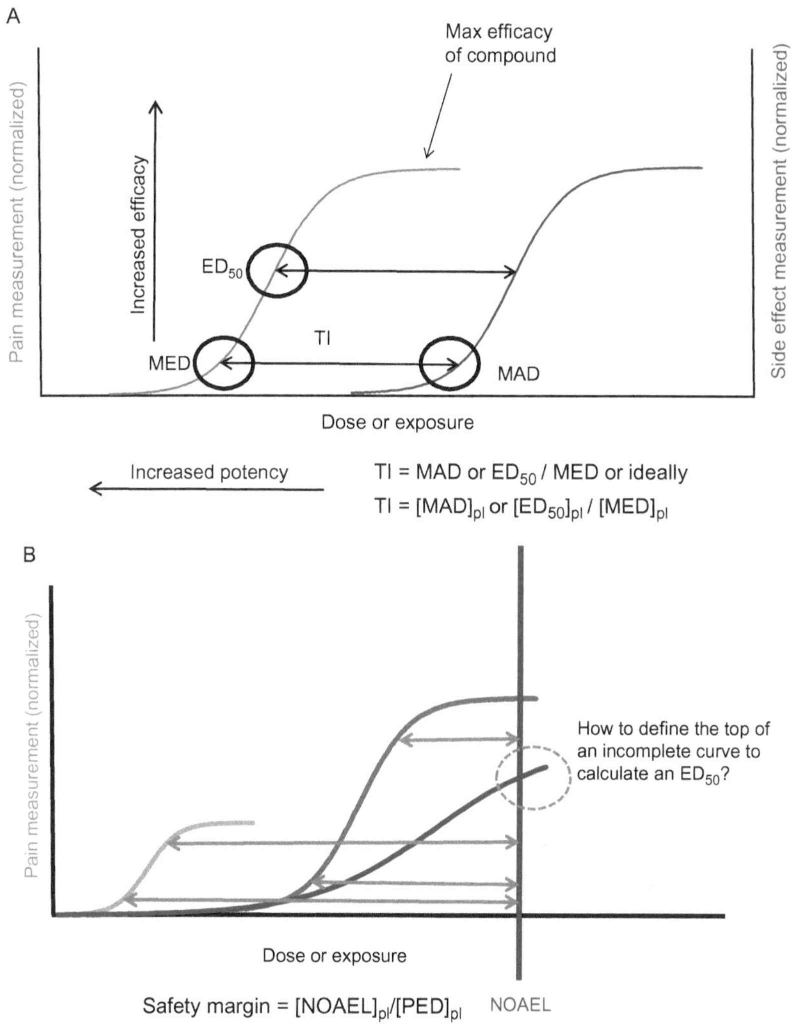

Figure 2 Efficacy and side effect dose–response curves and utility in establishing preclinical therapeutic index (TI). (A) Dose–response curves are stylized to show classic S-shaped pattern. For compounds to be considered potential drug candidates, side effect curves typically are right shifted relative to efficacy curves, with the separation used in the calculation of a TI. In this example, TI is calculated by dividing the minimally ataxic (or impairing) dose (MAD) or plasma concentration of drug at the MAD $[MAD]_{pl}$ by the minimally efficacious dose (MED) or median effective dose (ED_{50}) or their associated plasma concentration $[MED]_{pl}$. (B) Dose–response curves drawn to represent compounds with differing potency, efficacy, and hill slopes. These curves are compared to a dose defined as a safety barrier, the no observed adverse effect level (NOAEL), defined as the highest tested dose of a compound that shows no toxicologically significant effects. The safety margin/TI for each compound is derived by dividing the NOAEL dose (or resulting drug concentration in the animal) by the dose (or concentration) producing an ED_{80} (upper arrows) or an MED (lower arrows) response. The dotted circle highlights a dose–response curve where a true top (E_{max}) is not achieved, impacting the precision with which safety margins can be estimated.

usually accomplished by comparing the minimally efficacious dose (MED) or the median efficacious dose (ED_{50}) to the minimally adverse/impairing dose (MAD). The disadvantage of the use of MED, though directly measured, is that it is unlikely to accurately reflect either the dose or efficacy required of a drug to show efficacy in humans. This has led in many cases to the use of either ED_{50} or ED_{80}, i.e., pharmacologically effective doses (PED), for calculating TI and safety margins; however, PED, in addition to being a calculated rather than measured value, is often a contrived estimate unless the true top (maximal compound effect) and bottom (no effect) doses/exposures for a compound are measured. The curves in Fig. 2A are idealized; what is more often encountered when profiling compound efficacy and side effects is represented in Fig. 2B where, for any number of reasons, including compound solubility and PK characteristics, compound dose–response curves for efficacy and side effects are not similarly shaped, and accurately measuring the tops of the efficacy and side effect curves is impossible. As such, considering only one variable such as potency (ED_{50}) can be very misleading for compounds with different efficacies (E_{max}) and hill slopes. Also shown in Fig. 2B, compound advancement decisions always involve balancing of potency, efficacy, and safety; in this example, rather than measuring the separation of efficacy from a side effect model like rotarod impairment, a preclinical TI is calculated based on the results of toxicology studies that establish a clinically important safety margin. Here, the no observed adverse effect limit (NOAEL) is used; however, as the figure depicts, a wide array of safety margins can be calculated, depending on compound potency, efficacy, and the shape of calculated dose–response curve.

Which of these choices is best? The foregoing illustrates just one of the many challenges drug discovery programs face when making decisions whether to advance a compound for further development leading to clinical trial testing. For example, there may be cases where depending on the indication being targeted and the nature and severity of the side effect or potential toxicity, a highly potent, but significantly less efficacious, compound may be chosen for advancement. In the end, drug development decisions are ultimately made on the basis of patient risk to benefit. In addition, because preclinical datasets are as rich and complex as clinical datasets, attempts to reduce a compound's preclinical profile to a single value/descriptor (e.g., ED_{50}, half-life, or maximal efficacy) should be avoided, as this may lead to incorrect or misleading conclusions. It is paramount to understand how changing dose level affects the relevant outcome measures, whether efficacy or side effects, and this can be understood only by studying a broad range of doses. Together with the large array of *in vitro* assays, pharmaceutical profiling, and safety assays, preclinical behavioral pharmacology models ultimately enable focus of development resources onto those compounds with the greatest chance of achieving clinical success.

5. RECOMMENDATIONS/PATH FORWARD FOR THE FUTURE

Our goal is to identify both strengths and weaknesses of animal models of pain in order to spur additional discussion, leading to further innovation and progress. As part of the discussion, we propose recommendations for a path forward based on the two main components: the first pertains to the need for uniform reporting of methodologies and the second involves data analysis and interpretation.

We are not the first to call for uniform reporting standards and refer the reader to published recommendations (Rice et al., 2008, 2013; van der Worp et al., 2010) that specify the types of information that should be included when describing *in vivo* experiments. Note that neither those nor the recommendations in this chapter call for uniform experimental protocols but for uniform reporting standards and enhanced transparency. Variations in methodology across animal models of pain, such as injecting different volumes and concentrations of formalin, or ligation of the L5 rather than L5 and L6 spinal nerves, may ultimately represent a (small) step toward approximating the phenotypic heterogeneity of clinical trial subjects. Indeed, experimental details should be considered important variables (neither "right" nor "wrong") but must be clearly described for anyone wishing to repeat a study. Not only is replication a key component of the scientific method, it is absolutely critical for making rational, informed decisions in drug discovery. If data cannot be reproduced across laboratories or across separate studies (to a level allowing consistent conclusions to be drawn), enthusiasm to proceed further with development activities will be greatly diminished. In short, confirmation of experimental findings across laboratories is an often overlooked factor impacting predictive validity, yet one that has been noted to be disturbingly poor (Ioannidis, 2005; Prinz, Schlange, & Asadullah, 2011).

Although we agree on the importance of continued refinement of currently used models as well as development of new models and endpoints, we also assert that current approaches provide significantly more information than is often utilized. Efficacy determinations driven solely by accepting statistically significant increases in response thresholds can lead to false-positives and obscure understanding of relative efficacy. To this end, animal model data assessed through the lens of outcomes routinely reported in pain clinical trials such as effect size and responder rates can provide a broader and potentially more translatable understanding of efficacy.

The relevance of effect size is exemplified in analyses of the relationship between clinical trials and clinical practice as described in the IMMPACT group consensus statement on understanding the clinical importance of outcomes (Dworkin et al., 2008). Of specific relevance is the finding by Farrar, Young, LaMoreaux, Werth, and Poole (2001) that a 4-point change (on a 10-point Numeric Rating Scale) or a 50% decrease in pain ratings for an individual patient equates to patient ratings of "very much improved"; a 2-point change (30% decrease) equates to "much improved." These self-reported ratings illustrate a key component in determining successful interventions; a change in outcomes must not be only statistically significant but also a magnitude that will have a meaningful impact on patients' perceptions of efficacy. These data also suggest that 30% is near the cut-off for a pain score reduction that is perceived as clinically meaningful. An important question then becomes whether translation can be improved by making similar determinations in preclinical studies.

One approach to answering this is to perform back-translation studies in the animal models. For example, we can examine the efficacy of gabapentin for the treatment of pain associated with postherpetic neuralgia (PHN) and compare that to gabapentin efficacy in the spinal nerve ligation (SNL) model of neuropathic pain in rats. In patients that received gabapentin, average daily pain scores decreased approximately 33% from baseline, whereas pain scores in the placebo group decreased by 8% (Rowbotham, Harden, Stacey, Bernstein, & Magnus-Miller, 1998). Further, approximately 43% of patients rated their pain as "moderately or much improved," indicating treatment success in almost half of the patients. These data can provide a framework for judging the effect size of a meaningful drug effect in a successful clinical trial, but what does this effect look like in an animal model of neuropathic pain? We analyzed data from a study assessing gabapentin effects on SNL-induced mechanical allodynia (Algos Preclinical Services, internal data). In animals treated with 100 mg/kg gabapentin, the maximum possible effect (%MPE; analogous to %pain relief above) was calculated to be 65%. Further, 5 of 7 rats (71%) treated with this dose showed a %MPE of 50% or more (Table 1). Although the dosing regimens are different in the two studies, the relative exposures between rats and humans at the doses tested in these

Table 1 Comparison of the Efficacy of Gabapentin and Duloxetine in Clinical Trials and Preclinical Studies

Drug (Dose)	Indication or Model Tested	Species	% Reduction	50% Responder Rate
Gabapentin (<3600 mg/day)	PHN	Man	33.3	43.2[a]
Gabapentin (100 mg/kg)	SNL	Rat	65.4	71.4
Duloxetine (60 mg/day)	Knee OA	Man	41.38	27.9
Duloxetine (30 mg/kg)	MIA	Rat	58.1	60.0
Duloxetine (60 mg/kg)	MIA	Rat	81.3	100.0

[a]Value represents the percentage of patients that reported pain ratings to be "moderately or much improved."

studies are remarkably similar. As such, we can begin to understand how a clinically meaningful result in clinical practice and clinical trials (moderately or much improved) translates to a very robust effect in an animal model (65% MPE).

This analysis also can be extended to other pain models and drugs. In a clinical trial assessing duloxetine effects on pain associated with OA of the knee (Chappell et al., 2010), 24-h average pain scores decreased by approximately 41% in the duloxetine group and 29% in the placebo group. Further, approximately 28% of subjects in the duloxetine group reported pain relief of >50%, whereas 22% of subjects in the placebo group reported pain relief of at least 50%. In a study assessing duloxetine efficacy on hind limb weight bearing in the monosodium iodoacetate model of OA pain in rats (Marker, Pomonis, & Gottshall, 2010), duloxetine (30 mg/kg) produced a %MPE of 58%, while vehicle-treated animals showed no effects. Responder rates were high, with 6/10 rats showing %MPE >50% in the 30 mg/kg group (Table 1). While exposure levels required for efficacy are typically much higher in rats than in humans, note that 30 mg/kg is considered the minimally effective dose in rats and, as such, is consistent with the rodent greater effect size concept. And it is also worth noting that for compounds where rodent and human efficacious exposures vary, rodents consistently require higher exposures to see efficacy. As a result, preclinical models of pain are less, rather than more, likely to lead to advancement of false-positive drugs into clinical trials in contrast to what many commonly assume.

In both cases, the effect size in clinical trials is approximately half of that seen in animals. This does not mean that a metric of a twofold difference should be firmly applied to determine productivity. Instead, it simply demonstrates the importance of establishing biologically meaningful effects; the examples cited provide an objective, rational approach for helping determine what this might look like. These two studies also demonstrate the significant confound that can arise due to placebo effects in clinical trials that are generally absent in preclinical studies. Though clearly an oversimplification based on their complexity, if we subtract placebo effects from those of gabapentin in the PHN study, the % pain relief from gabapentin is 25%. In the duloxetine study, the same subtraction yields a % pain relief of 12%. In both cases, the pain relief attained was significant, and both products are widely used to treat various painful conditions. One might consider that in preclinical studies, an effect size (as calculated by %MPE or %reversal) of at least 60% at a nonimpairing/confounding dose may be required to predict clinical efficacy; however, a much lower % reversal often produces a statistically significant effect, emphasizing that effect size should be considered more important overall than statistical significance.

Another commonly used method for determining efficacy in clinical trials is number needed to treat (NNT). Briefly, NNT reflects the number of patients that must be treated with a given intervention in order to see one successful outcome, typically 50% pain relief. The NNT for gabapentin for treating PHN was calculated to be 3.2, indicating that just over three patients must be treated with the drug in order to see >50% pain relief in one patient. In our calculations from a dataset of over 200 animals, the NNT for gabapentin (SNL; 100 mg/kg) was calculated to be 2 (Algos Preclinical Services internal data), again showing that efficacy in animal models is consistently greater at comparable exposures than that observed in successful clinical trials.

Examples such as these suggest that accepting a "low bar" for efficacy in animal models of pain by focusing largely on achieving statistically significant effects may translate to low or no efficacy in clinical trials, supporting our contention that criteria for compound advancement into clinical trials should be appropriately stringent. The question this presents is how one can set an "efficacy threshold" preclinically that is analogous to a meaningful clinical effect. While subject to a number of caveats, this might be approximated by determining the efficacy (e.g., %reversal of hyperalgesia) for a test compound in an animal model of pain compared to efficacy observed with a clinical SOC drug dosed to achieve an exposure equivalent to the human efficacious exposure. The efficacy observed with this dose/exposure now effectively sets the "efficacy bar" in models to a level known to be important to patients and moves away from a reliance solely on statistically significant reversals that can result in oversimplified conclusions that the treatment strategy "worked." Study population homogeneity in animal studies yields decreased variability, increasing the likelihood of detecting statistically significant effects for smaller effect sizes. In order to protect against Type 1 errors, preclinical studies should focus on effect size as well as statistical significance in order to make sound decisions on which compounds should be advanced.

As discussed previously, it is not only efficacy that needs to be considered when assessing the potential utility of novel compounds. A number of side effects (e.g., sedation, cognitive impairment, GI irritation) can confound conclusions of efficacy, and, as well, experimental parameters (potency, efficacy, exposure, etc.) can affect side effect assay results and interpretations. The saying "the dose makes the poison" is applicable here; no drug is without side effects or toxicity if given in large enough quantities. True efficacy does not exist in isolation, but is balanced by tolerability. As noted earlier, research and development programs typically determine a ratio of efficacy to side effects, or TI, calculated by dividing the minimal ataxic dose/exposure (or another mechanistically relevant side effect assay) by a pharmacologically effective dose/exposure. Most overtly, toxic effects can be identified well before development; however, confounding or intolerable side effects remain a major challenge for drug discovery programs. Sometimes, these side effects, if well-understood, can be overcome. For example, the well-documented hyperthermia seen after administration of TRPV1 antagonists was considered problematic (Gavva et al., 2008), but improved mechanistic understanding led to discovery of compounds with reduced hyperthermia that retained efficacy (Quiding et al., 2013). Unfortunately, side effects for many compounds have no clear mechanistic underpinning; these ultimately limit doses and, hence, efficacy that can be achieved clinically. As part of the drug discovery process, drug developers routinely compare under identical experimental conditions the TIs of test compounds to those of known compounds, whether SOC drugs or tool compounds targeting the same mechanism. Because differentiating a new pharmacotherapy from currently prescribed drugs requires a balance between improved efficacy and reduced or less aversive side effects, animal models of pain must be paired with assays assessing potential side effects in order to both confidently conclude preclinical efficacy and more accurately predict clinical success.

6. CONCLUSION

The goal of this chapter has been to stimulate discussion and debate and in doing so further progress the ultimate goal of all who work with animal models of pain, namely to better understand human disease and develop more effective therapies. It is important to recognize that animal model data are essential in the development of new analgesic drugs, whether small or large molecule, and are used to determine efficacious exposure levels and derivative preclinical safety margins. These data also inform dose ranges in early human studies and are required prior to initiating human trials. The question then becomes which animal pain model(s) should be utilized to achieve these goals. We wholeheartedly support the concept of adding depth to traditional models and endpoints by considering supraspinally mediated contributions to pain in addition to spontaneous pain but argue the pain research community would err if such models and endpoints are developed as a means to discount or replace traditional ones. We propose assuming a more enlightened view of the value, appropriate uses, and limitations of both traditional models and novel models being developed. Furthermore, the drug discovery process needs robust, reproducible, and high-throughput assays that can be used to screen and to prioritize high numbers of compounds and focus on those with the best chance of successful development. More complex and involved/lower throughput assays and models, including large animal models, are better applied later in the process on fewer compounds and when one may be able to better align the clinical methodology and patient population being targeted. We also propose that existing datasets contain richer information than is often utilized and have suggested options for alternative data analyses that are more aligned to analysis of clinical datasets. It is our belief that these will improve conclusions of efficacy from preclinical studies and should also help move us further from the temptation to reduce complex datasets to simplistic assessments of "worked" or "didn't work," inappropriate terminology for either preclinical or clinical datasets. Finally, public–private partnership consortia such as the European IMI (Innovative Medicines Initiative) and the US-sponsored ACTTION/PPRECISE groups, as well as others, in addition to their efforts in calling for uniform standards for experimental reporting, might expand their leadership roles to foster discussions on enhancing data analysis techniques. This could include helping to open doors into the analysis (and publication) of neutral/negative/failed preclinical studies and clinical trial data (Sena, van der Worp, Bath, Howells, & Macleod, 2010), more extensive meta-analyses of preclinical data across laboratories, promoting better alignment of animal model evoked endpoints with QST measures, and the potential adoption of additional readouts such as effect size in preclinical models. Together, these efforts may serve to span what many perceive at present to be an unbridgeable gap between preclinical research and clinical trial success.

CONFLICT OF INTEREST

G.T.W. is an employee of Purdue Pharma L.P., J.D.P. is an employee of American Preclinical Services, LLC, and J.D.K. has no conflicts of interest to declare.

REFERENCES

Andrews, N., Legg, E., Lisak, D., Issop, Y., Richardson, D., Harper, S., et al. (2012). Spontaneous burrowing behaviour in the rat is reduced by peripheral nerve injury or inflammation associated pain. *European Journal of Pain*, *16*, 85–495.

Baron, R., Förster, M., & Binder, A. (2012). Subgrouping of patients with neuropathic pain according to pain-related sensory abnormalities: A first step to a stratified treatment approach. *Lancet Neurology*, *11*, 999–1005.

Blackburn-Munro, G. (2004). Pain-like behaviours in animals—How human are they? *Trends in Pharmacological Sciences*, *25*, 299–305.

Blackshaw, L. A. (2012). Visceral pain readouts in experimental medicine. *Neurogastroenterology and Motility*, *24*, 891–894.

Brown, D. C., Boston, R. C., Coyne, J. C., & Farrar, J. T. (2008). Ability of the canine brief pain inventory to detect response to treatment in dogs with osteoarthritis. *Journal of the American Veterinary Medicine Association*, *233*, 1278–1283.

Chappell, A. S., Desaiah, D., Liu-Seifert, H., Zhang, S., Skljarevski, V., Belenkov, Y., et al. (2010). Placebo-controlled study of the efficacy and safety of duloxetine for the treatment of chronic pain due to osteoarthritis of the knee. *Pain Practice*, *11*, 33–41.

Dworkin, R. H., Turk, D. C., Wyrwich, K. W., Beaton, D., Cleeland, C. S., Farrar, J. T., et al. (2008). Interpreting the clinical importance of treatment outcomes in chronic pain clinical trials: IMMPACT recommendations. *Journal of Pain*, *9*, 105–121.

Farrar, J. T., Young, J. P., LaMoreaux, L., Werth, J. L., & Poole, R. M. (2001). Clinical importance of changes in chronic pain intensity measured on an 11-point numerical pain rating scale. *Pain*, *94*, 149–158.

Gavva, N. R., Treanor, J. J., Garami, A., Fang, L., Surapaneni, S., Akrami, A., et al. (2008). Pharmacological blockade of the vanilloid receptor TRPV1 elicits marked hyperthermia in humans. *Pain*, *136*, 202–210.

Granmo, M., Jensen, T., & Schouenborg, J. (2013). Nociceptive transmission to rat primary somatosensory cortex—Comparison of sedative and analgesic effects. *PLoS ONE*, *8*, e53966.

Henze, D. A., & Urban, M. O. (2010). Large animal models for pain therapeutic development. In S. A. Simon, & M. A. L. Nicolelis (Series Eds.) & L. Kruger, & A. R. Light (Vol. Eds.), *Translational pain research: From mouse to man* (pp. 371–391). Boca Raton, FL: CRC Press/Taylor & Francis Group.

Hill, R. (2000). NK1 (substance P) receptor antagonists—Why are they not analgesic in humans? *Trends in Pharmacological Sciences*, *21*, 244–246.

Huang, W., Calvo, M., Karu, K., Olausen, H. R., Bathgate, G., Okuse, K., et al. (2013). A clinically relevant rodent model of the HIV antiretroviral drug stavudine induced painful peripheral neuropathy. *Pain*, *154*, 560–575.

Huggins, J. P., Smart, T. S., Langman, S., Taylor, L., & Young, T. (2012). An efficient randomised, placebo-controlled clinical trial with the irreversible fatty acid amide hydrolase-1 inhibitor PF-04457845, which modulates endocannabinoids but fails to induce effective analgesia in patients with pain due to osteoarthritis of the knee. *Pain*, *153*, 1837–1846.

Hummel, M., Lu, P., Cummons, T. A., & Whiteside, G. T. (2008). The persistence of a long-term negative affective state following the induction of either acute or chronic pain. *Pain*, *140*, 436–445.

Huntjens, D. R., Spalding, D. J., Danhof, M., & Della Pasqua, O. E. (2009). Differences in the sensitivity of behavioural measures of pain to the selectivity of cyclo-oxygenase inhibitors. *European Journal of Pain, 13*, 448–457.

Ioannidis, J. P. A. (2005). Why most published research findings are false. *PLoS Medicine, 2*, e124.

Joshi, S. K., & Honore, P. (2006). Animal models of pain for drug discovery. *Expert Opinion in Drug Discovery, 1*, 341–352.

King, T., Vera-Portocarrero, L., Gutierrez, T., Vanderah, T. W., Dussor, G., Lai, J., et al. (2009). Unmasking the tonic-aversive state in neuropathic pain. *Nature Neuroscience, 12*, 1364–1366.

Kola, I., & Landis, J. (2004). Can the pharmaceutical industry reduce attrition rates? *Nature Reviews. Drug Discovery, 3*, 711–715.

Langford, D. J., Bailey, A. L., Chanda, M. L., Clarke, S. E., Drummond, T. E., Echols, S., et al. (2010). Coding of facial expressions of pain in the laboratory mouse. *Nature Methods, 7*, 447–449.

Lau, W., Dykstra, C., Thevarkunnel, S., Silenieks, L. B., de Lannoy, I. A. M., Lee, D. K. H., et al. (2013). A back translation of pregabalin and carbamazepine against evoked and non-evoked endpoints in the rat spared nerve injury model of neuropathic pain. *Neuropharmacology, 73*, 204–215.

Leys, L. J., Chu, K. L., Xu, J., Pai, M., Yang, H. S., Robb, H. M., et al. (2013). Disturbances in slow-wave sleep are induced by models of bilateral inflammation, neuropathic, and postoperative pain, but not osteoarthritic pain in rats. *Pain, 154*, 1092–1102.

Mao, J. (2012). Current challenges in translational pain research. *Trends in Pharmacological Sciences, 33*, 568–573.

Marker, C. L., Pomonis, J. D., & Gottshall, S. L. (2010). Abstract: Measuring use-related pain in a rat model of osteoarthritis. In *13th IASP world congress on pain, Montreal, Canada.*

Mogil, J. S. (2009). Animal models of pain: Progress and challenges. *Nature Reviews. Neuroscience, 10*, 283–294.

Negus, S. S., Vanderah, T. W., Brandt, M. R., Bilsky, E. J., Becerra, L., & Borsook, D. (2006). Pre-clinical assessment of candidate analgesic drugs: Recent advances and future challenges. *Journal of Pharmacology and Experimental Therapeutics, 319*, 507–514.

Oertel, B. G., & Lötsch, J. (2013). Clinical pharmacology of analgesics assessed with human experimental pain models: Bridging basic and clinical research. *British Journal of Pharmacology, 168*, 534–553.

Pande, A. C., Pyke, R. E., Greiner, M., Cooper, S. A., Benjamin, R., & Pierce, M. W. (1996). Analgesic efficacy of the kappa-receptor agonist, enadoline, in dental surgery pain. *Clinical Neuropharmacology, 19*, 92–97.

Pereira Do Carmo, G., Stevenson, G. W., Carlezon, W. A., & Negus, S. S. (2009). Effects of pain- and analgesia-related manipulations on intracranial self-stimulation in rats: Further studies on pain-depressed behavior. *Pain, 144*, 170–177.

Piesla, M. J., Leventhal, L., Strassle, B. W., Harrison, J. E., Cummons, T. A., Lu, P., et al. (2009). Abnormal gait, due to inflammation but not nerve injury, reflects enhanced nociception in preclinical pain models. *Brain Research, 1295*, 89–98.

Prinz, F., Schlange, T., & Asadullah, K. (2011). Believe it or not: How much can we rely on published data on potential drug targets? *Nature Reviews. Drug Discovery, 10*, 328–329.

Quiding, H., Jonzon, B., Svensson, O., Webster, L., Reimfelt, A., Karin, A., et al. (2013). TRPV1 antagonistic analgesic effect: A randomized study of AZD1386 in pain after third molar extraction. *Pain, 154*, 808–812.

Rice, A. S. C., Cimino-Brown, D., Eisenach, J. C., Kontinen, V. K., Lacroix-Fralish, M. L., Machin (on behalf of the Preclinical Pain Consortium), I., et al. (2008). Animal models and the prediction of efficacy in clinical trials of analgesic drugs: A critical appraisal and call for uniform reporting standards. *Pain, 139*, 243–247.

Rice, A. S. C., Morland, R., Huang, W., Currie, G. L., Sena, E. S., & Macleod, M. R. (2013). Transparency in the reporting of in vivo pre-clinical pain research: The relevance and implications of the ARRIVE (Animal Research: Reporting In Vivo Experiments) guidelines. *Scandinavian Journal of Pain*, *4*, 58–62.
Rowbotham, M., Harden, N., Stacey, B., Bernstein, P., & Magnus-Miller, L. (1998). Gabapentin for the treatment of postherpetic neuralgia. *Journal of the American Medical Association*, *280*, 1837–1842.
Sena, E. S., van der Worp, H. B., Bath, P. M. W., Howells, D. W., & Macleod, M. R. (2010). Publication bias in reports of animal stroke studies leads to major overstatement of efficacy. *PLoS Biology*, *8*, e1000344.
Silva, A., Andersen, M. L., & Tufik, S. (2008). Sleep pattern in an experimental model of osteoarthritis. *Pain*, *140*, 446–455.
Stevenson, G. W., Cormier, J., Mercer, H., Adams, C., Dunbar, C., Negus, S. S., et al. (2009). Targeting pain-depressed behaviors in preclinical assays of pain and analgesia: Drug effects on acetic acid-depressed locomotor activity in ICR mice. *Life Sciences*, *85*, 309–315.
Sufka, K. (1994). Conditioned place preference paradigm: A novel approach for analgesic drug assessment against chronic pain. *Pain*, *58*, 355–366.
Taneja, A., Di lorio, V. L., Danhof, M., & Della Pasqua, O. (2012). Translation of drug effects from experimental models of neuropathic pain and analgesia to humans. *Drug Discovery Today*, *17*, 837–849.
van der Kam, E. L., Vry, J. D., Schiene, K., & Tzschentke, T. M. (2008). Differential effects of morphine on the affective and the sensory component of Carrageenan-induced nociception in the rat. *Pain*, *136*, 373–379.
van der Worp, H. B., Howells, D. W., Sena, E. S., Porritt, M. J., Rewell, S., O'Collins, V., et al. (2010). Can animal models of disease reliably inform human studies? *PLoS Medicine*, 7, e1000245.
Vierck, C. J., Hansson, P. T., & Yezierski, R. P. (2008). Clinical and pre-clinical pain assessment: Are we measuring the same thing? *Pain*, *135*, 7–10.
Walton, M. B., Cowderoy, E., Lascelles, D., & Innes, J. F. (2013). Evaluation of construct and criterion validity for the 'Liverpool Osteoarthritis in Dogs' (LOAD) clinical metrology instrument and comparison to two other instruments. *PLoS ONE*, *8*, e58125.
Whiteside, G. T., Adedoyin, A., & Leventhal, L. (2008). Predictive validity of animal pain models? A comparison of the pharmacokinetic–pharmacodynamic relationship for pain drugs in rats and humans. *Neuropharmacology*, *54*, 767–775.
Whiteside, G. T., Pomonis, J. D., & Kennedy, J. D. (2013). An industry perspective on the role and utility of animal models of pain in drug discovery. *Neuroscience Letters*, *55*, 65–72.

CHAPTER TWELVE

The Potential of Traditional Chinese Medicine in the Treatment and Modulation of Pain

Guan-hua Du*,†,1, Tian-yi Yuan*,†, Li-da Du‡, Yong-xiang Zhang§,¶,1

*State Key Laboratory of Bioactive Substances and Functions of Natural Medicines, Institute of Materia Medica, Chinese Academy of Medical Sciences and Peking Union Medical College, Beijing, PR China
†Beijing Key Laboratory of Drug Targets Identification and Drug Screening, Institute of Materia Medica, Chinese Academy of Medical Sciences and Peking Union Medical College, Beijing, PR China
‡School of Biomedical Sciences, Chinese University of Hong Kong, Hong Kong, PR China
§Department of Neuroimmunopharmacology, Beijing Institute of Pharmacology and Toxicology, Beijing, PR China
¶State Key Laboratory of Toxicology and Medical Countermeasures, Beijing, PR China
[1]Corresponding authors: e-mail address: dugh@imm.ac.cn; zhangyx@bmi.ac.cn

Contents

Advances in Pharmacology, Volume 75
ISSN 1054-3589
http://dx.doi.org/10.1016/bs.apha.2016.01.001

Abstract

Pain is an unpleasant sensory and emotional experience associated with various diseases. Extensive research has been conducted to find appropriate methods of relieving pain and improving the quality of life. However, the most commonly used pain-relieving agents such as opioid therapeutics are often associated with harmful side effects; moreover, users are prone to become addicted to these agents and may develop tolerance. Often, nonopioid therapeutics is only marginally effective, thus leading to a significant unmet medical need. Scientists have studied herbal medicines, finding more than 800 kinds of traditional Chinese medicine (TCM) to be effective in relieving pain while also creating several monomeric compounds to develop novel analgesic drugs. In this review, we summarize the representative TCM currently available for the treatment and modulation of pain. Ten different natural products, mainly herbs, used in Chinese medicine to relieve pain are discussed in light of the theories of TCM and modern pharmacology. We hope that this review will provide valuable information for future studies on the potential of TCM in alleviating pain.

ABBREVIATIONS

5-HT 5-hydroxytryptamine
DA brain dopamine
DHCB dehydrocorybulbine
ET endothelin
GABA γ-aminobutyric acid
IL-1β interleukin-1β
MSL methyl salicylate 2-*O*-β-D-lactoside
NO nitric oxide
NSAIDs nonsteroidal antiinflammatory drugs
RA rheumatoid arthritis
TCM traditional Chinese medicine
THP tetrahydropalmatine

1. INTRODUCTION

Traditional Chinese medicine (TCM), including Chinese herbal medicine, has been in use across Asia for thousands of years in the treatment of diseases, with a long history of development and continued use. TCM has had a significant influence on the Chinese, and its practical efficacy has been verified through extensive use. Many of the herbs used in ancient China are being investigated, with various reported therapeutic effects on different diseases. Analgesia is one of the most promising pharmacological effects of TCM (Miyaoka & Monga, 2009; Trinh, Cui, & Wang, 2010).

TCM defines pain similarly to modern medicine in that it is an unpleasant sensory and emotional experience associated with actual or potential tissue damage. Typically, pain serves to warn the individual to withdraw from potentially harmful situations (Gorczyca, Filip, & Walczak, 2013; Hague & Shenker, 2014). However, this protective reaction may become intolerable, significantly interfering with an individual's quality of life and general functioning. Thus, alleviating pain is an important task in health care as well as a challenge to drug administration.

Opioids remain the gold standard for the treatment of severe acute and chronic pain; they are the most common antinociceptive drugs found to be effective in 70–80% of patients. However, the undesirable side effects and addictive nature of such drugs have already been established (Cheatle, 2015; Reardon, Anger, & Szumita, 2015). Nonsteroidal antiinflammatory drugs (NSAIDs) are another class of analgesics that are used to alleviate low or moderate pain. This class of drugs also causes side effects such as gastrointestinal dysfunction (Pellicano, 2014; Wehling, 2014). Thus, it has become important to develop efficacious analgesics for both acute and chronic pain without producing tolerance, dependence, or other side effects. It is also worth noting that several herbs and formulations in TCM used to treat different types of pain do not produce dependence or tolerance.

TCM considers pain to be a form of self-defense or self-regulation against exogenous pathogenic factors. According to TCM, the pathologies of pain include the blockage of blood flow; signal transduction; and accumulation of secretions due to different factors, such as inflammations, blood stasis, and cold. Based on this theory of pain, several effective physical treatment methods are used in clinical setting such as acupuncture (Hesse, Henkel, Zygmunt, Mustea, & Usichenko, 2015; Xue, Sun, Li, & Liu, 2015), massage, exercise (Martinez et al., 2015), moxibustion (Ma, Yang, et al., 2015), and cupping for chronic pain. These methods are effective, safe, and easy to use.

The efficacy of TCM is well known, providing reference values for modern medicine in China. Over 2000 years ago, the Chinese collected and recorded herbs of medicinal value. These records eventually developed into books, such as "Shen Nong's herbal classic," the earliest monograph on medicine that has had a profound impact on Chinese culture and modern Chinese medicine. The conditions were not ideal in ancient times, when herbal medicines were identified and put to use, as no effective treatments or analgesics were available. Since then, the theory and practical use of TCM analgesia has evolved, and many of these natural pain-relieving agents are used in modern clinical medicine.

Some TCM formulations used either alone or in combination can be used to relieve acute pain and chronic pain. Recent studies have shown the significant efficacy of several single herbs, compounds, or extracts of TCM against different kinds of pain.

Some analgesic TCM formulations, such as *Papaver somniferum* L. (Ying Su), *Corydalis rhizoma* (Yan Hu Suo) and similar herbal medicines, act on the central nervous system (CNS) and eliminate pain. Many TCM formulations alleviate pain by treating the underlying disease. For example, most analgesic TCM formulations such as Szechuan Lovage Rhizome (Chuan Xiong) and Radix Angelicae Pubescentis (Du Huo) have antiinflammatory effects and promote blood circulation. These formulations alleviate pain by reducing inflammation and blood stasis and treat the underlying disease. Analgesic TCM formulations not only act on a single target but always have multiple mechanisms. Common analgesic agents usually act by blocking pain signaling and merely relieve the symptoms. Targeting the underlying condition causing pain is the most important difference between TCMs and common analgesic agents.

Recently, some small molecules purified from TCM were found to have strong analgesic effects. Some of these molecules are more effective than opioids with reduced adverse reactions. Thus, TCM may provide the basis for further development of novel analgesics. As TCM may differ in the diagnosis or assessment and treatment of pain, we discuss analgesic TCM formulations in the context of modern science methodology. Based on this background, several forms of TCM are included in this review, as well as their efficacy, active constituents, and mechanisms. The aim of this study is to systematically summarize and analyze Chinese herbal medicines investigated in pain models and provide future references for basic and clinical studies.

2. TCM AND HERBAL MEDICINES WITH ANALGESIC EFFECTS

2.1 *C. rhizoma* (延胡索, Yan Hu Suo)

Yan Hu Suo is the dry tuber of the perennial herbaceous plant *Corydalis yanhusuo* W.T. Wang, which belongs to the Papaveraceae family. According to Chinese theories of medicine, Yan Hu Suo effectively unclogs blood vessels, dissolves blood stasis, and alleviates pain (Wang, Fu, Zhou, & Wang,

2014). According to legend, Princess Jingmu of the Ming Dynasty (more than 500 years ago) developed epigastric pain when eating soba noodles while angry. A famous Chinese doctor, Li Shizhen, was consulted, who recalled a statement from Lei Gong's treatise on the preparation (Lei Gong Pao Zhi Lun) recommending Yan Hu as quickly as possible in the event of cardiodynia. Thus, the princess was given Yan Hu Suo soaked in warm wine, which stopped the vomiting and relieved her stomachache. This story was recorded in the Compendium of Matera Medica (Ben Cao Gang Mu), with Yan Hu Suo being subsequently used as an analgesic. Yan Hu Suo and its active ingredients have been extensively studied in clinical and preclinical trials. Several kinds of preparations or formulations containing Yan Hu Suo have a potent analgesic effect.

2.1.1 Chemical and Analgesic Activities

More than 30 alkaloids have been extracted from Yan Hu Suo, such as tetrahydropalmatine (THP), corydaline, berberine, dehydrocorybulbine (DHCB), and coptisine (Guo, Cai, Su, & Li, 2014). Among these alkaloids, THP, corydaline, and DHCB have been considered the main active components responsible for the analgesic effect (Fig. 1; Ma, Yue, Cao, Li, & Ge, 2013).

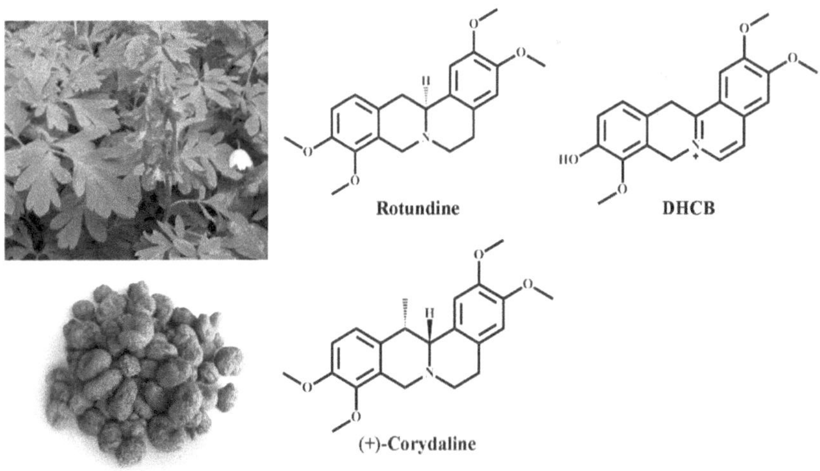

Figure 1 Photos of *Corydalis rhizoma* and its medicinal components, including its main analgesic components.

THP has been confirmed to be the principal active component in Yan Hu Suo. This compound has been successfully prepared via total synthesis, and it is used to treat headache, dysmenorrhea, and labor pain. In the pharmaceutical industry, the more potent enantiomer Levo-THP, with the trade name of Rotundine in China, was synthetically produced as an alternative to anxiolytic and sedative drugs of the benzodiazepine group and analgesics such as opiates.

The exact mechanism of action of Rotundine is under investigation. Some studies have shown that inhibition of the ascending reticular activating system and the action of dopamine (DA) receptors in the brain might be responsible for the analgesic effects of Rotundine. The central role of DA in pain modulation has been suggested previously (Hu & Jin, 1999b). Furthermore, researchers have shown that Rotundine produces antinociception by blocking the supraspinal D2 receptor. Rotundine has a low addictive potential and diminished tolerance as it scarcely related to opioid receptors. Rotundine has been preferred for alleviating moderate pain (Chu, Jin, Friedman, & Zhen, 2008; Wu, Jiang, Wu, & Cao, 1990). Furthermore, the combination of Rotundine and pethidine produces an enhanced analgesic effect, thus reducing the dose of pethidine required and the incidence of drug dependence (Li, Yang, Zhang, Lu, & Wu, 2009). Research has also shown that Rotundine can be used to treat addiction to both cocaine and opiates, and it has been preliminarily tested in human models (Wang & Mantsch, 2012; Yang et al., 2008). Rotundine is also a potent muscle relaxant, as it acts as a blocker of calcium channels and an activator of potassium channels. These properties have been used to demonstrate the therapeutic value of Rotundine for heart disease and liver damage (Huang et al., 1999; Min, Bai, Shu, & Ren, 2006; Xu et al., 1996).

Like Rotundine, corydaline also belongs to the class of tetrahydroprotoberberines (THPBs). Both compounds have a similar structure and bioactivity. Corydaline enhances the activity of the descending pain modulation system of the brain stem by the blockade of D2 receptors in the striatum and nucleus accumbens; it also sequentially inhibits the inputs of peripheral pain afferent information (Hu & Jin, 1999a; Wu et al., 2014). Some reports have indicated that corydaline has a weaker effect than Rotundine (Lu et al., 2012; Ma et al., 2008).

DHCB has a similar structure to that of THP and is a potent antagonist of DA receptors. DHCB is only marginally active at opioid receptors, but it induces potent, dose-dependent antinociception at nonsedative doses (Wu, Xu, Zhang, Zhang, & Chen, 2015). The effect of DHCB is independent of the activation of opioid receptors, as it is insensitive to the opioid antagonist naloxone. DHCB acts as an effective analgesic agent in both inflammatory and neuropathic pain models without inducing tolerance after repeated administration. DHCB shows higher affinity to D2-like receptors than to D1-like DA receptors. However, DHCB produces weaker sedative effects than THP at analgesic doses (Kim, Ryu, Lee, & Kim, 2014; Zhang et al., 2014).

2.1.2 Pharmacology of Yan Hu Suo

Yan Hu Suo is primarily used to treat pain induced by blood stasis and qi stagnation. It has a weaker analgesic effect but fewer side effects than Ying Su, which belongs to the same family. Modern pharmacology suggests that the mechanisms of action of Yan Hu Suo are related to the DA system, as mentioned previously. This herbal medicine unclogs blood vessels and dissolves blood stasis to alleviate pain (Wang et al., 2014). To date, Yan Hu Suo has mostly been used for its analgesic properties. However, it is effective against neurodynia, dysmenorrhea, and cancer pain, as well as a form of local anesthesia. In the writhing, hot-plate, and electric stimulation tests conducted *in vivo*, Yan Hu Suo and its extracts exhibited a potent central analgesic effect (Liu, Li, Zhu, Wang, & Wang, 1990; Tian et al., 2014). In addition, higher doses of Yan Hu Suo produce hypnotic and sedative effects or stable potency (Sun et al., 2012; Zhao et al., 2014; Zhu, 1991).

2.1.3 Formulae with Yan Hu Suo

Yan Hu Suo has also been used in various Chinese medicinal formulations. Jin Ling Zi San, which is composed of Yan Hu Suo and Chuan Lian Zi (Szechwan chinaberry fruit), is used to treat stomachache, chest pain, hernia, and dysmenorrhea. Yuan Hu Zhi Tong, which contains Yan Hu Suo and Bai Zhi (*Angelica dahurica*), has similar effects to Jin Ling Zi San, sold in the form of patented tablets in China. Apart from these oral preparations, some external preparations and injections also contain Yan Hu Suo. Yan Hu Suo is the first analgesic TCM formulation recognized in the world over with low addictive potential and tolerance.

2.2 *A. dahurica* Radix (白芷, Bai Zhi)

Bai Zhi is the root of the perennial herbaceous plant *A. dahurica* (Fisch. ex Hoffm.) Benth. and Hook. f. or *A. dahurica* (Fisch. ex Hoffm.) Benth. and Hook. f. var. *formosana* (Boiss.) Shan and Yuan of the Umbelliferae family. This herbal medicine, which contains multiple coumarins, is widely

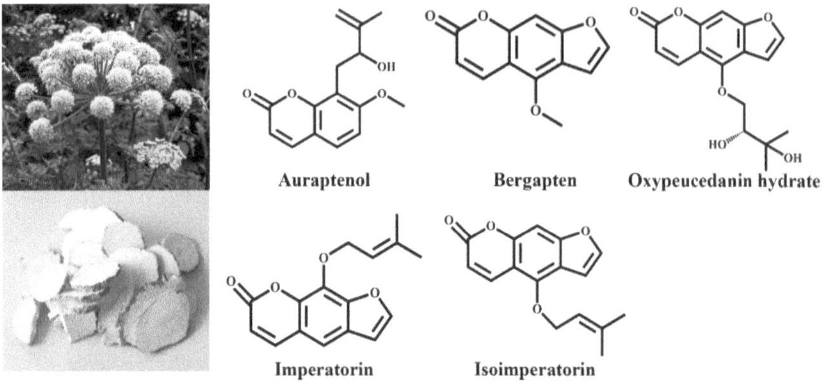

Figure 2 Photos of *Angelica dahurica* Radix and its medicinal components, including its main analgesic components.

used in China for its medicinal value. In ancient China, as early as the Jin Dynasty, Zhang Cong Zheng, a renowned doctor, proposed that diseases were caused by external harmful factors, or pathogens, that entered the human body. He listed Bai Zhi as a herbal medicine that purges the body of any negative toxins. Currently, Bai Zhi is mostly used to treat wind–cold external syndrome and pain syndromes such as headache, toothache, and arthralgia (Fig. 2).

2.2.1 Chemicals and Analgesic Activities

Bai Zhi is generally used with Yan Hu Suo to alleviate pain. Both exhibit a synergistic effect, enhance analgesia, and produce fewer adverse effects when used in combination. The well-known Yan Hu Zhi Tong is primarily composed of these two herbs, used for the treatment of gastralgia, costalgia, headache, and dysmenorrhea in TCM. The alkaloids present in Yan Hu Suo have been shown to have potent analgesic effects, as mentioned earlier. The total coumarins and volatile oil derived from Bai Zhi can enhance the analgesic effects of Yan Hu Suo, as it improves the plasma concentration of THP, as proven in some studies (Liao et al., 2010; Ma, Gu, et al., 2015; Ma, Yang, et al., 2015; Ma, Zhang, et al., 2015).

Various coumarins and volatile oils extracted from Bai Zhi are the primary active ingredients. The total volatile oil and water decoction of Bai Zhi are effective in several animal pain models (Nie & Shen, 2002). Furanocoumarins extracted from Bai Zhi, including oxypeucedanin hydrate, imperatorin, isoimperatorin, and bergapten, exhibit potent analgesic ability (Chen, Sun, et al., 2014). The mechanisms of the analgesic action of Bai Zhi remain to be elucidated. Some studies from China have shown its possible action on opioid, γ-aminobutyric acid (GABA), or DA receptors (Wang, Liu, Chen, Zhao, & Hu, 2001; Yuan et al., 2004).

2.2.2 Formulae with Bai Zhi

Cancer pain is a significant symptom of malignant disease with a major impact on the patients' quality of life (Schug & Chandrasena, 2015). Zhi Xi Fang mainly consists of Bai Zhi, Xi Xin (*Asarum sieboldii*), and Chuan Xiong (*Ligusticum wallichii*), which has a significant effect on cancer pain (Zhang, Sun, Chen, & Zhou, 2015). It was first developed to treat neuropathic pain in the clinical setting. Recently, Zhi Xi Fang was found to be effective in the rat bone cancer pain model, which may be related to the inhibition of the proliferation and activation of gliocytes as well as the activation of Toll-like receptors and nuclear factor kappa B (NF-κB) (Zhang, Wei, Bian, Bai, & Zhou, 2015). Thus, Bai Zhi possibly alleviates pain by relieving inflammation.

Migraine is a neurological disease characterized by recurrent moderate to severe headaches. The Tou Feng Yu pill is composed of three Chinese herbal drugs: Bai Zhi, Chuan Xiong (*L. wallichii*), and green tea (*Camellia sinensis folium*). It is used to treat migraine, as it regulates the levels of neurotransmitters, neuropeptides, and other bioactive substances. It also leads to a significant decrease in the levels of plasma calcitonin gene-related peptide (CGRP), serum nitric oxide (NO), and brain DA. It is known to increase the levels of plasma endothelin (ET), brain 5-hydroxytryptamine (5-HT), and norepinephrine (NE) (Li, Shen, Meng, Zhang, & Lai, 2011). Qu Feng Ding Tong, another herbal formulation consisting of Bai Zhi, Qiang Huo (*Notopterygium incisum*), and Xu Chang Qing (Paniculate swallowwort root), has also been found to be effective in treating migraine. The mechanism of action appears to be the downregulation of 5-HT in the brain (Li, Ji, & Bai, 2015). In conclusion, Bai Zhi produces an analgesic effect by downregulating the release of proinflammatory factors as well as neurotransmitters (Kang et al., 2008; Wang, Cao, et al., 2013).

2.3 Notoginseng Radix and Rhizoma (三七, San Qi)

San Qi is the root of the perennial herbaceous plant *Panax notoginseng* (Burk.) F.H. Chen of the Araliaceae family. In ancient China, San Qi was known for its hemostatic ability after growing for 3–7 years, hence the name San Qi

(San and Qi denoting three and seven in Chinese, respectively). As the family name of the doctor who discovered this herbal medicine was Tian, San Qi is generally also called Tian Qi. Although San Qi was primarily used to staunch bleeding, recently, its efficacy was proven in several diseases. In Latin, the term "Panax" means "cure-all," which is indicative of its medicinal value. It is the major ingredient of Yun Nan Bai Yao, a popular hemostatic proprietary herbal remedy, used by the Viet Cong during the Vietnam War to treat the wounded (Fig. 3).

Currently, San Qi is used to alleviate various kinds of pain due to blood stasis. San Qi is commonly used to prepare herbal plasters for pain relief in Chinese medicine, especially back pain (Chang et al., 2007; Chow, Lai, Tang, & Leung, 2013). It increases blood circulation and reduces inflammation by inhibiting the production of several bioactive substances such as tumor necrosis factor-α (TNF-α), interleukin-1β (IL-1β), inducible nitric oxide (iNO), and matrix metalloproteinase-13 (MMP-13) (Jin et al., 2007; Ling, Nheu, Dai, Guo, & Komesaroff, 2008; Rhule, Navarro, Smith, & Shepherd, 2006). To date, the ginsenoside Rb1 is considered to be the major effective constituent of San Qi. This herbal medicine alleviates pain primarily by reducing inflammation, increasing blood circulation, clearing blood clots, and reducing swelling, which can also cause pain. San Qi has achieved beneficial treatment effects in clinics (Ma, Qin, Wei, & Yu, 2014). However, its mechanisms of analgesic action must be investigated further, especially in relation to its effects on the nervous system.

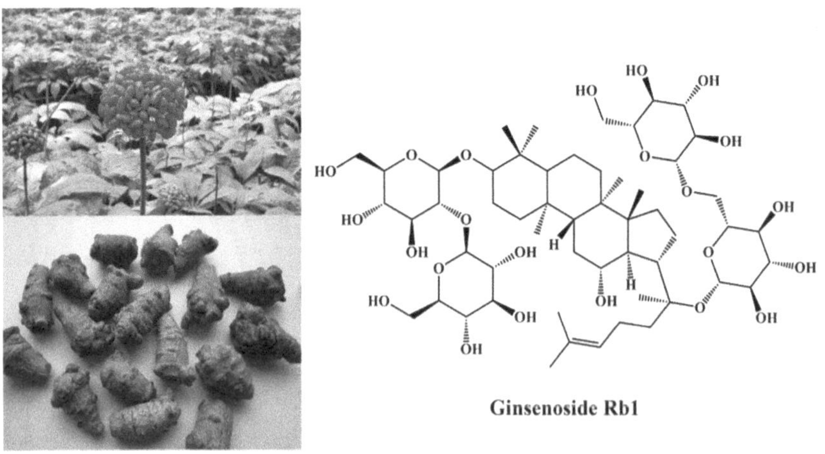

Figure 3 Photos of Notoginseng Radix and Rhizoma and its medicinal components, including its main analgesic components.

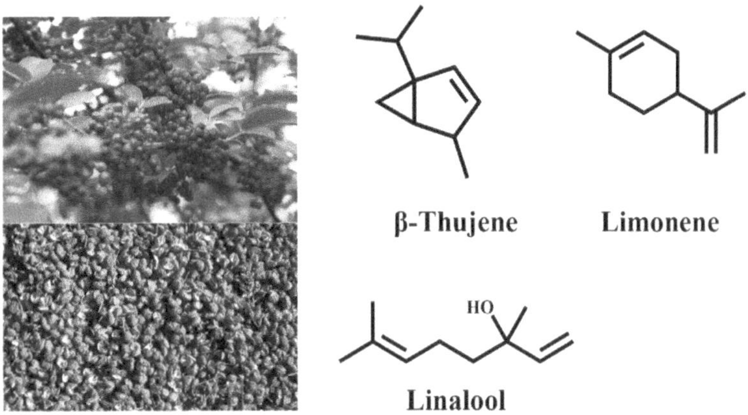

Figure 4 Photos of Zanthoxyli Pericarpium and its medicinal components, as well as its main analgesic components.

2.4 Zanthoxyli Pericarpium (花椒, Hua Jiao)

Hua Jiao is the mature pericarp of *Zanthoxylum schinifolium* Sieb. and Zucc. or *Zanthoxylum bungeanum* Maxim. of the Rutaceae family. Also known as Chinese prickly ash, this plant is used as a condiment and in TCM for detoxification and treatment of vomiting and stomachache (Li et al., 2014). The essential oil constitutes the main active ingredient of Hua Jiao, which consists of linalool, limonene, β-thujene, etc. This essential oil has a profound effect on acute or chronic inflammation and inhibits the pain induced by inflammation (Fig. 4).

The root of a specific kind of Hua Jiao, named *Zanthoxylum simulans* Hance, is also used for pain relief, particularly as an adjuvant in surgery anesthesia. The active ingredients include edulinine and skimmianine, which produce potent analgesic and central inhibition effects (Wei, Hong, Chang, Li, & Gu, 1988).

2.5 Paeoniae Radix Alba (白芍, Bai Shao)

Bai Shao, also known as Chinese peony, is a TCM formulation used to treat inflammatory disorders. It is the root of the perennial herbaceous plant *Paeonia lactiflora* Pall. of the buttercup family. Bai Shao is one of the effective components in a TCM preparation named Gui Zhi Fu Ling Tang. These formulae have been used in clinics in China for several years for the treatment of pain caused by gynecopathy, especially dysmenorrhea. Paeoniflorin is the major active component extracted from Bai Shao with

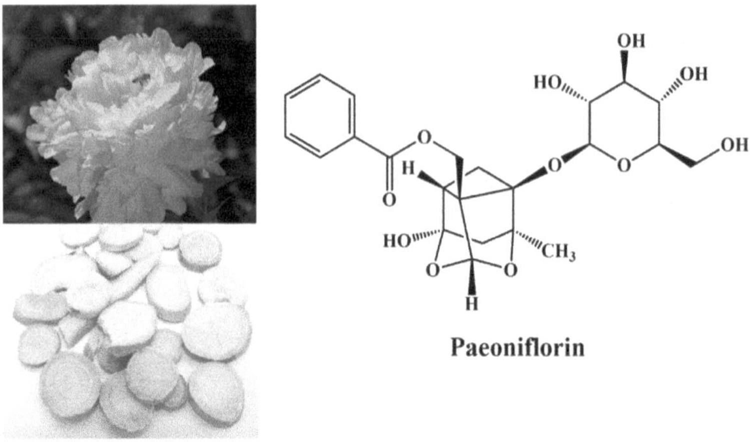

Figure 5 Photos of Paeoniae Radix Alba and its medicinal components, including its main analgesic components.

proven efficacy against gynecological disorders, pain, and hyperactivity of liver-yang, among other disorders (Jian, Yu, & Wang, 2010; Kim et al., 2009; Zhu et al., 2015). In recent studies, Bai Shao was proven to be effective in the treatment of rheumatoid arthritis (RA), systemic lupus erythematosus, hepatitis, and other inflammatory/autoimmune diseases (Zhang & Dai, 2012). Bai Shao is effective in relieving pain in RA models, which is the most common symptom of RA. Multiple pathways may be involved in the analgesic effect of Bai Shao, one of them being its anticholinergic action. The effect of Bai Shao might also be mediated by adenosine A1 receptors, κ-opioid receptors, and α2-adrenoceptors (Lee et al., 2008; Zhang et al., 2009; Zhang, Li, et al., 2008). In addition to its action on the CNS, Bai Shao may also produce antiinflammatory effects that contribute to its analgesic effects. It can inhibit the production of inflammatory mediators and proinflammatory cytokines. It also inhibits chemokine production from endothelial cells, induces the production of antioxidants, and decreases microvascular permeability (Wang, Zhang, Wu, & Wei, 2011; Zheng & Wei, 2005). Furthermore, a recent study has shown that paeoniflorin directly suppresses morphine-induced microglial activation, thus potentiating the acute analgesic effects of morphine and attenuating antinociceptive tolerance to chronic administration (Jiang et al., 2015) (Fig. 5).

2.6 *Gelsemium elegans* (钩吻, Gou Wen)

Gelsemium is a small flowering plant belonging to the family Loganiaceae, which comprises five species. Of these, *G. elegans* Benth., also known as

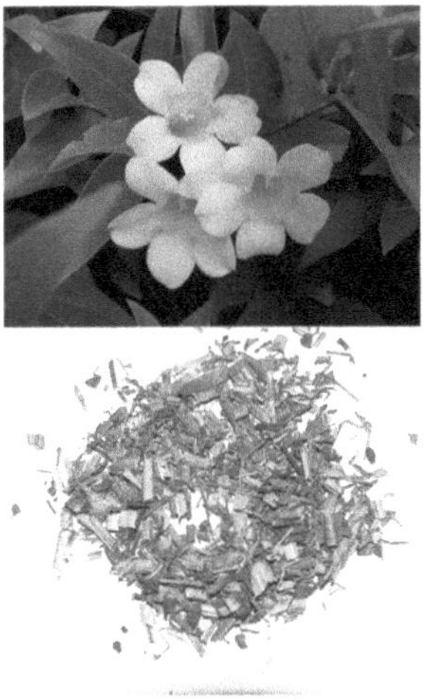

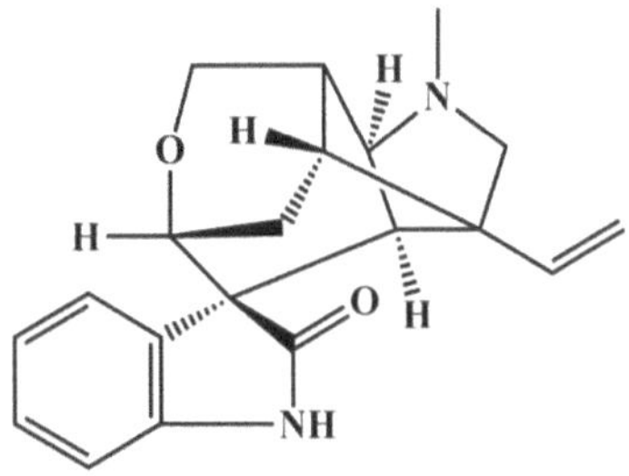

Gelsemine

Figure 6 Photos of *Gelsemium elegans* and its medicinal components, as well as its main analgesic components.

Gou Wen, is native to East Asia and particularly China. This plant was known to be responsible for the death of Shen Nong, a pioneer of Chinese medicine. The whole plant of Gou Wen is poisonous, in particular its tender leaves or green shoots (Jin et al., 2014), thus earning the name Duan Chang Cao in China (Dutt, Thakur, Dhar, & Sharma, 2010; Zhang, Gong, Huang, Guo, & Wang, 2013).

Approximately 200 compounds have been isolated from Gou Wen, including alkaloids, iridoids, steroids, and coumarins (Jin et al., 2014; Zhang, Wang, Yuan, & Li, 2008). Recently, researchers have shown the potent analgesic effect of one such alkaloid, known as gelsemine. This compound exhibits potent and specific antinociceptive effects to alleviate chronic pain by acting at the spinal α3 glycine receptors and the allopregnanolone analgesic pathway in the CNS. Gou Wen and its active extracts have shown analgesic effects in a variety of inflammatory, neuropathic, diabetic, and cancer pain models. However, they do not induce tolerance in cases of neuropathic and bone cancer pain even after being administered multiple times daily. Despite the toxicity of this Chinese medicine, Gou Wen and its active ingredient can be used for long-term clinical therapy in the future (Rujjanawate, Kanjanapothi, & Panthong, 2003; Fig. 6).

2.7 *Strychni semen* (马钱子, Ma Qian Zi)

Ma Qian Zi is composed of the dried seeds of *Strychnos nux-vomica* L., and is widely used in TCM to increase blood circulation and relieve rheumatic pain. Recent studies have shown the great potential of Ma Qian Zi as a promising pain-relieving agent. Brucine and brucine *N*-oxide are the main active constituents of Ma Qian Zi, which are effective in various pain and inflammatory models (Chen, Lin, et al., 2014; Chen, Qu, et al., 2014; Chen, Sun, et al., 2014). Both central and peripheral mechanisms are involved in the pain-modulating and antiinflammatory effects of Ma Qian Zi and its active ingredients. These compounds have been proven to reduce the levels of 5-HT in the blood plasma of arthritic rats, while increasing the levels of 5-hydroxytryindole-3-acetic acid (5-HIAA) accordingly. They also inhibit cyclooxygenase-2 (COX-2) in the metabolic pathway of arachidonic acid (AA) and reduce the release of prostaglandin (PG) E2 in inflammatory tissue while also reducing the vascular permeability (Tripathi et al., 2004). Some researchers state that brucine is a more morphine-like analgesic drug, whereas brucine *N*-oxide is a more NSAID-like drug, which inhibits the synthesis or release of PGs. Both of these compounds inhibit the activities of COX and MAO simultaneously (Yin, Wang, Yin, & Cai, 2003). Ma Qian Zi and Gou Wen belong to the same family, Loganiaceae. It is well established that Ma Qian Zi also has potent toxicity (Chen, Lin, et al., 2014; Chen, Qu, et al., 2014; Chen, Sun, et al., 2014; Ma, Gu, et al., 2015; Ma, Yang, et al., 2015; Ma, Zhang, et al., 2015). Therefore, developing less toxic active compounds from this herbal medicine will be useful in treating pain in the clinical setting (Fig. 7).

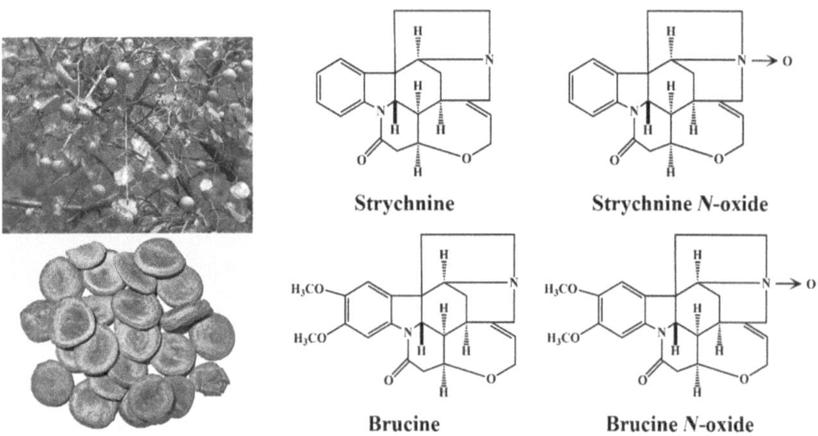

Figure 7 Photos of *Strychni semen* and its medicinal components, including its main analgesic components from this herb medicine.

2.8 Sophorae Flavescentis Radix (苦参, Ku Shen)

Ku Shen is the root of deuto shrub *Sophora flavescens* Ait. of the Leguminosae family. This medicinal herb is cultivated and used across China. It is one of the oldest herbs used in TCM to clear heat and dry dampness, purge fire, remove toxicity, eliminate parasites, and induce diuresis. Modern studies have confirmed the various pharmacological activities of Ku Shen such as its antitumor (Wang, You, et al., 2015; Xiao, Wang, Wang, & Shen, 2013), antiviral (Liu, Zhu, Shi, & Yang, 2003), and antiinflammatory (Ji, Cui, Liang, Guan, & Li, 2013) effects. Recent evidence has pointed to the pain-relieving effect of some compounds from Ku Shen in several animal models (Fig. 8).

Several compounds present in Ku Shen have shown an analgesic effect, including matrine, oxymatrine, sophocarpine, and oxysophocarpine. Matrine has been shown to alleviate pain induced by anticancer drugs, and produce an antinociceptive effect on vincristine-induced painful neuropathy mouse models (Dun et al., 2014) as well as an antinociceptive effect on neuropathic pain induced by chronic constriction injury (Wang, Cao, et al., 2013; Wang, Li, Dun, Xu, Hao, et al., 2013; Wang, Li, Dun, Xu, Jin, et al., 2013). The mechanisms of action of matrine remain to be elucidated. Some studies have indicated that matrine exerts

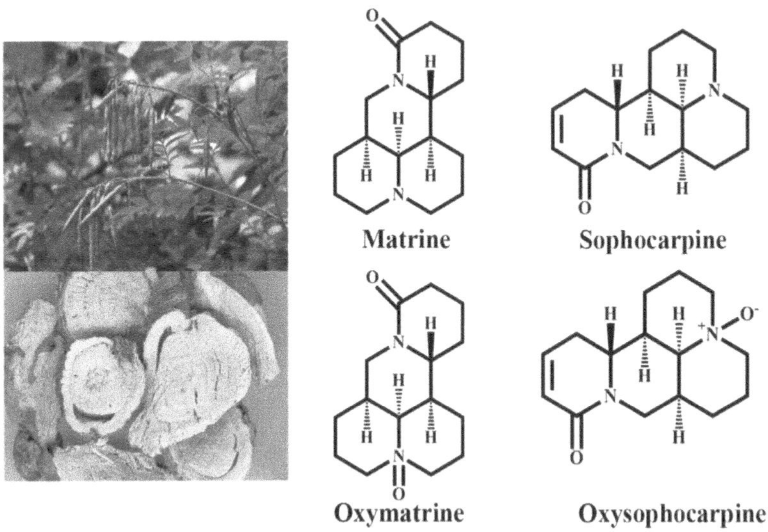

Figure 8 Photos of Sophorae Flavescentis Radix and its medicinal components as well as its main analgesic components.

antinociceptive effects via the opioid receptors (Kamei et al., 1997), while other reports have shown that it can increase cholinergic activation in the CNS rather than act on opioid receptors directly (Yin & Zhu, 2005). Oxymatrine has a similar effect to matrine, which occurs by affecting the calcium channel, GABA release (Lu, Yang, Deng, Wu, & Liu, 2015), and regulation of NR2B-containing NMDA receptor-ERK/CREB signaling (Liu et al., 2012; Wang, Cao, et al., 2013; Wang, Li, Dun, Xu, Hao, et al., 2013; Wang, Li, Dun, Xu, Jin, et al., 2013) in neuropathic pain models. In multiple pain animal models, sophocarpine and oxysophocarpine have shown effective antiinflammatory effect by inhibiting the expression of PG E2 and cytokines (Gao et al., 2009; Yang et al., 2015). These compounds also act on the CNS, for example, by increasing the expression of GABAAα1 receptors (Xu et al., 2013). To date, Ku Shen and matrine have been approved by the China Food and Drug Administration in the treatment of viral infections or gynecological disorders. We believe that Ku Shen has great potential as a novel analgesic agent due to its multiple targets of action. However, the exact mechanisms of action of Ku Shen must be investigated in depth. The therapeutic effect of Ku Shen and its active ingredient on pain also require further evaluation.

2.9 Papaveris Pericarpium (罂粟壳, Ying Su Qiao)

Ying Su Qiao is the dry mature proper exciple of *P. somniferum* L. of the Papaveraceae family. *P. somniferum*, the opium poppy, is the plant species from which opium and poppy seeds are derived. Opium is the source of some drugs, including morphine, codeine, and papaverine. It is well known for its potent analgesic effect (McQuay, 1999) and is a highly addictive narcotic drug. In many countries, including China, the cultivation and processing of *P. somniferum* are restricted and illegal (Trang et al., 2015). To date, only Ying Su Qiao, a part of *P. somniferum*, has been used in TCM to treat cough, diarrhea, and pain in the abdomen. Ying Su Qiao is also rich in morphine, codeine, and papaverine, but the content and purity of these compounds are not as high as opium (Cao, Li, He, Li, & Liu, 2007). Therefore, Ying Su Qiao is not commonly used as a pain-relieving agent in the clinical setting. Ying Su Qiao is also used as food flavoring (Dong & Wang, 2000). However, the active compounds in this medicinal herb should be explored further. The long-term use of Ying Su Qiao can lead to addiction and dependence (Fig. 9).

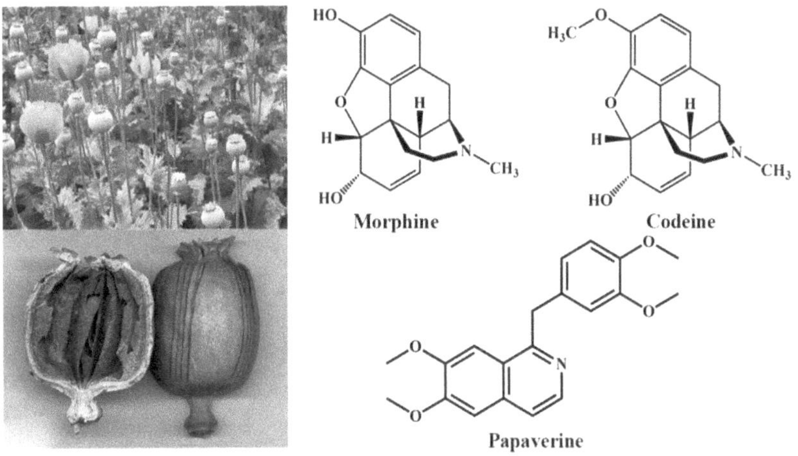

Figure 9 Photos of Papaveris Pericarpium and its medicinal components, including its main analgesic components.

2.10 Belladonnae Herba (颠茄草, Dian Qie Cao)

Dian Qie Cao is the entire dry plant of *Atropa belladonna* L. of the Solanaceae family. Dian Qie Cao is a toxic plant containing tropane alkaloids such as atropine, scopolamine, and hyoscyamine, which can cause delirium and hallucinations (Consroe, 1973; Glatstein, Danino, Wolyniez, & Scolnik, 2014). These compounds are also used as pharmaceutical anticholinergic agents (Qiang et al., 2014). Dian Qie Cao has long been used as medicine, cosmetic product, and poison. Before the Middle Ages in Europe, it was used as an anesthetic for surgery. The active compounds in Dian Qie Cao are antagonists of muscarinic receptors (M-receptors). The blockage of the reaction between acetylcholine and M-receptors could inhibit glandular secretion and relieve smooth muscle spasms (Xiao et al., 2009). Therefore, it is generally used to relieve spasms inducing pain such as headaches induced by cerebral vascular spasm (Stieg, 1977). Although Dian Qian Cao relieves pain through different mechanisms, because of its potent effect on the CNS, it is not currently in use as an analgesic (Fig. 10).

2.11 Other Analgesic TCM Formulations

More than 800 kinds of Chinese medicines have been reported to exhibit analgesic effects for various kinds of pain. Of these, more than 400 are single Chinese herbs, which are used widely in the clinical setting. Moreover, several other pain-relieving Chinese medicinal herbs should also be acknowledged. The TCM herbs found to be effective in animal models or in clinical

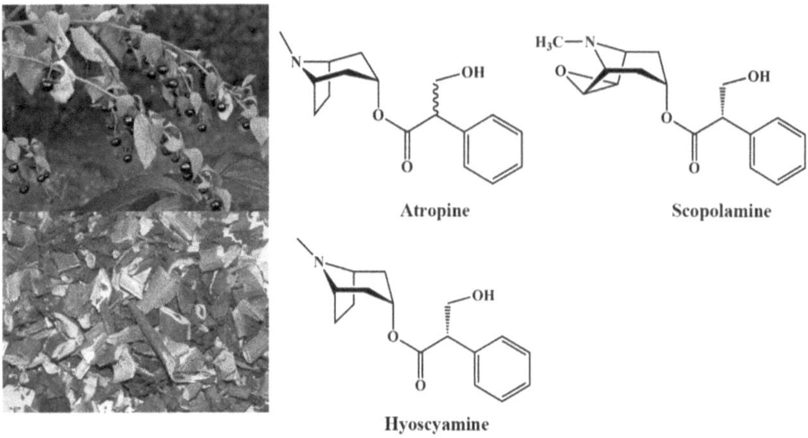

Figure 10 Photos of Belladonnae Herba and its medicinal components, and its main analgesic components.

settings are summarized in Table 1. Based on modern pharmacological principles, analgesic TCM formulations can be divided into six groups: central analgesia, anesthetic analgesia, antiinfection analgesia, antipyretic analgesia, spasmolytic analgesia, and anticoagulant analgesia. Based on the principles of TCM, analgesic TCM formulations can be divided into five classes: those regulating vital energy and promoting blood flow (理气活血), those increasing circulation and removing stasis (活血化瘀), those warming the meridian to relieve pain (温经止痛), those dispelling cold to relieve pain (散寒止痛), and those activating the meridians to relieve pain (通络止痛). Yan Hu Suo is most widely used in TCM to increase blood circulation, dissolve blood stasis, and promote the flow of qi. Medicinal herbs such as Flos Carthami (Hong Hua) (Zhou, Tang, Xu, Zhou, & Wang, 2014), Resina Draconis (Xue Jie) (Liu et al., 2013), Radix Salviae Miltiorrhiza (Dan Shen) (Wang, Wang, Xiong, Mao, & Li, 2006), and Herba Lamiophlomis (Du Yi Wei) (Zhu et al., 2014) are effective in relieving swelling and pain in traumatic injuries and inflammatory diseases as they increase circulation and inhibit stasis. TCM herbs that activate the meridians for pain relief are generally used to treat dysmenorrhea, for example, Radix Aconiti (Chuan Wu) (Wang, Sun, et al., 2015; Wang, You, et al., 2015), Radix Aconiti Lateralis Praeparata (Fu Zi) (Schroder et al., 2013), and Rhizoma Cyperi (Xiang Fu) (Choi et al., 2012). They dispel wind and eliminate dampness (祛风除湿), in addition to warming the uterus and inhibiting strong uterine contraction. In TCM, dispelling wind and

Table 1 Traditional Chinese Medicine for Analgesia

Name	Latin Name	Source	Indications
Yan Hu Suo	Rhizoma Corydalis	Lei Gong Pao Zhi Lun (Lei's Treaties on Preparation of Drugs)	Pain due to blood stasis and qi stagnation, heart disease, liver damage, drug addiction
Ying Su Qiao	Papaveris Pericarpium	Ben Cao Gang Mu (Compendium of Materia Medica)	Chronic diarrhea and dysentery, chronic cough due to lung deficiency, abdomen and stomach pain, joint pain
Bai Zhi	Radix Angelicae Dahuricae	Shen Nong Ben Cao Jing (Shen Nong's Herbal)	Pain such as headache, toothache, arthralgia; wind–cold external syndrome; anti-inflammation; antifungal; laxative; sedative
San Qi	Radix Notoginseng	Ben Cao Gang Mu (Compendium of Materia Medica)	Bleeding, traumatic injury, swelling, and pain due to blood stasis
Hua Jiao	Pericarpium Zanthoxyli	Shen Nong Ben Cao Jing (Shen Nong's Herbal)	Vomiting and diarrhea due to cold–damp, detoxification, ascariasis with abdominal pain, stomachache, eczema, and pruritus vulvae
Bai Shao	Radix Paeoniae Alba	Shen Nong Ben Cao Jing (Shen Nong's Herbal)	Irregular menstruation, hypochondriac pain, abdominal pain, muscular contracture pain, dizziness, and vertigo
Gou Wen	*Gelsemium elegans*	Ben Jing (Herbal Classic)	Swelling, pain, eczema, deep-rooted boil, traumatic injury, rheumatic arthralgia
Ma Qian Zi	*Strychnos nux-vomica* L.	Ben Cao Gang Mu (Compendium of Materia Medica)	Traumatic injuries, abscess, carbuncle, swelling and pain, arthralgia, numbness, and paralysis

Continued

Table 1 Traditional Chinese Medicine for Analgesia—cont'd

Name	Latin Name	Source	Indications
Chuan Xiong	Szechuan Lovage Rhizome	Shen Nong Ben Cao Jing (Shen Nong's Herbal)	Headache, arthralgia
Dang Gui	Radix Angelicae Sinensis	Shen Nong Ben Cao Jing (Shen Nong's Herbal)	Pain, irregular menstruation, amenorrhea, dysmenorrhea, ulcer, constipation
Du Huo	Radix Angelicae Pubescentis	Shen Nong Ben Cao Jing (Shen Nong's Herbal)	Arthralgia
Hong Hua	Flos Carthami	Xin Xiu Ben Cao (Newly Revised Materia Medica)	Dysmenorrhea, abdominal pain, traumatic injury, sore, abscess, swelling
Xiang Fu	Rhizoma Cyperi	Ming Yi Bie Lu (miscellaneous records of famous physicians)	Dysmenorrhea, breast distending pain
Wu Zhu Yu	Fructus Evodiae	Shen Nong Ben Cao Jing (Shen Nong's Herbal)	Pain due to congealing cold
Rou Gui	Cortex Cinnamomi	Shen Nong Ben Cao Jing (Shen Nong's Herbal)	Pain due to congealing cold, blood stasis syndrome
Qiang Huo	Rhizoma seu Radix Notopterygii	Shen Nong Ben Cao Jing (Shen Nong's Herbal)	Arthralgia
Xue Jie	Resina Draconis	Lei Gong Pao Zhi Lun (Lei's Treaties on Preparation of Drugs)	Traumatic injuries, stagnant pain of heart and abdomen, sores, and ulcers
Dan Shen	Radix Salviae Miltiorrhizae	Shen Nong Ben Cao Jing (Shen Nong's Herbal)	Blood stasis, sores, abscesses, carbuncles, and swellings

Du Yi Wei	Herba Lamiophlomis	Sichuan Zhong Yao Zhi (Chinese Material Medica of Sichuan)	Traumatic injury rheumatic arthritis
Chuan Wu	Radix Aconiti	Shen Nong Ben Cao Jing (Shen Nong's Herbal)	Arthralgia syndrome due to wind, cold, and dampness; various pains due to cold congealing; pain due to traumatic injury
Fu Zi	Radix Aconiti Lateralis Praeparata	Shen Nong Ben Cao Jing (Shen Nong's Herbal)	Pain syndrome of cold type
Xu Chang Qing	Radix Cynanchi Paniculati	Ben Jing (Herbal Classic)	Stomachache, toothache, edema, traumatic injury, rheumatic arthritis, dysmenorrhea
Fang Ji	Radix Stephaniae Tetrandrae	Shen Nong Ben Cao Jing (Shen Nong's Herbal)	Arthralgia
Wu Yao	Radix Linderae	Ben Cao Shi Yi (A Supplement to the Compendium of Materia Medica)	Thoracic and abdominal pain
Chuan Lian Zi	Fructus Toosendan	Shen Nong Ben Cao Jing (Shen Nong's Herbal)	Pain due to qi stagnation and ascariasis with abdominal pain
Pu Gong Ying	Herba Taraxaci	Xin Xiu Ben Cao (Newly Revised Materia Medica)	Sores and abscess, swollen and sore throat, swelling and pain of gum, red eyes with swelling and pain
Long Dan Cao	Radix Gentianae	Shen Nong Ben Cao Jing (Shen Nong's Herbal)	Headache, sore throat, arthralgia
Ku Shen	Radix Sophorae Flavescentis	Shen Nong Ben Cao Jing (Shen Nong's Herbal)	Dysentery, jaundice, itching, sores, abscess, sore throat, swollen and painful gum, leukorrhagia
Dian Qie Cao	Belladonnae Herba	Yao Cai Xue (Pharmacognosy)	Nausea, vomiting, night sweat, cholecystalgia, salivation, gastric and duodenal ulcer

eliminating dampness are believed to ease discomfort, as wind and dampness are considered to cause cold and pain. Thus, TCM formulations that eliminate wind and dampness are effective in treating pain, cold, and rheumatism. Fructus Evodiae (Wu Zhu Yu) (Matsuda, Wu, Tanaka, Iinuma, & Kubo, 1997), Cortex Cinnamomi (Rou Gui) (Ahn et al., 2014), and Rhizoma seu Radix Notopterygii (Qiang Huo) (Qin & Jiao, 1987) are effective in dispelling wind, cold, and xeransis, as well as treating pain induced by cold wind. Finally, Ma Qian Zi is well known for its activating effect on meridians (经络, the network of channels in the human body) to alleviate pain. Furthermore, some TCM formulations are derived from animals such as earthworms (Di Long), *Scolopendra* (Wu Gong) (Li, Chen, & Gan, 1996), and Eupolyphaga seu Steleophaga (Tu Bie Chong) (Xie et al., 2001), which are known to activate meridians to alleviate pain.

2.12 TCM Compounds in Pain Management

Compared with single Chinese herbs, TCM compounds have a great efficacy in pain treatment when used in combination. Several formulations have been recorded in ancient medical books such as Ephedra Decoction and Dang Gui Shao Yao San. The use of novel TCM formulations has been confirmed in clinical trials and experimental studies including Jia Yuan Qing pills and Gui Zhi Fu Ling capsules. The TCM compounds commonly used to treat pain are summarized in Table 2.

3. THE DISCOVERY OF ACTIVE COMPONENTS IN TRADITIONAL CHINESE ANALGESICS

For more than 7000 years, various extracts of natural products, mostly plants, have been used as potent analgesics. These extracts contain several components that are responsible for their analgesic effects. Thus, the extracts in TCM can be used to produce novel analgesic compounds with a combination of several technologies including analytical purification, pharmacological analysis, and drug screening.

In modern medicine, drugs directed at multiple targets are clearly more efficacious. This "network pharmacology" has gained importance, challenging the traditional principle of drug discovery of "one gene, one target, one drug" (Wu & Wu, 2015). TCM formulations typically have several targets and are therefore effective in the treatment of various diseases. Thus, TCM herbs have a long-standing history of clinical use.

Table 2 Traditional Chinese Medicine Compounds for Treatment of Pain

Prescription	Source	Component	Indications	References
Ma Huang Tang (Ephedra Decoction)	Shang Han Lun (Treatise on Febrile Disease)	Herba ephedrae, almond, cassia twig, *Glycyrrhiza uralensis*	Headache, backache, arthralgia, wind–cold, asthma, dystocia	He et al. (2014) and Zheng, Zhou, Wan, Chen, and He (2015)
Shao Yao Gan Cao Decoction	Shang Han Lun (Treatise on Febrile Disease)	Peony and licorice	Nourishing liver, relaxing spasm, relieving pain	Bi, Gong, and Di (2014) and Hu et al. (2011)
Dang Gui Shao Yao San	Jin Kui Yao Lue (Medical treasures of the Golden Chamber)	Radix angelicae sinensis, *Paeonia veitchii*, *Poria cocos*	Dysmenorrhea, edema, chronic pelvic inflammation, functional uterine bleeding, orthodontic pain	Hsu and Lin (1996) and Shen et al. (2005)
Jia Yuan Qing pills	Novel	Porcellio laevis latreille, *Corydalis rhizoma*, Radix cynanchi paniculata	Cancer pain	Tian et al. (2014) and Tian et al. (2015)
Tou Feng Yu pills	Chuan Xiong Cha Tiao powder Tai Ping Hui Min He Ji Ju Fang	*Angelica dahurica*, Rhizome Ligustici, and Folium *Camellia sinensis*	Migraine, fever, nasal congestion	Li et al. (2011)
Tong Luo San Jie gel	San Qi He Bi Zhen	*Piper kadsura*, *Trachelospermum jasminoides*, *Dioscorea nipponica* Makino, *Corydalis yanhuso* W.T. Wang, *Melia toosendan* Sieb. et Zucc, *Boswellia carterii* Birdw., and *Commiphora myrrha* Engl.	Rheumatism, rheumatoid arthritis, sciatica, scapulohumeral periarthritis	Wang et al. (2012)

Continued

Table 2 Traditional Chinese Medicine Compounds for Treatment of Pain—cont'd

Prescription	Source	Component	Indications	References
Xiao Zheng Zhi Tong paste	Novel	Xuejie (Dragon's blood), Yanhusuo (*Corydalis rhizoma*), Ruxiang (olibanum), Moyao (Myrrha), Qingdai (natural indigo), and Bingpian (*Borneolum syntheticum*)	Cancer pain	Bao, Gao, et al. (2015) and Bao, Wang, et al., (2015)
Die Sun Miao Fang	Die Sun Miao Fang	*Angelica sinensis*, Radix rehmanniae, *Areca catechu* and Radix paeoniae rubra	Activate blood, remove stasis, promote qi circulation, and relieve pain	Zheng, Fu, et al. (2015)
Tian Shu formula	Da Chuan Xiong Fang Xuan Ming Lun Fang	Rhizoma chuanxiong, *Gastrodia elata*	Migraine	Li, Zhang, et al. (2015), Wang, Zhang, et al. (2013), and Xia et al. (2013)

Pain can be differentiated into mechanical pain, inflammatory pain, and neuropathic pain, wherein inflammatory pain is associated with tissue damage and the infiltration of immune cells. Current pain management strategies mostly involve the use of antiinflammatory and antinociceptive agents. The most prevalent antiinflammatory drugs are NSAIDs, including the COX inhibitors. Several TCM formulations and their active ingredients exhibit antiinflammatory and analgesic effects, wherein pain is relieved as inflammation is reduced. NSAIDs constitute the first-line therapy for low or moderate pain.

DL0309 is a novel antiinflammatory drug discovered in our laboratory (Zhang, He, Ding, & Du, 2006). It is one of the active compounds with structure frame as methyl salicylate 2-*O*-β-D-lactoside (MSL) derived from *Gaultheria yunnanensis* (Franch) Rehder (*G. yunnanensis*), which is used in TCM to treat rheumatism and arthritis pain. In our earlier work, we aimed to identify the active ingredient in this medicinal herb, which exhibited antiinflammatory and analgesic effects. With the help of experts in phytochemistry, we recorded the presence of MSL, as the chemical structure of MSL is related to salicylic acid. This compound was named as DL0309, which was found to have various effects after considerable research. DL0309 demonstrated antiinflammatory and analgesic effects on a murine model of croton oil-induced ear swelling and acetic acid-induced writhing response. The compound acts as an antiinflammatory agent by inhibiting the activity of NF-κB in macrophages, microglia, and astrocytes (Lan, Liu, Sun, Zhang, & Du, 2011; Zhang, Sun, et al., 2012; Zhang, Sun, Xin, et al., 2015). DL0309 also inhibits the inflammatory response of fibroblast-like synoviocytes and joint destruction in murine models of arthritis (Xin et al., 2014). DL0309 is still being investigated in our laboratory; it is considered to be a potent antiinflammatory and analgesic drug. In addition, this compound produces fewer adverse drug reactions than aspirin. This drug serves as a successful example of discovering the analgesic component of TCM. Monomers are obtained and identified through advanced extraction and separation technology. The compounds of medicinal value are studied after comparing their structures with existing drugs.

However, in most studies, related structures are not always found. Thus, screening models are needed to identify the expected compounds. Presently, new advances in separation techniques have facilitated the extraction and purification of lipids, carbohydrates, and polar compounds that could not be effectively isolated in the past (Gao et al., 2007; Zhang & Dai, 2012;

Zhang, Liu, et al., 2012; Zhang, Sun, et al., 2012). After several single Chinese herbs are separated and isolated, in vitro evaluation to determine the target compounds is urgently needed. As opioids are still the gold standard for the treatment of pain, screening models for μ-opioid receptor agonists are still widely used (Podolsky et al., 2013; Serohijos et al., 2011). However, drugs that activate μ-opioid receptors, such as morphine and its various derivatives, are potentially addicting. Alternative approaches include the use of novel compounds that target delta (δ) or kappa (κ) opioid receptors, or those that interact with two or more of the opioid receptors (Stein, 2016; Wang, Sun, Tao, Chi, & Liu, 2010). The advantage of TCM formulations is that they typically have multiple targets including opioid receptors. The use of Chuan Wu, the mother root of *Aconitum carmichaelii* Debeauxv, has been reported with potent antinociceptive effects under inflammatory conditions via the activation of kappa opioid receptor by releasing dynorphin and inhibiting TRPV1. This herb has been widely used in TCM as a pain reliever for more than two millennia (Wang, Sun, et al., 2015; Wang, You, et al., 2015). In addition to the drug screening models based on μ-, κ-, and δ-opioid receptors, other in vitro models might also contribute to the discovery of active components from TCM such as DA receptor-expressing cells (Zhang et al., 2014), adenosine A1 receptors, adrenergic receptors, and spinal α3 glycine receptors. These targets have been described previously, although most have not been widely used as drugs screening models.

In vitro drug screening models help researchers discover targets rapidly and conveniently. However, animal models are more objective in reflecting the pharmacological function of drugs. Several classical animal models of pain are also suitable for evaluating analgesic agents from TCM. Experimental models of pain sensitivity include tests of response thresholds to high-intensity stimuli (acute pain tests) and changes in spontaneous or evoked behavioral responses in animals with peripheral injury or inflammation (persistent pain models) (Bannon & Malmberg, 2007). Acute pain tests include the thermal tail-flick and Hargreaves tests, the hot-plate test, and the mechanical von Frey test, among others. The writhing and inflammatory formalin pain tests are persistent pain models. Specific models such as the spinal nerve ligation model are available for mimicking neuropathic pain (Liu et al., 2016), as well as the bone cancer pain model established by Medhurst et al. (2002). Single Chinese medicine compounds and active ingredients can be evaluated in all of these animal pain models (Geng, 2009).

Modern technologies can help develop new TCM formulations more accurately and conveniently, particularly in the discovery of new analgesic TCM formulations from plant species. Herbs from the same family, genus, and species may share similar active components and characteristics with generally the same functions. For example, *P. somniferum* L. (Ying Su) is a well-known analgesic agent with highly addictive potential, which limits its clinical use. Yan Hu Suo, which belongs to the same family, also produces an analgesic effect. Although Yan Hu Suo has a weaker effect than Ying Su, its side effects are greatly reduced. Effective TCM formulations for pain relief can be discovered through a study of Chinese medical literature and ancient books, which record the experiences of renowned doctors in ancient China and can provide further insight on the discovery of novel analgesic agents in TCM.

4. MECHANISMS OF ANALGESIA OF TCMs

4.1 Theories of Analgesia in TCM

The theories of the mechanism of action in TCM differ significantly from those of modern pharmacology, in that the former theories are multiple and complicated. Traditional Chinese doctors believed that the pain was caused by qi stagnation and blood stasis. TCM formulations that can increase blood circulation and remove blood stasis are considered to be effective analgesics.

At present, analgesic drugs in TCM can be divided into four categories based on their mechanisms of action: those that promote blood circulation, disperse stasis, dispel the cold, and dredge collaterals. In this case, TCM formulations are empirically used in the clinical setting based on the accumulated experience. The lack of understanding of the active ingredients and the specific mechanisms may prevent TCM formulations from being developed further and becoming generally accepted. Therefore, fundamental research into the mechanisms of TCM has become crucial.

In general, TCM formulations have multiple targets that form a complicated network. Advances in analgesic TCM agents have led many Chinese scientists to study the mechanisms of action of TCM drugs in the treatment of pain.

4.2 Mechanisms of TCM in Modern Pharmacological Theory

Some TCM formulations act on receptors in the CNS, thus exerting a central analgesic effect. In addition, most analgesic TCM agents alleviate pain by inhibiting inflammation. Modern research has shown the pivotal role of Chinese medicinal herbs and compounds derived from TCM in the regulation of pain-related signaling pathways. In addition, these compounds most likely have an impact on the expression of related proteins to alleviate pain.

Pain is a highly complicated pathological process that is regulated by multiple signaling molecules. Mitogen-activated protein kinase (MAPK) pathways including those of ERK, c-Jun/SAPK, and p38MAPK are involved in the development of pain (Wang et al., 2011). Nerve injury and bone cancer result in the rapid-onset and long-lasting expression of WNTs, as well as the activation of WNT/frizzled/β-catenin signaling in primary sensory neurons. The blockade of WNT signaling pathways is known to inhibit the production and persistence of neuropathic pain (Itokazu, Hayano, Takahashi, & Yamashita, 2014; Tang, 2014; Zhang, Huang, et al., 2013). TRPV1 is a nonselective positive ion channel primarily expressed in sensory neurons, belonging to the transient receptor potential (TRP) family. This receptor can be activated by mechanical irritation, chemical irritation, or endogenous ligands to mediate pain and cause injury to body functions. Several TCM formulations have been found to have analgesic effects via the interaction with TRPV1, such as Wu Zhu Yu and Rou Gui (Liu, Lv, & Zhang, 2014).

5. CONCLUSION

In conclusion, TCM formulations are effective analgesics. In TCM, it is believed that "stagnation of qi and blood may bring about pain," which has been the underlying principle for the use of analgesic TCM formulations. Although the theories of TCM are generally abstract and complicated, we believe the mechanisms of action of analgesic TCM formulations can be well explained by modern science. First, potent analgesic agents in TCM typically contain active compounds that directly target the nervous system such as Yan Hu Suo and Gou Wen. Second, most of these agents have a similar effect to NSAIDs, relieving pain via the inhibition of inflammation. Unlike modern medicine, drugs used in TCM alleviate pain by treating the underlying diseases. Thus, TCM aims to address the etiology of pain instead of merely relieving symptoms; hence, a permanent cure may be achieved. For example, the treatment of dysmenorrhea is usually dependent on PG synthetase inhibitors such as ibuprofen and ketone. These drugs merely relieve the symptoms but do not treat the underlying dysmenorrhea. TCM formulations used in the treatment of this disease, for instance, Yan Hu Suo and Dang Gui, attempt to treat the pathogenesis to treat the pain (Chen, Lin, et al., 2014; Chen, Qu, et al., 2014; Chen, Sun, et al., 2014). The advantages of these formulations in pain treatment are their low addictive potential and tolerance. In addition, China has abundant resources of medicinal herbs and a sound foundation of TCM, although its global market share (less than 5%) in plant extractions is small. The active ingredients require further investigations. The development of TCM has tremendous socioeconomic value. The advanced technology available currently can help evaluate the efficacy of ancient Chinese medicinal herbs with modern science, which can then be used globally. However, in-depth experimental studies are urgently needed to determine their active components and elucidate their mechanisms. TCM can lead to the discovery of novel analgesic drugs with greater efficacy and lower toxicity.

CONFLICT OF INTEREST

The authors declare that they have no conflict of interest.

ACKNOWLEDGMENTS

This study was supported by the national scientific and technological major special project "Significant Creation of New Drugs" (2013ZX09103001-008, 2012ZX09103101-078) and the National Natural Science Foundation of China (No. 81102444, 81202538).

REFERENCES

Ahn, B. S., Kim, S. K., Kim, H. N., Lee, J. H., Lee, J. H., Hwang, D. S., et al. (2014). Gyejigachulbu-tang relieves Oxaliplatin-induced neuropathic cold and mechanical hypersensitivity in rats via the suppression of spinal glial activation. *Evidence-based Complementary and Alternative Medicine*, *2014*, 436482.

Bannon, A. W., & Malmberg, A. B. (2007). Models of nociception: Hot-plate, tail-flick, and formalin tests in rodents. *Current Protocols in Neuroscience*. Chapter 8, Unit 8 9.

Bao, Y., Gao, Y., Du, M., Hou, W., Yang, L., Kong, X., et al. (2015). Topical treatment with xiaozheng zhitong paste (XZP) alleviates bone destruction and bone cancer pain in a Rat model of prostate cancer-induced bone pain by modulating the RANKL/RANK/OPG signaling. *Evidence-based Complementary and Alternative Medicine*, *2015*, 215892.

Bao, Y., Wang, G., Gao, Y., Du, M., Yang, L., Kong, X., et al. (2015). Topical treatment with Xiaozheng Zhitong Paste alleviates bone cancer pain by inhibiting proteinase-activated receptor 2 signaling pathway. *Oncology Reports*, *34*(3), 1449–1459.

Bi, X., Gong, M., & Di, L. (2014). Review on prescription compatibility of shaoyao gancao decoction and reflection on pharmacokinetic compatibility mechanism of traditional Chinese medicine prescription based on in vivo drug interaction of main efficacious components. *Evidence-based Complementary and Alternative Medicine*, *2014*, 208129.

Cao, Q., Li, S., He, C., Li, K., & Liu, F. (2007). Extraction and determination of papaverin in pericarpium papaveris using aqueous two-phase system of poly(ethylene glycol)-(NH4)

2SO4 coupled with high-performance liquid chromatography. *Analytica Chimica Acta, 590*(2), 187–194.

Chang, S. H., Choi, Y., Park, J. A., Jung, D. S., Shin, J., Yang, J. H., et al. (2007). Anti-inflammatory effects of BT-201, an n-butanol extract of Panax notoginseng, observed in vitro and in a collagen-induced arthritis model. *Clinical Nutrition, 26*(6), 785–791.

Cheatle, M. D. (2015). Prescription opioid misuse, abuse, morbidity, and mortality: Balancing effective pain management and safety. *Pain Medicine, 16*(Suppl. 1), S3–S8.

Chen, H. Y., Lin, Y. H., Su, I. H., Chen, Y. C., Yang, S. H., & Chen, J. L. (2014). Investigation on Chinese herbal medicine for primary dysmenorrhea: Implication from a nationwide prescription database in Taiwan. *Complementary Therapies in Medicine, 22*(1), 116–125.

Chen, J., Qu, Y., Wang, D., Peng, P., Cai, H., Gao, Y., et al. (2014). Pharmacological evaluation of total alkaloids from nux vomica: Effect of reducing strychnine contents. *Molecules, 19*(4), 4395–4408.

Chen, X., Sun, W., Gianaris, N. G., Riley, A. M., Cummins, T. R., Fehrenbacher, J. C., et al. (2014). Furanocoumarins are a novel class of modulators for the transient receptor potential vanilloid type 1 (TRPV1) channel. *Journal of Biological Chemistry, 289*(14), 9600–9610.

Choi, J. G., Kang, S. Y., Kim, J. M., Roh, D. H., Yoon, S. Y., Park, J. B., et al. (2012). Antinociceptive effect of Cyperi rhizoma and Corydalis tuber extracts on neuropathic pain in rats. *Korean Journal of Physiology and Pharmacology, 16*(6), 387–392.

Chow, D. H., Lai, A., Tang, F. H., & Leung, M. C. (2013). Effects of Panax ginseng-containing herbal plasters on compressed intervertebral discs in an in vivo rat tail model. *Chinese Medicine, 8*(1), 4.

Chu, H., Jin, G., Friedman, E., & Zhen, X. (2008). Recent development in studies of tetrahydroprotoberberines: Mechanism in antinociception and drug addiction. *Cellular and Molecular Neurobiology, 28*(4), 491–499.

Consroe, P. F. (1973). Treatment of acute hallucinogenic drug toxicity: Specific pharmacological intervention. *American Journal of Hospital Pharmacy, 30*(1), 80–84.

Dong, N., & Wang, H. Y. (2000). Determination of Pericarpium papaveris in foods accompanied with some fragrant substances by high performance liquid chromatography. *Se Pu, 18*(6), 554–555.

Dun, L., Li, Y., Xu, Y., Zhou, R., Ma, L., Jin, S., et al. (2014). Antinociceptive effect of matrine on vincristine-induced neuropathic pain model in mice. *Neurological Science, 35*(6), 815–821.

Dutt, V., Thakur, S., Dhar, V. J., & Sharma, A. (2010). The genus Gelsemium: An update. *Pharmacognosy Reviews, 4*(8), 185–194.

Gao, M., Deng, C., Lin, S., Hu, F., Tang, J., Yao, N., et al. (2007). Recent developments and contributions from Chinese scientists in multidimensional separations for proteomics and traditional Chinese medicines. *Journal of Separation Science, 30*(6), 785–791.

Gao, Y., Li, G., Li, C., Zhu, X., Li, M., Fu, C., et al. (2009). Anti-nociceptive and anti-inflammatory activity of sophocarpine. *Journal of Ethnopharmacology, 125*(2), 324–329.

Geng, X. H. (2009). *Research methodology of analgesic*. Beijing: People Health Publishing House.

Glatstein, M., Danino, D., Wolyniez, I., & Scolnik, D. (2014). Seizures caused by ingestion of Atropa belladonna in a homeopathic medicine in a previously well infant: Case report and review of the literature. *American Journal of Therapy, 21*(6), e196–e198.

Gorczyca, R., Filip, R., & Walczak, E. (2013). Psychological aspects of pain. *Annals of Agricultural and Environmental Medicine, Spec no. 1*, 23–27.

Guo, Z., Cai, R., Su, H., & Li, Y. (2014). Alkaloids in processed Rhizoma corydalis and crude Rhizoma corydalis analyzed by GC/MS. *Journal of Analytical Methods in Chemistry, 2014*, 281342.

Hague, M., & Shenker, N. (2014). How to investigate: Chronic pain. *Best Practice & Research. Clinical Rheumatology*, *28*(6), 860–874.
He, Y., Gai, Y. Q., Zhou, H. F., Sun, Y. W., Jin, W. F., & Wan, H. T. (2014). Study on multi-target optimization of prescription dose of Mahuang decoction. *Zhongguo Zhong Yao Za Zhi*, *39*(7), 1270–1275.
Hesse, T., Henkel, B., Zygmunt, M., Mustea, A., & Usichenko, T. I. (2015). Acupuncture for pain control after Caesarean section: A prospective observational pilot study. *Acupuncture in Medicine*. Aug 25, pii: acupmed-2015-010852. [Epub ahead of print].
Hsu, H. Y., & Lin, C. C. (1996). A preliminary study on the radioprotection of mouse hematopoiesis by dang-gui-shao-yao-san. *Journal of Ethnopharmacology*, *55*(1), 43–48.
Hu, J. Y., & Jin, G. Z. (1999a). Effect of tetrahydropalmatine analogs on Fos expression induced by formalin-pain. *Zhongguo Yao Li Xue Bao*, *20*(3), 193–200.
Hu, J. Y., & Jin, G. Z. (1999b). Supraspinal D2 receptor involved in antinociception induced by l-tetrahydropalmatine. *Zhongguo Yao Li Xue Bao*, *20*(8), 715–719.
Hu, R. W., Shen, L., Feng, Y., Xu, D. S., Ruan, K. F., Lin, X., et al. (2011). Pharmacokinetics study on characteristic ingredients of different-dose herbs of shaoyao-gancao decoction. *Yao Xue Xue Bao*, *46*(3), 329–332.
Huang, K., Dai, G. Z., Li, X. H., Fan, Q., Cheng, L., Feng, Y. B., et al. (1999). Blocking L-calcium current by l-tetrahydropalmatine in single ventricular myocyte of guinea pigs. *Zhongguo Yao Li Xue Bao*, *20*(10), 907–911.
Itokazu, T., Hayano, Y., Takahashi, R., & Yamashita, T. (2014). Involvement of Wnt/beta-catenin signaling in the development of neuropathic pain. *Neurosciences Research*, *79*, 34–40.
Ji, R., Cui, W., Liang, R. W., Guan, Z. Y., & Li, R. F. (2013). Effect of radix sophorae flavescentis (RSF) mixture on mast cells in jejunal mucosa of mice infected by Cryptosporidium. *Zhongguo Xue Xi Chong Bing Fang Zhi Za Zhi*, *25*(3), 280–283.
Jian, Z. Y., Yu, J. B., & Wang, W. Q. (2010). RP-HPLC determination of main chemical components in different parts and different harvest periods of Paeonia lactiflora. *Yao Xue Xue Bao*, *45*(4), 489–493.
Jiang, C., Xu, L., Chen, L., Han, Y., Tang, J., Yang, Y., et al. (2015). Selective suppression of microglial activation by paeoniflorin attenuates morphine tolerance. *European Journal of Pain*, *19*(7), 908–919.
Jin, U. H., Park, S. G., Suh, S. J., Kim, J. K., Kim, D. S., Moon, S. K., et al. (2007). Inhibitory effect of Panax notoginseng on nitric oxide synthase, cyclo-oxygenase-2 and neutrophil functions. *Phytotherapy Research*, *21*(2), 142–148.
Jin, G. L., Su, Y. P., Liu, M., Xu, Y., Yang, J., Liao, K. J., et al. (2014). Medicinal plants of the genus Gelsemium (Gelsemiaceae, Gentianales)—A review of their phytochemistry, pharmacology, toxicology and traditional use. *Journal of Ethnopharmacology*, *152*(1), 33–52.
Kamei, J., Xiao, P., Ohsawa, M., Kubo, H., Higashiyama, K., Takahashi, H., et al. (1997). Antinociceptive effects of (+)-matrine in mice. *European Journal of Pharmacology*, *337*(2–3), 223–226.
Kang, O. H., Chae, H. S., Oh, Y. C., Choi, J. G., Lee, Y. S., Jang, H. J., et al. (2008). Anti-nociceptive and anti-inflammatory effects of Angelicae dahuricae radix through inhibition of the expression of inducible nitric oxide synthase and NO production. *American Journal of Chinese Medicine*, *36*(5), 913–928.
Kim, S. H., Lee, M. K., Lee, K. Y., Sung, S. H., Kim, J., & Kim, Y. C. (2009). Chemical constituents isolated from Paeonia lactiflora roots and their neuroprotective activity against oxidative stress in vitro. *Journal of Enzyme Inhibition and Medicinal Chemistry*, *24*(5), 1138–1140.
Kim, J. H., Ryu, Y. B., Lee, W. S., & Kim, Y. H. (2014). Neuraminidase inhibitory activities of quaternary isoquinoline alkaloids from Corydalis turtschaninovii rhizome. *Bioorganic and Medicinal Chemistry*, *22*(21), 6047–6052.

Lan, X., Liu, R., Sun, L., Zhang, T. T., & Du, G. H. (2011). Methyl salicylate 2-O-beta-D-lactoside, a novel salicylic acid analogue, acts as an anti-inflammatory agent on microglia and astrocytes. *Journal of Neuroinflammation*, *8*, 98.

Lee, B., Shin, Y. W., Bae, E. A., Han, S. J., Kim, J. S., Kang, S. S., et al. (2008). Antiallergic effect of the root of Paeonia lactiflora and its constituents paeoniflorin and paeonol. *Archives of Pharmacal Research*, *31*(4), 445–450.

Li, X., Chen, H., & Gan, M. (1996). Anti-inflammatory and analgesic effects of scolopendra from different habitats. *Zhongguo Zhong Yao Za Zhi*, *21*(8), 498–499. 512.

Li, R. J., Ji, X., & Bai, X. Q. (2015). Observation of Qufeng-qingre-dingtong decoction on analgesia effects and the content of ET-1, 5-HT in migraine rats. *Hebei Journal of Traditional Chinese Medicine*, *8*, 1118–1183.

Li, J. C., Shen, X. F., Meng, X. L., Zhang, Y., & Lai, X. R. (2011). Analgesic effect and mechanism of the three TCM-herbal drug-combination Tou Feng Yu pill on treatment of migraine. *Phytomedicine*, *18*(8-9), 788–794.

Li, R., Yang, J. J., Shi, Y. X., Zhao, M., Ji, K. L., Zhang, P., et al. (2014). Chemical composition, antimicrobial and anti-inflammatory activities of the essential oil from Maqian (Zanthoxylum myriacanthum var. pubescens) in Xishuangbanna, SW China. *Journal of Ethnopharmacology*, *158*(Pt. A), 43–48.

Li, X. Q., Yang, T. F., Zhang, K. X., Lu, Y., & Wu, J. R. (2009). Study of synergistic analgesic action of rotundine combined with subthreshold dose of dolantin. *Acta academiae medicinae Xu Zhou*, *05*, 319–320.

Li, Y., Zhang, J., Zhang, L., Chen, X., Pan, Y., Chen, S. S., et al. (2015). Systems pharmacology to decipher the combinational anti-migraine effects of Tianshu formula. *Journal of Ethnopharmacology*, *174*, 45–56.

Liao, Z. G., Liang, X. L., Zhu, J. Y., Zhao, G. W., Yang, M., Wang, G. F., et al. (2010). Correlation between synergistic action of Radix Angelica dahurica extracts on analgesic effects of Corydalis alkaloid and plasma concentration of dl-THP. *Journal of Ethnopharmacology*, *129*(1), 115–120.

Ling, S., Nheu, L., Dai, A., Guo, Z., & Komesaroff, P. (2008). Effects of four medicinal herbs on human vascular endothelial cells in culture. *International Journal of Cardiology*, *128*(3), 350–358.

Liu, H. Y., Li, Y. X., Hao, Y. J., Wang, H. Y., Dai, X. Y., Sun, T., et al. (2012). Effects of oxymatrine on the neuropathic pain induced by chronic constriction injury in mice. *CNS Neuroscience and Therapeutics*, *18*(12), 1030–1032.

Liu, L., Li, G., Zhu, F., Wang, L., & Wang, Y. (1990). Comparison of analgesic effect between locally vinegar-processed preparation of fresh rhizoma Corydalis and traditionally vinegar-processed rhizoma Corydalis. *Zhongguo Zhong Yao Za Zhi*, *15*(11), 666–667. 702.

Liu, H., Lin, S., Xiao, D., Zheng, X., Gu, Y., & Guo, S. (2013). Evaluation of the wound healing potential of resina draconis (dracaena cochinchinensis) in animal models. *Evidence-based Complementary and Alternative Medicine*, *2013*, 709865.

Liu, X., Liu, H., Xu, S., Tang, Z., Xia, W., Cheng, Z., et al. (2016). Spinal translocator protein alleviates chronic neuropathic pain behavior and modulates spinal astrocyte-neuronal function in rats with L5 spinal nerve ligation model. *Pain*, *157*(1), 103–116.

Liu, X. L., Lv, C., & Zhang, W. S. (2014). Advance in studies on TRPV1 and analgesic effect of traditional Chinese medicines. *Zhongguo Zhong Yao Za Zhi*, *39*(10), 1757–1760.

Liu, J., Zhu, M., Shi, R., & Yang, M. (2003). Radix Sophorae flavescentis for chronic hepatitis B: A systematic review of randomized trials. *American Journal of Chinese Medicine*, *31*(3), 337–354.

Lu, Z., Sun, W., Duan, X., Yang, Z., Liu, Y., & Tu, P. (2012). Chemical constituents from Corydalis yanhusuo. *Zhongguo Zhong Yao Za Zhi*, *37*(2), 235–237.

Lu, X. Q., Yang, L., Deng, Y. O., Wu, S. X., & Liu, Y. G. (2015). The analgesia of oxymatrine affecting calcium channel and GABA release. *Zhongguo Zhong Xi Yi Jie He Za Zhi*, *35*(5), 603–607.

Ma, L., Gu, R., Tang, L., Chen, Z. E., Di, R., & Long, C. (2015). Important poisonous plants in Tibetan ethnomedicine. *Toxins (Basel)*, 7(1), 138–155.

Ma, T. H., Qin, Y. X., Wei, Z. M., & Yu, B. L. (2014). Effect of Panax notoginseng in patients with multiple fractured ribs and pulmonary contusions caused by the 2008 Wenchuan earthquake. *Forschende Komplementärmedizin*, *21*(6), 360–364.

Ma, Z. Z., Xu, W., Jensen, N. H., Roth, B. L., Liu-Chen, L. Y., & Lee, D. Y. (2008). Isoquinoline alkaloids isolated from Corydalis yanhusuo and their binding affinities at the dopamine D1 receptor. *Molecules*, *13*(9), 2303–2312.

Ma, Y. X., Yang, X. Y., Guo, G., Du, D. Q., Yu, Y. P., & Gao, S. Z. (2015). Research of herb-partitioned moxibustion for primary dysmenorrhea patients based on the LC-MS metabonomics. *Evidence-Based Complementary and Alternative Medicine*, *2015*, 621490.

Ma, Y. G., Yue, X. K., Cao, G., Li, J., & Ge, W. H. (2013). Determination of main active components in crude and processed Corydalis Rhizoma samples from different habitats. *Zhong Yao Cai*, *36*(11), 1754–1758.

Ma, Y., Zhang, Y. C., Tao, Y., Chen, X. M., Wang, P., Xu, H. Y., et al. (2015). Research of Yuanhu Zhitong prescription based on strategy of integrative pharmacology. *Zhongguo Zhong Yao Za Zhi*, *40*(6), 1048–1054.

Martinez, N., Martorell, C., Espinosa, L., Marasigan, V., Domenech, S., & Inzitari, M. (2015). Impact of Qigong on quality of life, pain and depressive symptoms in older adults admitted to an intermediate care rehabilitation unit: A randomized controlled trial. *Aging Clinical and Experimental Research*, *27*(2), 125–130.

Matsuda, H., Wu, J. X., Tanaka, T., Iinuma, M., & Kubo, M. (1997). Antinociceptive activities of 70% methanol extract of Evodiae fructus (fruit of Evodia rutaecarpa var. bodinieri) and its alkaloidal components. *Biological and Pharmaceutical Bulletin*, *20*(3), 243–248.

McQuay, H. (1999). Opioids in pain management. *Lancet*, *353*(9171), 2229–2232.

Medhurst, S. J., Walker, K., Bowes, M., Kidd, B. L., Glatt, M., Muller, M., et al. (2002). A rat model of bone cancer pain. *Pain*, *96*(1-2), 129–140.

Min, Q., Bai, Y. T., Shu, S. J., & Ren, P. (2006). Protective effect of dl-tetrahydropalmatine on liver injury induced by carbon tetrachloride in mice. *Zhongguo Zhong Yao Za Zhi*, *31*(6), 483–484. 521.

Miyaoka, R., & Monga, M. (2009). Use of traditional Chinese medicine in the management of urinary stone disease. *International Brazilian Journal of Urology*, *35*(4), 396–405.

Nie, H., & Shen, Y. J. (2002). Effect of essential oil of Radix Angelicae Dahuricae on beta-endorphin, ACTH, NO and proopiomelanocortin of pain model rats. *Zhongguo Zhong Yao Za Zhi*, *27*(9), 690–693.

Pellicano, R. (2014). Gastrointestinal damage by non-steroidal anti-inflammatory drugs: Updated clinical considerations. *Minerva Gastroenterologica e Dietologica*, *60*(4), 255–261.

Podolsky, A. T., Sandweiss, A., Hu, J., Bilsky, E. J., Cain, J. P., Kumirov, V. K., et al. (2013). Novel fentanyl-based dual mu/delta-opioid agonists for the treatment of acute and chronic pain. *Life Sciences*, *93*(25-26), 1010–1016.

Qiang, W., Wang, Y. X., Zhang, Q. Z., Li, J. D., Xia, K., Wu, N. B., et al. (2014). Expression pattern of genes involved in tropane alkaloids biosynthesis and tropane alkaloids accumulation in Atropa belladonna. *Zhongguo Zhong Yao Za Zhi*, *39*(1), 52–58.

Qin, C. L., & Jiao, Y. (1987). Effects of aqueous extracts of rhizoma seu radix Notopterygii (Notopterygium incisum Ting ex H. T. Chang) on experimental arrhythmias. *Zhong Yao Tong Bao*, *12*(12), 45–47. 60.

Reardon, D. P., Anger, K. E., & Szumita, P. M. (2015). Pathophysiology, assessment, and management of pain in critically ill adults. *American Journal of Health-System Pharmacy, 72*(18), 1531–1543.

Rhule, A., Navarro, S., Smith, J. R., & Shepherd, D. M. (2006). Panax notoginseng attenuates LPS-induced pro-inflammatory mediators in RAW264.7 cells. *Journal of Ethnopharmacology, 106*(1), 121–128.

Rujjanawate, C., Kanjanapothi, D., & Panthong, A. (2003). Pharmacological effect and toxicity of alkaloids from Gelsemium elegans Benth. *Journal of Ethnopharmacology, 89*(1), 91–95.

Schroder, S., Beckmann, K., Franconi, G., Meyer-Hamme, G., Friedemann, T., Greten, H. J., et al. (2013). Can medical herbs stimulate regeneration or neuroprotection and treat neuropathic pain in chemotherapy-induced peripheral neuropathy? *Evidence-Based Complementary and Alternative Medicine, 2013*, 423713.

Schug, S. A., & Chandrasena, C. (2015). Pain management of the cancer patient. *Expert Opinion on Pharmacotherapy, 16*(1), 5–15.

Serohijos, A. W., Yin, S., Ding, F., Gauthier, J., Gibson, D. G., Maixner, W., et al. (2011). Structural basis for mu-opioid receptor binding and activation. *Structure, 19*(11), 1683–1690.

Shen, A. Y., Wang, T. S., Huang, M. H., Liao, C. H., Chen, S. J., & Lin, C. C. (2005). Antioxidant and antiplatelet effects of dang-gui-shao-yao-san on human blood cells. *American Journal of Chinese Medicine, 33*(5), 747–758.

Stein, C. (2016). Opioid receptors. *Annual Review of Medicine, 14*(67), 433–451.

Stieg, R. L. (1977). Double-blind study of belladonna-ergotamine-phenobarbital for interval treatment of recurrent throbbing headache. *Headache, 17*(3), 120–124.

Sun, S., Chen, Z., Li, L., Sun, D., Tian, Y., Pan, H., et al. (2012). The two enantiomers of tetrahydropalmatine are inhibitors of P-gp, but not inhibitors of MRP1 or BCRP. *Xenobiotica, 42*(12), 1197–1205.

Tang, S. J. (2014). Synaptic activity-regulated Wnt signaling in synaptic plasticity, glial function and chronic pain. *CNS & Neurological Disorders Drug Targets, 13*(5), 737–744.

Tian, Y., Teng, L. R., Song, J. J., Meng, Q. F., Lu, J. H., Zhang, W. W., et al. (2014). Studies on the analgesic activities of Jia-Yuan-Qing pill and its safety evaluation in mice. *Protoplasma, 251*(5), 1245–1253.

Tian, Y. E., Teng, L. R., Wang, Z. Z., Zhao, M., Meng, Q. F., Lu, J. H., et al. (2015). Study of the analgesic activities, chronic toxicity and addictive potential of Jia-Yuan-Qing pill in rats. *Experimental and Therapeutic Medicine, 9*(6), 2349–2355.

Trang, T., Al-Hasani, R., Salvemini, D., Salter, M. W., Gutstein, H., & Cahill, C. M. (2015). Pain and poppies: The good, the bad, and the ugly of opioid analgesics. *Journal of Neuroscience, 35*(41), 13879–13888.

Trinh, K., Cui, X., & Wang, Y. J. (2010). Chinese herbal medicine for chronic neck pain due to cervical degenerative disc disease. *Spine (Phila Pa 1976), 35*(24), 2121–2127.

Tripathi, Y. B., Reddy, M. M., Pandey, R. S., Subhashini, J., Tiwari, O. P., Singh, B. K., et al. (2004). Anti-inflammatory properties of BHUx, a polyherbal formulation to prevent atherosclerosis. *Inflammopharmacology, 12*(2), 131–152.

Wang, Y., Cao, S. E., Tian, J., Liu, G., Zhang, X., & Li, P. (2013). Auraptenol attenuates vincristine-induced mechanical hyperalgesia through serotonin 5-HT1A receptors. *Scientific Reports, 3*, 3377.

Wang, P., Fu, X. J., Zhou, Y., & Wang, Z. G. (2014). Effect of 5 warm-hot nature Chinese drugs for promoting blood circulation and removing blood stasis on 5-HT, NE, and endocrine hormones of rats of cold coagulation and blood stasis syndrome. *Zhongguo Zhong Xi Yi Jie He Za Zhi, 34*(11), 1365–1368.

Wang, H. Y., Li, Y. X., Dun, L., Xu, T., Hao, Y. J., Liu, H., et al. (2013a). Antinociceptive effects of matrine on neuropathic pain induced by chronic constriction injury. *Pharmaceutical Biology, 51*(7), 844–850.

Wang, H., Li, Y., Dun, L., Xu, Y., Jin, S., Du, J., et al. (2013b). Antinociceptive effects of oxymatrine from Sophora flavescens, through regulation of NR2B-containing NMDA receptor-ERK/CREB signaling in a mice model of neuropathic pain. *Phytomedicine*, *20*(11), 1039–1045.

Wang, K. T., Liu, H. T., Chen, X. G., Zhao, Y. K., & Hu, Z. D. (2001). Identification and determination of active components in Angelica dahurica Benth and its medicinal preparation by capillary electrophoresis. *Talanta*, *54*(4), 753–761.

Wang, J. B., & Mantsch, J. R. (2012). l-tetrahydropalamatine: A potential new medication for the treatment of cocaine addiction. *Future Medicinal Chemistry*, *4*(2), 177–186.

Wang, W., Mei, X. P., Wei, Y. Y., Zhang, M. M., Zhang, T., Wang, W., et al. (2011). Neuronal NR2B-containing NMDA receptor mediates spinal astrocytic c-Jun N-terminal kinase activation in a rat model of neuropathic pain. *Brain, Behavior, and Immunity*, *25*(7), 1355–1366.

Wang, C., Sun, D., Liu, C., Zhu, C., Jing, X., Chen, S., et al. (2015). Mother root of Aconitum carmichaelii Debeaux exerts antinociceptive effect in Complet Freund's Adjuvant-induced mice: Roles of dynorpin/kappa-opioid system and transient receptor potential vanilloid type-1 ion channel. *Journal of Translational Medicine*, *13*, 284.

Wang, Y. H., Sun, J. F., Tao, Y. M., Chi, Z. Q., & Liu, J. G. (2010). The role of kappa-opioid receptor activation in mediating antinociception and addiction. *Acta Pharmacologica Sinica*, *31*(9), 1065–1070.

Wang, G., Wang, L., Xiong, Z. Y., Mao, B., & Li, T. Q. (2006). Compound salvia pellet, a traditional Chinese medicine, for the treatment of chronic stable angina pectoris compared with nitrates: A meta-analysis. *Medical Science Monitor*, *12*(1), SR1–SR7.

Wang, W., You, R. L., Qin, W. J., Hai, L. N., Fang, M. J., Huang, G. H., et al. (2015). Antitumor activities of active ingredients in Compound Kushen Injection. *Acta Pharmacologica Sinica*, *36*(6), 676–679.

Wang, J., Zhang, R., Dong, C., Jiao, L., Xu, L., Liu, J., et al. (2012). Topical treatment with Tong-Luo-San-Jie gel alleviates bone cancer pain in rats. *Journal of Ethnopharmacology*, *143*(3), 905–913.

Wang, L., Zhang, J., Hong, Y., Feng, Y., Chen, M., & Wang, Y. (2013). Phytochemical and pharmacological review of da chuanxiong formula: A famous herb pair composed of chuanxiong rhizoma and gastrodiae rhizoma for headache. *Evidence-based Complementary and Alternative Medicine*, *2013*, 425369.

Wang, Q. T., Zhang, L. L., Wu, H. X., & Wei, W. (2011). The expression change of beta-arrestins in fibroblast-like synoviocytes from rats with collagen-induced arthritis and the effect of total glucosides of paeony. *Journal of Ethnopharmacology*, *133*(2), 511–516.

Wehling, M. (2014). Non-steroidal anti-inflammatory drug use in chronic pain conditions with special emphasis on the elderly and patients with relevant comorbidities: Management and mitigation of risks and adverse effects. *European Journal of Clinical Pharmacology*, *70*(10), 1159–1172.

Wei, B. W., Hong, G. X., Chang, Z. Q., Li, G. S., & Gu, K. J. (1988). Edulinine analgesia and its mechanism of action. *Yao Xue Xue Bao*, *23*(10), 783–785.

Wu, G., Jiang, J. W., Wu, G. C., & Cao, X. D. (1990). Effects of four dopamine agonists on l-tetrahydropalmatine-induced analgesia and electroacupuncture analgesia in rabbits. *Zhongguo Yao Li Xue Bao*, *11*(3), 196–200.

Wu, H., Waldbauer, K., Tang, L., Xie, L., McKinnon, R., Zehl, M., et al. (2014). Influence of vinegar and wine processing on the alkaloid content and composition of the traditional Chinese medicine Corydalis Rhizoma (Yanhusuo). *Molecules*, *19*(8), 11487–11504.

Wu, X. M., & Wu, C. F. (2015). Network pharmacology: A new approach to unveiling traditional Chinese medicine. *The Chinese Journal of Natural Medicines*, *13*(1), 1–2.

Wu, X. S., Xu, J., Zhang, X. M., Zhang, T. J., & Chen, C. Q. (2015). Research progress on chemical constituents and pharmacological activities of Yuanhu Zhitong Prescription. *Chinese Traditional and Herbal Drugs*, *46*(7), 1081–1095.

Xia, W., Zhu, M., Zhang, Z., Kong, D., Xiao, W., Jia, L., et al. (2013). Effect of Tianshu capsule in treatment of migraine: A meta-analysis of randomized control trials. *Journal of Traditional Chinese Medicine, 33*(1), 9–14.

Xiao, H., Liao, Z., Meng, X., Yan, X., Chen, S., & Mo, Z. (2009). Effects of the selective muscarinic receptor antagonist penehyclidine hydrochloride on the respiratory tract. *Pharmazie, 64*(5), 337–341.

Xiao, Z. M., Wang, A. M., Wang, X. Y., & Shen, S. R. (2013). Effects of ethanol extract of Radix Sophorae Flavescentis on activity of colon cancer HT29 cells. *African Journal of Traditional, Complementary, and Alternative Medicines, 10*(5), 352–355.

Xie, F., Li, X., Sun, K., Chu, Y., Cao, H., Chen, N., et al. (2001). An experimental study on drugs for improving blood circulation and removing blood stasis in treating mild chronic hepatic damage. *Journal of Traditional Chinese Medicine, 21*(3), 225–231.

Xin, W., Huang, C., Zhang, X., Xin, S., Zhou, Y., Ma, X., et al. (2014). Methyl salicylate lactoside inhibits inflammatory response of fibroblast-like synoviocytes and joint destruction in collagen-induced arthritis in mice. *British Journal of Pharmacology, 171*(14), 3526–3538.

Xu, T., Li, Y., Wang, H., Xu, Y., Ma, L., Sun, T., et al. (2013). Oxysophocarpine induces anti-nociception and increases the expression of GABAAalpha1 receptors in mice. *Molecular Medicine Reports*, 7(6), 1819–1825.

Xu, C., Sun, M. Z., Li, Y. R., Yang, B. F., Wang, L. J., & Li, J. M. (1996). Inhibitory effect of tetrahydropalmatine on calcium current in isolated cardiomyocyte of guinea pig. *Zhongguo Yao Li Xue Bao, 17*(4), 329–331.

Xue, F. S., Sun, C., Li, R. P., & Liu, G. P. (2015). Acupuncture for pain relief after total knee arthroplasty: A call for clarification. *Regional Anesthesia and Pain Medicine, 40*(5), 640–641.

Yang, Y., Li, Y. X., Wang, H. L., Jin, S. J., Zhou, R., Qiao, H. Q., et al. (2015). Oxysophocarpine ameliorates Carrageenan-induced inflammatory pain via inhibiting expressions of prostaglandin E2 and cytokines in mice. *Planta Medica, 81*(10), 791–797.

Yang, Z., Shao, Y. C., Li, S. J., Qi, J. L., Zhang, M. J., Hao, W., et al. (2008). Medication of l-tetrahydropalmatine significantly ameliorates opiate craving and increases the abstinence rate in heroin users: A pilot study. *Acta Pharmacologica Sinica, 29*(7), 781–788.

Yin, W., Wang, T. S., Yin, F. Z., & Cai, B. C. (2003). Analgesic and anti-inflammatory properties of brucine and brucine *N*-oxide extracted from seeds of Strychnos nux-vomica. *Journal of Ethnopharmacology, 88*(2-3), 205–214.

Yin, L. L., & Zhu, X. Z. (2005). The involvement of central cholinergic system in (+)-matrine-induced antinociception in mice. *Pharmacology Biochemistry and Behavior, 80*(3), 419–425.

Yuan, C. S., Mehendale, S. R., Wang, C. Z., Aung, H. H., Jiang, T., Guan, X., et al. (2004). Effects of Corydalis yanhusuo and Angelicae dahuricae on cold pressor-induced pain in humans: A controlled trial. *Journal of Clinical Pharmacology, 44*(11), 1323–1327.

Zhang, X. J., Chen, H. L., Li, Z., Zhang, H. Q., Xu, H. X., Sung, J. J., et al. (2009). Analgesic effect of paeoniflorin in rats with neonatal maternal separation-induced visceral hyperalgesia is mediated through adenosine A(1) receptor by inhibiting the extracellular signal-regulated protein kinase (ERK) pathway. *Pharmacology Biochemistry and Behavior, 94*(1), 88–97.

Zhang, W., & Dai, S. M. (2012). Mechanisms involved in the therapeutic effects of Paeonia lactiflora Pallas in rheumatoid arthritis. *International Immunopharmacology, 14*(1), 27–31.

Zhang, J. Y., Gong, N., Huang, J. L., Guo, L. C., & Wang, Y. X. (2013). Gelsemine, a principal alkaloid from Gelsemium sempervirens Ait., exhibits potent and specific antinociception in chronic pain by acting at spinal alpha3 glycine receptors. *Pain, 154*(11), 2452–2462.

Zhang, B., He, X. L., Ding, Y., & Du, G. H. (2006). Gaultherin, a natural salicylate derivative from Gaultheria yunnanensis: Towards a better non-steroidal anti-inflammatory drug. *European Journal of Pharmacology, 530*(1-2), 166–171.

Zhang, Y. K., Huang, Z. J., Liu, S., Liu, Y. P., Song, A. A., & Song, X. J. (2013). WNT signaling underlies the pathogenesis of neuropathic pain in rodents. *Journal of Clinical Investigation, 123*(5), 2268–2286.

Zhang, X. J., Li, Z., Leung, W. M., Liu, L., Xu, H. X., & Bian, Z. X. (2008). The analgesic effect of paeoniflorin on neonatal maternal separation-induced visceral hyperalgesia in rats. *The Journal of Pain, 9*(6), 497–505.

Zhang, X., Liu, Y., Guo, Z., Feng, J., Dong, J., Fu, Q., et al. (2012). The herbalome—An attempt to globalize Chinese herbal medicine. *Analytical and Bioanalytical Chemistry, 402*(2), 573–581.

Zhang, B., Sun, S. X., Chen, Y. C., & Zhou, C. X. (2015a). Effect of zhixin formula on gliocyte protein expressions, TLRs and NF-kappaB in bone cancer pain model rats. *Zhongguo Zhong Xi Yi Jie He Za Zhi, 35*(6), 704–711.

Zhang, T. T., Sun, L., Liu, R., Zhang, D., Lan, X., Huang, C., et al. (2012). A novel naturally occurring salicylic acid analogue acts as an anti-inflammatory agent by inhibiting nuclear factor-kappaB activity in RAW264.7 macrophages. *Molecular Pharmaceutics, 9*(3), 671–677.

Zhang, X., Sun, J., Xin, W., Li, Y., Ni, L., Ma, X., et al. (2015b). Anti-inflammation effect of methyl salicylate 2-O-beta-D-lactoside on adjuvant induced-arthritis rats and lipopolysaccharide (LPS)-treated murine macrophages RAW264.7 cells. *International Immunopharmacology, 25*(1), 88–95.

Zhang, Y., Wang, C., Wang, L., Parks, G. S., Zhang, X., Guo, Z., et al. (2014). A novel analgesic isolated from a traditional Chinese medicine. *Current Biology, 24*(2), 117–123.

Zhang, Z., Wang, P., Yuan, W., & Li, S. (2008). Steroids, alkaloids, and coumarins from Gelsemium sempervirens. *Planta Medica, 74*(15), 1818–1822.

Zhang, B., Wei, D. M., Bian, Y. Y., Bai, K. K., & Zhou, C. X. (2015). Impact of Xinzhi Formula on the expression of glial cell protein and nuclear factor kB in bone cancer pain rats. *Journal of Traditional Chinese Medicine, 56*(2), 148–151.

Zhao, N., Chen, Y., Zhu, J., Wang, L., Cao, G., Dang, Y., et al. (2014). Levo-tetrahydropalmatine attenuates the development and expression of methamphetamine-induced locomotor sensitization and the accompanying activation of ERK in the nucleus accumbens and caudate putamen in mice. *Neuroscience, 258*, 101–110.

Zheng, C. S., Fu, C. L., Pan, C. B., Bao, H. J., Chen, X. Q., Ye, H. Z., et al. (2015). Deciphering the underlying mechanisms of Diesun Miaofang in traumatic injury from a systems pharmacology perspective. *Molecular Medicine Reports, 12*(2), 1769–1776.

Zheng, Y. Q., & Wei, W. (2005). Total glucosides of paeony suppresses adjuvant arthritis in rats and intervenes cytokine-signaling between different types of synoviocytes. *International Immunopharmacology, 5*(10), 1560–1573.

Zheng, M., Zhou, H., Wan, H., Chen, Y. L., & He, Y. (2015). Effects of herbal drugs in Mahuang decoction and their main components on intestinal transport characteristics of Ephedra alkaloids evaluated by a Caco-2 cell monolayer model. *Journal of Ethnopharmacology, 164*, 22–29.

Zhou, X., Tang, L., Xu, Y., Zhou, G., & Wang, Z. (2014). Towards a better understanding of medicinal uses of Carthamus tinctorius L. in traditional Chinese medicine: A phytochemical and pharmacological review. *Journal of Ethnopharmacology, 151*(1), 27–43.

Zhu, X. Z. (1991). Development of natural products as drugs acting on central nervous system. *Memórias do Instituto Oswaldo Cruz, 86*(Suppl. 2), 173–175.

Zhu, B., Gong, N., Fan, H., Peng, C. S., Ding, X. J., Jiang, Y., et al. (2014). Lamiophlomis rotata, an orally available Tibetan herbal painkiller, specifically reduces pain hypersensitivity states through the activation of spinal glucagon-like peptide-1 receptors. *Anesthesiology, 121*(4), 835–851.

Zhu, S., Yu, X., Wu, Y., Shiraishi, F., Kawahara, N., & Komatsu, K. (2015). Genetic and chemical characterization of white and red peony root derived from Paeonia lactiflora. *Journal of Natural Medicines, 69*(1), 35–45.

INDEX

Note: Page numbers followed by "*f*" indicate figures, and "*t*" indicate tables.

M

N

O

P

Kolibri 360 GmbH
Ferdinand-Jühlke-Straße 7
99095 Erfurt, Deutschland
produktsicherheit@kolibri360.de